# Critiquing Nursing Research

# Critiquing Nursing Research

## John R Cutcliffe and Martin Ward

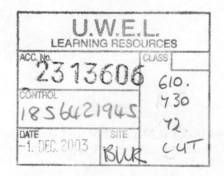

Quay
Books

MA Healthcare Ltd

Quay Books Division, MA Healthcare Limited, Jesses Farm,
Snow Hill, Dinton, Wiltshire, SP3 5HN

British Library Cataloguing-in-Publication Data
A catalogue record is available for this book

© MA Healthcare Limited 2003
ISBN 1 85642 194 5

Printed in the UK by Bath Press, Bath

# Contents

# Foreword

The Royal College of Nursing Institute is proud to have been associated with the establishment of the Network for Psychiatric Nursing Research (NPNR) in the mid-1990s. As host for this Department of Health (England) funded innovation, the spirit and commitment shown by the originators of the idea, were very much in synchrony with the aspirations and vision of the Institute.

The authors of this book have provided us with a detailed outline of how the network developed, what it was trying to achieve and how it has refined its purposes. Responding to the policy imperative of the evidence-based practice movement, the founders of NPNR have been able to combine the essential ingredients of effective utilisation of evidence into practice; namely, the ability to critique research with a practitioner/researcher network of interested, committed individuals. This combination of critical appraisal skill development (covering both conventional quantitative and qualitative approaches) with dissemination and networking strategies is still quite a rare phenomenon. And the efforts of all those volunteers, who have contributed their intellectual and clinical expertise by way of being involved in critiquing research, or attending NPNR conferences, should also be acknowledged.

But the last words rightly rest with the authors themselves on the future direction of this timely and important initiative. Acknowledging the changing policy and practice landscape, the evolution of a much more integrated, interprofessional, person-centred research agenda and the impact of technology on research dissemination and implementation methods, Cutcliffe and Ward comment:

> ... Our future success lies in combining all the evidence resources at our disposal, including research, with the spontaneity of our intuitive actions and subjecting both to the same level of critical evaluation. In short, raising the level of our professional thinking to a more mature status.

This book offers one perspective on this journey.

Alison Kitson RN, PhD, FRCN
Executive Director, Nursing
Royal College of Nursing
April 2003

# Preface

The reasons for writing this book are best summarised under three points:

* There is a distinct absence of books that focus specifically on critiquing nursing research.
* There is an increasing requirement for nurses to become conversant with research, understand its link with the use of evidence to underpin practice and move towards being an evidence-based discipline.
* A crucial aspect of this increased 'mindfulness' of research is an awareness of the contemporary research issues facing nursing and the wider policy, multi-disciplinary and political contexts in which these issues are embedded.

Consequently, we feel that having read this book readers should gain an appropriate knowledge and awareness pertaining to these three points. Nurses should be more familiar with some of the approaches and techniques involved in critiquing nursing research and be able to utilise some of these skills and techniques in their own efforts to critique. Accordingly, they will be better placed to make informed judgements regarding the quality of the research paper and the value of the evidence reported. Finally, they should also be able to locate the critiqued paper(s) within the wider policy, multi-disciplinary and political contexts.

The book is divided into four integrated sections.

Section one contains chapters which set the context and background to critiquing nursing research, explain the purpose and value of the critiquing process and describes the evolution of the Network for Psychiatric Nursing Research (NPNR) and its National Journal Club.

Section two is comprised of a range of approaches used to critique nursing research and identifies the strengths and limitations of these approaches. Each approach is also accompanied by two examples of critiques, which are based on critiques undertaken by the NPNR National Journal Club.

In section three, the NPNR National Journal Club's approach to critiquing nursing research is described. Since this is a developmental approach, we provide two additional examples for each of the four stages identified (a total of sixteen different critiques of nursing research papers are included throughout the book).

The final section contains a chapter which discusses contemporary trends and themes in psychiatric/mental health nursing research and considers the complex relationship between psychiatric/mental health nursing research and multi-disciplinary, collaborative research in the formal area of 'psychiatric care'. It also looks at the responsibilities for research of both nurse researchers and non-researchers.

The reader will notice that the papers reviewed using the NPNR National Journal Club approach are presented after the reviews undertaken using a range of models. This sequence of reviews was carried out purposefully in this 'order' since we wanted an approach to evolve and develop out of the National Journal Club work. Having done so, we were able to compare and contrast our approach with this range of approaches.

John R Cutcliffe and Martin Ward
November 2002

# Acknowledgements

This book could not have been produced without the sterling commitment and efforts of the National Journal Club co-ordinators and members. Accordingly, this book is a 'tribute' to all your hard work.

Furthermore, we offer our thanks to Annelie Guard and the previous administrators of the Network for Psychiatric and Nursing Research for their support in maintaining the National Journal Club.

John R Cutcliffe and Martin Ward
November 2002

# Section one: Background to psychiatric/ mental health nursing research and critiquing research

# 1

# The growth of evidence-based practice, and the importance of critiquing research

*Man's search for meaning is the primary motivation in his life and not a secondary rationalization of instinctive drives.*

(Victor Frankl, 1945)

## The movement towards evidence-based practice

A son asks his father, 'How does petrol make your car work, daddy?' The father, not wishing to confuse the little boy, and not really knowing himself, replies, 'Well, when the engine gets thirsty you put the petrol in and the engine drinks it. When it has had enough it feels better and it runs again — just like you'. The boy, not wholly convinced of this asks further questions so his father brings out a mechanics manual, then an encyclopaedia then takes the boy next door to talk to his neighbour. Finally, in exasperation, the father connects to the Internet and finds a programme that gives the answer the boy needs, at the level he needs it and in a way that not only makes sense to him but also is technically correct for his age and degree of understanding.

Many years later the boy, despite his father, becomes a mechanic. One day a customer asks him, 'How does petrol make my car work?' If the son had learnt from his father and gone no further than making things up as he went along he would not have an answer to satisfy the customer's question. Fortunately, his studies and his training have taught him differently and he is able to provide an answer that equips the customer with the appropriate information. What is the moral of this story? Never listen to your parents? No, that there is always an answer to every question but sometimes you have to go to extraordinary lengths to find it and it is not possible to progress your understanding of life until you do. How does this help us come to a conclusion about the significance of evidence-based mental health care and perhaps, more importantly, how can its implementation help individual practitioners? To answer these questions it is necessary to look back at the history of psychiatric/mental health nursing and its relationship to service development and care delivery.

As a separate speciality, mental health nursing has perhaps only a hundred-year history. It was not until the 1910s that, for political reasons, those who cared for the mentally ill were seen as separate from those who cared for the physically ill. The science upon which these practitioners based their actions came from a combined source: general nursing and psychiatry. As a consequence, the only thing that differentiated these practitioners from other nurses was the diagnosis of their patients. Two world wars, the increase in psychotherapeutic psychiatry, the introduction of psychotropic medications and a greater public awareness of mental illness, shaped their professional actions into something akin to specialist care. However, they were under educated, made very few clinical decisions and had little power other than that of the subversive nature. By the late 1950s, their work was dominated by psychiatrists. Despite having their own syllabus for basic training most of their textbooks were written for them by psychiatrists, psychiatrists sat on their examination boards and dictated their working conditions and gave them clinical orders.

During this time it would have been very difficult for a mental health nurse to describe what s/he actually did. Yet, do something they did, for there were in excess of 250,000 in-patient beds and nurses were the mainstay of the daily support these people received. Over time the situation changed as nurses began to improve their own understanding of their capabilities, sought higher education, undertook research into their actions and began to share their experiences by writing about them. As they became more articulate they developed professional confidence, took responsibility for their own professional actions and began to develop a body of evidence to support their decisions. In effect, they displayed some of the traits that have been associated with being a profession (although whether or not nursing is a profession falls outside of the scope of this book). They influenced the reduction of power differentials between themselves and other disciplines, contributed to general strategic and policy activities and became independent of the restricting influence of the science from which they had sprung. Crucially, nurses started to undertake and lead their own research and began to develop their own unique knowledge base.

During that period of time, mental health services matured, shedding thousands of beds, developing more therapeutic alternatives rather than relying on the myopic polemicism of community versus in-patient care and advancing policy which would try to meet the needs of the patient rather than those of the service (Johnson and Thornicroft, 1993; Burns and Priebe, 1999). It could almost be posited that as mental health care evolved, so too did its nurses. The effects are startling. Nurses now take an active part in strategic planning, undertake a large portfolio of personal and professional research, influence clinical care and work collaboratively with service users to develop the diversity of care options necessary to meet the needs of a very specialised target population.

## Evidence-based practice and evidence-based mental health care

Much of contemporary mental health nursing practice is complicated and demands high levels of sophisticated personal and clinical technology. All of it can be complex and demanding. As described above, this shift in emphasis away from loosely defined nursing practices dictated by the actions of psychiatry, to ones which form part of dedicated nursing interventions that are brought to bear as part of a collaborative multi-disciplinary effort, has taken place as a result of many things. One of those is the advent of evidence-based health care (Evidence-based Medicine Working Group, 1992; Sackett *et al*, 1996; Sackett *et al*, 1997). Consequently, it is necessary to examine the key components of evidence-based practice, namely: research; evidence and critiquing/critical reading of the literature, in addition to locating these within the context of the development of evidence-based mental health care.

## What is research?

The often quoted definition of research provided by the English Department of Health (DoH, 1994, p. 37) asserts research is, 'rigorous and systematic enquiry conducted on a scale and using methods commensurate with the issue to be investigated, and designed to lead to more generalised contributions to knowledge.'

Research involves a systematic search for knowledge, and mental healthcare research is concerned with uncovering knowledge that is important (and useful) for mental health practitioners. As intimated in the Department of Health's definition, there exists a wide range of research methods and methodologies, which are broadly grouped together under two paradigms: the quantitative and the qualitative paradigm. Each paradigm is concerned with the uncovering of new knowledge; however, the type of knowledge produced and the way the researchers go about uncovering this knowledge is different within each paradigm.

Kerlinger (1986), one of many advocates of the quantitative approach to research, asserts that the way to truth is through rigorous research, involving the identification of variables within hypotheses and subjecting them to experimental manipulation. Here 'hard evidence' is required in order to be certain that something is or is not true. To Kerlinger, this approach is at the peak of a hierarchy of how to know; further down were less respectable ways of knowing, including 'tenacity', 'authority' and '*a priori*'. The end result of each of these ways of knowing is knowledge; what differs is how the knowledge is acquired. Kerlinger has great respect for knowledge gained through the scientific quantitative method and less for knowledge gained through what he perceives as more subjective approaches. The importance of qualitative research, what Kerlinger would describe as 'subjective', and the different forms of evidence are explored in more detail below.

There are commonalities between research and other related forms of enquiry, but there are important differences. Muir-Gray (1997, p. 69) declares that, within the UK National Health Service Research and Development programme, these distinguishing features can be summarised as follows. Research should:

• provide new knowledge necessary for the improvement of the NHS
• produce results that are generalisable
• should follow well-defined study protocols, which have been peer reviewed
• have obtained formal approval from an ethical committee where appropriate
• have defined arrangements for project management
• produce findings that are open to critical examination and accessible to all who could benefit from them (and this would therefore involve publication).

Here too it is acknowledged that different approaches can be used to obtain knowledge, yet there is an intimation that quantitative approaches are favoured. Generalisation is invariably associated with randomised controlled trials and most researchers who use a qualitative approach would not claim that their findings are generalisable. It is possible in the above description to see plainly the influence of a quantitative way of knowing. The need to confirm and verify takes precedence within this approach. The result is hard numerical data representing reality, that is then often accepted as truth and enters the knowledge base of the profession.

## The historical dominance of quantitative research within mental health care

Examination of the research undertaken within the domain of psychiatry (and psychiatric nursing) indicates a historical emphasis on quantitative studies. It can be seen that from the mid-1950s onwards, a large percentage of the research available to mental health practitioners centred on the trailing of medications. These drug studies were numerous but often of limited quality (Bero and Rennie, 1996; Greenhalgh, 1997a). Significantly, at first psychiatry was only interested in quantitative studies and in particular, randomised controlled trials (RCTs). Examples of the use of RCTs in psychiatry begin to appear in the professional literature throughout the 1980s but from the early 1990s onwards there is a marked increase in their numbers (McFarlane *et al*, 1995; Kulpers *et al*, 1997; Stensky *et al*, 2000).

This is because much of medical research is quantitative in nature and RCTs were regarded in the UK as the 'gold standard' of robust clinical enquiry. However, since the early 1990s those working within psychiatry and mental health care have recognised the need to use the huge amount of other forms of research and other forms of evidence at its disposal to inform its work.

Reviews of RCTs become essential during this time (Haynes *et al*, 1996; Roth and Fonagy, 1996) because it would be impractical for practitioners to read everything that has been published for themselves. Not only that, but not all the RCTs report the same results (Chalmers and Altman, 1995). You may have a situation where half of a group of research projects indicate that treatment X is the best, while the other half suggest that treatment Y is of better value. If the practitioner only read the first group of projects s/he would be inclined to use treatment X, and likewise for those only reading papers which recommended treatment Y. Four things occurred during the 1990s to deal with the massive increase in available research material:

❖ The development of models to enable individuals to appraise critically or review single and groups of literature papers (Greenhalgh, 1997b; NHSE, 1999).

❖ The development of models to undertake systematic reviews of large amounts of literature (Cullum, 1994; NHS Centre for Reviews and Dissemination, 1996; Hek *et al*, 2000).

❖ The development of databases and review libraries that would make available completed reviews carried out by panels of clinical and research experts in the field (Lefebvre, 1994; Brazier and Begley, 1996).

❖ The development for researchers of guidelines that would inform the design and management of robust clinical trials (Medical Research Council, 2000).

In theory, these four activities should provide a framework to ensure that practitioners know how to review literature, access reviews of large amounts of literature and researchers have a better understanding of how to carry out and report on their work. The problem with this is that it assumes that all staff are able to access these skills, or are given them while they are undertaking their professional training and education, which patently is not the case. Furthermore, up until the 1990s, it was also (wrongly) assumed that the only critically sound research was that carried out using quantitative methods of enquiry and for both nursing and mental health, yet this was patently not the case (Sackett *et al*, 1997; Ward *et al*, 1999). As Smith (1998) points out, much of mental health care is not susceptible to quantitative research methods.

## The movement towards a more pluralistic approach

As a result, pressure for the inclusion of qualitative research studies and other forms of evidence to be included within the scope of evidence-based practice came from several sources, including professional academia, the social sciences, clinical psychology, nursing and medicine, particularly psychiatry. Their reasoning was obvious and contained two main arguments. Firstly, that quantitative research examines known phenomena, eg. one therapy against another, one or both of which have already been in use and are being compared to establish effectiveness against each other. Or, the statistical outcome value of a drug used to reduce symptoms for a recognised diagnostic entity, such as one of the forms of schizophrenia. However, qualitative researchers suggest that for this research to take place, the entity itself has to be placed in context otherwise it is unclear just what the drug or therapy is acting upon. As Dodd (2001) argues, indicating the need for preliminary exploratory, descriptive, contextual, phenomenological and anthropological studies, ie. those which describe entities, are the domain of qualitative research.

Secondly, and perhaps more importantly, qualitative research is not simply used to describe contexts for entities. There are known phenomena that in themselves are not susceptible to quantitative processes, eg. belief structures, feelings, interactions, etc. (and an argument has been suggested which purports that much of psychiatric/mental health nursing may be invisible or immeasurable and not accessible using quantitative methods). Qualitative methods are required in order to understand the nature and complexity of these phenomena. Mental health care is based upon the principles of human interactions and the ability of service users to develop personal strategies for living. True, for some there is a major role for medication and some other forms of physical therapy in this work, but essentially it is people intensive and deals with emotions, thoughts and adaptability. Similarly, as we have already described, such care is being delivered in ever changing environments and increasingly community settings, very often those of the patient's own home. For research to make sense of these entities and for that research to be of value to practitioners wanting to implement it into their own work it has to be environmentally and people focused. Qualitative researchers argue that these types of services, and the personal work that they undertake, are the domains of their methods.

## What is evidence? The different forms of evidence

As indicated in the previous section, some authors regard the findings or results produced from a quantitative research study to be 'hard evidence'. Appleby *et al* (1995), for example, intimate that evidence is reliant on the existence of (quantitative) research findings. However, as we similarly indicated in the previous section, it is important to acknowledge that a more pluralistic perspective exists. In their often quoted work, Sackett *et al* (1996) provide a definition of evidence-based practice that does not specifically mention quantitative research. They see it as, 'the conscientious, explicit and judicious use of current best evidence in making decisions about the care of individual patients.' Similarly, McKibbon and Walker (1994) offer an even less rigid definition of evidence-based practice, representing it as, 'an approach to health care that promotes the collection, interpretation and integration of valid, important and applicable patient-reported, clinician-observed, and research-derived evidence.'

As a consequence of accepting more pluralistic views of the nature of evidence, and perhaps as a way to explain the apparent contradictions in definitions of evidence-based practice (McKenna *et al*, 2000), hierarchies of evidence have been suggested, such as the hierarchy described in *Box 1.1*.

---

**Box 1.1: Hierarchy of evidence**

Level 1: meta-analysis of a series of randomised controlled trials
Level 2: at least one well-designed randomised control trial
Level 3: at least one controlled study without randomisation
Level 4: non-experimental descriptive studies

---

(Based on Muir-Gray, 1997)

It needs to be acknowledged that such hierarchies of evidence are by no means universally accepted, particularly within mental health care. An alternative, and well accepted view posits that research methods within quantitative and qualitative paradigms can be regarded as a 'tool kit'; a collection of methods that are purposefully designed to answer specific questions and discover particular types of knowledge. To attempt to place these designs (and the evidence they produce) into some artificial and linear hierarchy only serves to confuse and obfuscate. If what is needed to answer a particular problem (eg. the comparison of the therapeutic effects of two drugs) is a meta-analysis of the current studies in one particular area, then for that particular problem, that is clearly the best form of evidence. Concomitantly, if what is required to answer a particular problem (eg. what is the lived experience of experiencing violent incidents) is deep, thorough, sophisticated understanding, then for that particular problem, that is clearly the best form of evidence.

Certainly there has been a gradual acceptance among the scientific community within health care that there is a definite role for both methodological forms (Mueser *et al*, 1998; Fenton, 2000). Additionally, it is also recognised that it is necessary to undertake research that uses both quantitative as well as qualitative research and there is a growing trend for such approaches within mental health care (Gournay *et al*, 2001). Greenhalgh

(1999) described this as the dissonance between the 'science' of objective measurement and the 'art' of clinical proficiency and judgement. She attempted to integrate these different perspectives into clinical methods, albeit for psychiatry the approach was certainly consistent with nursing.

In addition to the evidence produced by qualitative research studies, the definitions of Sackett *et al* (1996) and McKibbon and Walker (1994), and Muir-Gray's (1997) hierarchy, each allude to additional forms of evidence, namely: reports (grey literature), opinions from experts/respected authorities, conference presentations, results from audits, continuous quality improvement initiatives and importantly, patient reported information. What such an extensive list clearly indicates is that the absence of formal research findings (from quantitative or qualitative studies) does not mitigate against evidence-based decisions. As McKenna *et al* (2000, p. 40) state, 'what is required is the best evidence available — not the best evidence possible.'

In her systematic approach to evidence-based practice, Peat (2001) describes an eight-stage process and an adapted version of this approach is contained in *Box 1.2*.

---

**Box 1.2: The systematic process of evidence-based practice (adapted from Peat, 2001)**

❖ Define the problem.

❖ Reduce the problem into a series of smaller questions, which can be addressed.

❖ Search for relevant literature, using both electronic and manual forms of literature search (including grey literature where it exists).

❖ Select the appropriate studies according to clear criteria.

❖ Critique or critically appraise each of these studies.

❖ Draw conclusions which help lead to clinical decisions, implement practice.

---

Among other helpful steps, Peat's (2001) approach clearly identifies the final of the three key elements of evidence-based practice: critiquing or critical reading of the literature.

## Critiquing or critical reading of the literature

There appear to be a range of terms that are used to indicate the activity of reading an article, manuscript or paper, in a critical manner, in order to gauge the quality of the research. Throughout this book, the terms, critiquing, critical reading and critical appraisal will be used interchangeably, all of which refer to the process identified in the previous sentence. Many authors have described this process of critiquing, for example, Sackett *et al*, 1996; Sajiwandani, 1996; Muir-Gray, 1997; Bury and Jerosch-Herold, 1998; Dawes, 1999 and Peat, 2001. Critical appraisal should always be systematic and, according to Bury and Jerosch-Herold (1998), it is a way of considering the truthfulness of a piece of research. Peat (2001) makes similar statements suggesting that critical appraisal is the process used to evaluate the scientific merit of a study, and she argues it has become an essential clinical tool. Critiquing a paper involves asking a series of questions of the paper in order to comment on the various components of the work. A critique should assist the reviewer in deciding on how relevant and applicable the results/findings are (Sajiwandani, 1996). Peat (2001) goes as far as to suggest that critical appraisal skills are essential for making decisions about whether or not to change practice on the basis of the published research.

Practitioners who are inexperienced in critiquing literature occasionally make the mistake of associating critique exclusively with criticism, rather than associating critique with highlighting **both** the strengths and limitations of the work. Bury and Jerosch-Herold (1998) clearly point out that one thing critical appraisal is not, is an attempt to pull a paper to pieces. If we accept the axiom that there is no such thing as the perfect piece of research, and that should be the starting point for the reviewer (Bury and Jerosch-Herold, 1998), then the reviewer should always be able to identify a limitation of the paper. The important point to consider here is that there are different degrees of limitation or flaw. It is the reviewer's responsibility to decide whether or not these limitations are such that they undermine the conclusion(s) in the paper.

The second premise that should also be the starting point is that there is always something to be learned from a paper. Bearing this premise in mind should lead to a more balanced and constructive review. However, this point needs clarification. When one endeavours to produce a balanced critique, this in no way means that there should be an equal number of strengths and limitations identified. To attempt to do so would be to produce a somewhat synthetic and artificial critique. It is accepted as axiomatic that some published work is of a higher quality than other work. It is entirely appropriate, if not prudent, to point out each of the limitations where they exist. However, and crucially, it is equally important and appropriate to point out each of the strengths where they exist. It is entirely possible, if not likely, that some reviews will have a greater emphasis on the limitations of the paper, and some reviews will have a greater emphasis on the strengths of the paper.

# The importance of critiquing research

It is an unrealistic and untenable position to expect that every nurse is able to, or indeed wants to, undertake research to influence practice. Much of research is alien to many nurses. Understanding complex and sophisticated research methods, tools and procedures is just not something for which their training has prepared them. In truth, to be able to undertake good research requires a secondary training, as a researcher. For the vast majority of nurses such a luxury is neither required, nor wanted.

Increasingly, research information and evidence drawn from other sources, is influencing the path of care. Consequently, it is incumbent and necessary that all nurses recognise that they have a part to play in the development, understanding and implementation of that knowledge. Nurses are still expected to read scientific journals and to make sense of what they read. The little boy at the beginning of the chapter was dependent upon his father finding the information he needed to answer his question. That dependence made him vulnerable to misinformation and ultimately, ignorant of the truth. Similarly, nurses need to be able to access the skills to find out for themselves rather than be dependent upon others for giving them the information they seek.

There exists a wide range of cogent reasons why nurses should be able to critique research literature. These reasons benefit the nurse who is undertaking the critique, the researcher or researchers who undertook the study, and the people (if any) who read the critique. Being able to critique the literature effectively:

- helps the researcher to refine the study or to develop a better study in the future
- allows the reader to make sense of things for themselves without having to rely upon other people to do it for them, therefore giving him/her more independence and substantially increasing his/her knowledge base (because the knowledge belongs to them)
- helps another potential researcher to decide whether or not to base his/her study on the critiqued work
- reduces the possibility of misinterpretations being passed on by word of mouth, and so stopping good research being implemented or bad research being inappropriately used
- helps facilitate the scientific/academic potential of a researcher towards excellence in developing his/her research skills
- potentially increases the research reading audience, and as such, increases the rejection of badly conducted or poorly written research papers
- helps exchange information, facilitate debate around the research issues arising from the critique

- gives more nurses the opportunity to explore research and evidence-based literature to find innovative ways of expanding their own work practices
- increases the possibility of mental health nursing becoming more evidence-based and hopefully, providing a greater degree of best practice and care diversity for clients
- gives nurses the contemporary, up-to-date knowledge and evidence they need to support their decision making within the wider multi-disciplinary team.

It has to be said that the techniques for effectively reviewing literature and research need to be learnt, but they are infinitely more accessible to the novice or non-researcher than the intricacies of research. They do not teach you how to do research but they can teach you how to make sense of it, accept the high quality and reject low quality research. By allowing the reader to become more discerning and select effective literature through the process of critiquing, increases his/her enjoyment of the whole process of enquiry. A process that we have already said has been the basis for professional development in the absence of any real research skill.

## The argument against the use of evidence-based practice

Evidenced-based practice has its critics. Certainly, few credible practitioners would argue with the notion of producing the right care for the right condition or problem at the right time. However, this is not where the criticism lies. The difficulty rests with the nature of the evidence itself (and the debate surrounding what constitutes credible evidence), and how this evidence is used to influence practice, with mental health care in particular being one of the main areas where this causes concern.

Taking the first point, that of the nature of evidence. Using the example of case management for serious mental illness, Tyrer (2000) argues that much of the research into different forms of case management has shown inconclusive results because we have been trying to identify which organisational method is best. Citing the work of Burns *et al* (2000), Thornicroft *et al* (1998) and Wykes *et al* (1998), Tyrer concludes that research needs to concentrate on establishing the impact of evidence-based interventions used within service user contacts, not the number of contacts themselves. Although this is not a problem with the philosophy of evidence-based practice itself, it does highlight something of the issues surrounding what constitutes 'appropriate' evidence.

A further example of this situation exists in the use of new medications, specifically atypical antipsychotics. Geddes *et al* (2000), for example, published the findings of a systematic review of drug trials which stated that because of their actions, atypical antipsychotics could be analysed as a single entity; in effect, aggregating their scores. Despite admitting that there was poor quality of research into antipsychotic drugs, they still subjected that research to sophisticated statistical techniques and concluded, 'conventional drugs should remain the first treatment'. Whereas Prior *et al* (2001) made an impassioned plea to clinicians to think very carefully before accepting these results and accused Geddes and his colleagues of 'bad science and worse medicine', pointing out that the six drugs reviewed had both different ranges of benefits and side-effects.

The second issue, that of the use of evidence, is perhaps even more contentious for it might suggest a degree of ignorance among some practitioners of both research methods and the application of findings into practice. If practitioners remain relatively unskilled at critiquing research, it is possible to implement evidence that is not only poor in quality and unrepresentative of that available, but it may have detrimental effects when inappropriately implemented into practice. True, for nursing to have a genuine representative voice within the multi-disciplinary team it has to be able to use evidence to support its decisions and be able to articulate that evidence to others (Barker and Walker, 2000). If the evidence used is of dubious quality then, the nursing contribution to joint decision making is likely to be as devalued as if it used no evidence at all.

Further problems have been highlighted by McKenna *et al* (2000). They especially draw attention to the position that evidence should guide practice, rather than dictate it. Drawing on Barbara Carper's (1978) seminal work, they make the case that, at certain times, nurses may draw on different types of knowledge to underpin their practice. Of the four different types of knowledge that Carper describes (eg. empirical, ethical, aesthetic and personal), empirical knowledge refers to knowledge derived from research. There may be occasions when the nurse may draw upon the other forms of knowledge, despite the presence of research-based knowledge. As we have described earlier, such decisions can still be regarded as evidence-based decisions, given the different forms of evidence.

## What is the future?

There can be little doubt that evidence-based mental health care, in whatever form it takes, will be with us in the future. The need for rational decision making, based upon appropriate evidence, has the potential to be both cost and outcome effective. The difficulties in implementing such a dramatic cultural change must be addressed in a logical and systematic way. These difficulties are summarised in *Box 1.3*.

---

**Box 1.3: Summary of difficulties in implementing evidence-based practice**

❖ Ensuring that research priorities are set which produce the evidence which reflects the needs of both users and organisations.

❖ Carrying out the right research to produce the evidence required and not just the easy or quick research to give inconclusive and superficial information.

❖ Selecting the most appropriate research method/methodology for the questions being asked.

❖ Teaching practitioners how to read and critique research and evaluate the findings.

❖ Linking the aspirations of all mental healthcare disciplines to the same agenda, in effect, establishing multi-disciplinary research and change programmes.

❖ Maintaining a balance between the evidence base which informs practice and the practitioners own skill base, to ensure that they can practice effectively when the supporting empirical evidence exists, in addition to being able to perform effectively in its absence.

❖ Recognising that research is not the only source of evidence.

❖ Recognising and embracing the pluralistic approach to research methods/designs and the different types of knowledge they produce.

❖ Teaching the skills of putting research into practice, ie. rigorous and systematic practice development.

❖ Developing networks which keep practitioners informed, on both formal and informal levels, of innovation and practice development success.

---

Within the existing care system there are already mechanisms and organisational procedures which both support and necessitate the use of evidence. The National Institute for Clinical Excellence (NICE), a Government body established in 1999, was set up to link the clinical needs of patients with available technologies. This includes drugs, therapies and interventions. The clinical effectiveness of these activities has to be founded upon evidence suggesting such impact, thus making research crucial to decisions made by the organisation. The role of NICE is to decide which innovations to use and to recommend them to UK Ministers so that resources can be best managed within the health service as a whole. In theory, this body should be best positioned to sift through the evidence and make decisions about appropriate change. In practice, this will be difficult. The organisation has already been criticised for the way it carries out its work and, to a certain degree, these criticisms reflect the fundamental problems that many practitioners have with the way that evidence is used to inform clinical decision making. Smith (2001) argued that NICE is a good thing when it recommends treatments based on evidence but not so when it denies them, despite the evidence to suggest that they should be recommended. He felt that such a position was based solely upon financial constraints, ie. because the treatment would be too expensive, in effect, making a lie of evidence.

The right research needs to be carried out to ensure that we have the most conclusive evidence however, additionally, the decisions provoked by that evidence have to be seen to be reflecting the technologies available and should not be governed by the prohibitions of cost. Whether it is possible to do this or not is debatable.

## Conclusion

The growth and popularity of evidence-based practice over the last ten years is proof that health professionals generally strive to be as effective as possible. True, there are problems associated with the methods used to develop the evidence base, assess its effectiveness and use it to develop practice. However, the fact remains that clinical decision making has to keep pace with innovation and we can no longer introduce ideas into practice simply on the basis that they seemed like a good idea at the time. Mental health nurses must learn to move with the times and that means availing themselves of the skills to find and make sense of the evidence available to them.

Nurses have to continue to develop their own research activities. This will provide them with a knowledge base with which to underpin their actions and give greater credibility to their decision-making processes, especially within the confines of the multi-disciplinary team. The opportunities are enormous and perhaps nursing is only constricted by its own collective imagination. Ultimately, nursing will either make a genuine contribution to the evidence base movement or simply become passive observers of change. Individuals alone cannot affect this cultural shift. Nurses have to work together, share knowledge of both successes and failures and be prepared to take responsibility for their own actions. Networking their experiences is one significant way of achieving this and the next chapter deals with one way of doing this.

## References

Appleby J *et al* (1995) *Acting on the Evidence*. Research paper. National Association for Health Authorities and Trusts, London

Barker PJ, Walker L (2000) Nurse perceptions of multidisciplinary team working in acute psychiatric settings. *J Psychiatr Ment Health Nurs* 7(6): 539–46

Bero LA, Rennie D (1996) Influences on the quality of published drug studies. *Int J Health Technology Assessment* 12: 209–37 urses had was through their own personal development programmes and/or the gaining of higher degrees (Hunt and Hicks, 1983). In fact, Chung and Nolan (1994) show that mental health nurses were positively discouraged from questioning the nature and development of psychiatric knowledge up until the middle of the 1980s. Natural enquiry and the desire to get things done effectively have to a certain degree overcome these obstacles (Ward, 2000a) but, despite this, in the late twentieth century mental health nursing was still attempting to make sense of what it did, and for whom (Barker, 1999; Clarke, 1999).

That period of time also saw nurses themselves question practices that had been their responsibility for as long as mental health nursing had been available; such things as, close or special observations, control and restraining techniques, the use of 'as required' PRN medications following untoward or violent incidents, the use of seclusion and the efficacy of counselling and/or cathartic interactions. It also experienced alarm at the way that nursing was being used to plug the gaps in acute in-patient care (Ward *et al*, 1999) in the light of increasing shortages of suitably qualified staff (Ward, 2000b). Such self-doubt and questioning could have brought about a crisis within mental health nursing but it was not to be the case. As usual, individual nurses and opinion drivers rallied the others and new roles were accepted with the same enthusiasm as old ones, new organisational activities were tackled with resignation and purpose and new responsibilities were accepted, if at times, not fully appreciated. More importantly, mental health nursing began to undertake a large portfolio of research in its attempt to not only make sense of the work that it did but to provide the evidence to support its own actions and clinical decision making.

## Development of the NPNR

It was in the light of these activities that the Network for Psychiatric Nursing Research was born. Its rationale came from several quarters, but perhaps the most important was the 1994 review of mental health nursing (Department of Health, 1994) which cited MIDIRS (Midwives' Information Resource Service) as a good example of a speciality specific database and networking system. The review was very positive that mental health nursing should remain a speciality rather than be subsumed into generic nursing and recommended that part of this process included the development of its own information and networking system. At the time of evidence being presented to the review body, 1993, there was no obvious networking available for mental health nurses and much of its research was fragmented and, at times, personalised. Nurses tended to undertake research for higher degrees with the result that it was often not published and consequently prone to replication. There was no way of gauging the quality

Brazier H, Begley CM (1996) Selecting a database for literature searches in nursing: MEDLINE or CINAHL? *J Adv Nursing* 24(4): 868–75

Burns T, Fiander M, Kent A *et al* (2000) Effects of case-load on the process of care of patients with severe psychotic illness. Report from the UK700 trial. *Br J Psychiatry* 177: 427–33

Burns T, Priebe S (1999) Mental health care failure in England (editorial). *Br J Psychiatry* 174: 191–2

Bury T, Jerosch-Herold C (1998) Reading and critical appraisal of the literature. In: Bury T, Mead M, eds. *Evidence-based healthcare: A practical guide for therapists*. Butterworth Heinemann, Oxford: 136–61

Carper BA (1978) Fundamental patterns of knowing in nursing. *Adv Nurs Science* 1(1): 13–23

Chalmers I, Altman DG (eds) (1995) *Systematic Reviews*. BMJ Publishing Group, London

Cullum N (1994) Critical reviews of the literature. In: Hardey M, Mulhall A, eds. *Nursing Research. Theory and Practice*. Chapman and Hall, London

Dawes M (1999) Introduction to critical appraisal. In: Dawes M, Davies P, Gray A, Hunt J, Seers K and Snowbail R, eds. *Evidence-based practice: A primer for healthcare professionals*. Churchill Livingstone, Edinburgh: 47–8

Department of Health (1994) *Working in Partnership: The Report from the Mental Health Review Team*. HMSO, London

Dodd T (2001) Clues about evidence for mental health care in community settings — assertive outreach. *Ment Health Practice* 4: 10–14

Evidence-Based Medicine Working Group (1992) Evidence-based medicine: a new approach to teaching the practice of medicine. *J Am Med Assoc* 268: 2420–22

Fenton WS (2000) Evolving perspectives on individual psychotherapy for schizophrenia. *Schizophr Bull* 26: 47–72

Frankl V (1959) *Man's Search for Meaning*. Hodder and Stoughton, London

Geddes J, Freemantle N, Harrison P *et al* (2000) Atypical antipsychotics in the treatment of schizophrenia: systematic overview and meta-regression analysis. *Br Med J* 321: 1371–6

Greenhalgh T (1997a) How to read a paper: Papers that report drug trials. *Br Med J* 315: 480–3

Greenhalgh T (1997b) *How to Read a Paper*. BMJ Publishing Group, London

Greenhalgh T (1999) Narrative based medicine in an evidenced-based world. *Br Med J* 318: 323–5

Gournay K, Plummer S, Gray R (2001) The dream team at the institute. *Ment Health Practice* 4: 15–17

Haynes R, McKibben K, Kanani R (1996) Systematic reviews of RCTs of the effects of patient adherence and outcomes of interventions to assist patients to follow prescriptions for medications. Cochrane Library (Updated 30 August 1996). BMJ Publications, London

Hek G, Langton H, Blunden G (2000) Systematically searching and reviewing literature. *Nurse Researcher* 7(3): 40–57

Johnson S, Thornicroft G (1993) The sectorisation of psychiatric services in England and Wales. *Soc Psychiatry Psychiatr Epidemiol* 28: 45–7

Kerlinger FNB (1986) *Foundations of Behavioural Research*. 3rd edn. Holt, Rinehart and Winston, New York

Kulpers E, Garety P, Fowler D *et al* (1997) London – East Anglia randomised controlled trial of cognitive-behavioural therapy for psychosis 1: Effects of the treatment phase. *Br J Psychiatry* 171: 319–27

Lefebvre C (1994) The Cochrane Collaboration: the role of the UK Cochrane Collaboration in identifying evidence. Health Libraries Review 11

McFarlane RW, Lukens E, Link B *et al* (1995) Multiple family groups and psychoeducation in the treatment of schizophrenia. *Arch Gen Psychiatry* **52**: 679–87

McKenna HP, Cutcliffe JR, McKenna P (2000) Evidence-based practice: demolishing some myths. *Nurs Standard* **14**(16): 39–42

McKibbon KA, Walker CJ (1994) Beyond ACP Journal Club: how to harness Medline for therapy problems. *Ann Intern Med* **121**(1): 125–7

Medical Research Council (2000) *A Framework for Clinical Trials of Complex Health Interventions*. Medical Research Council, London

Mueser K, Bond G, Drake R *et al* (1998) Models of community care for severe mental illness: a review of research on case management. *Schizophrenia Bull* **24**: 37–74

Muir-Gray JA (1997) *Evidence-based Health Care*. Churchill Livingstone, Edinburgh

NHS Centre for Reviews and Dissemination (1996) Undertaking Systematic Reviews of Research on Effectiveness CRD Report No 4. Centre for Reviews and Research on Effectiveness, York

NHSE (1999) *Critical Appraisal Skills Programme*. NHSE, Anglia and Oxford

Peat J (with Mellis C, Williams K and Xuan W) (2001) *Health Science Research: A Handbook of Quantitative Methods*. Sage, London

Prior C, Clements J, Rowett M *et al* (2001) Atypical antipsychotics in the treatment of schizophrenia. *Br Med J* **322**(924)

Roth A, Fonagy P (1996) *What Works for Whom? A Critical Review of Psychotherapy Research*. Guilford Press, New York

Sackett DL, Rosenberg W, Muir-Gray J *et al* (1996) Evidence-based medicine: what it is and what it isn't. *Br Med J* **312**: 71–2

Sackett DL *et al* (1997) *Evidenced-based medicine: How to Practice and Teach*. Churchill Livingstone, EBM London

Sajiwandani J (1996) Ensuring the trustworthiness of quantitative research through critique. *Nursing Times Research* **1**(2): 135–42

Smith M (2001) The failings of NICE. *Br Med J* **322**: 489

Smith P (1998) *Nursing Research: Setting new agendas*. Arnold, London

Stensky T, Turkington D, Kingdon D *et al* (2000) A randomised controlled trial of cognitive-behavioural therapy for persistent symptoms of schizophrenia resistent to medication. *Arch Gen Psychiatry* **57**:165–72

Thornicroft G, Wykes T, Holloway F *et al* (1998) From efficacy to effectiveness in community mental health services. PRiSM Psychosis Study 10. *Br J Psychiatry* **173**: 423–7

Tyrer P (2000) Are small case-loads beautiful in severe mental illness? *Br J Psychiatry* **177**: 386–7

Ward MF, Cutcliffe J, Gournay K (1999) *A review of research and practice development undertaken by nurses, midwives and health visitors to support people with mental health problems*. United Kingdom Central Council for Nurses, Midwives and Health Visitors, London

Wykes T, Leese M, Taylor R *et al* (1998) Effects of community services on disability and symptoms. PRiSM Psychosis Study 4. *Br J Psychiatry* **173**: 385–90

# 2

# The Network for Psychiatric Nursing R (NPNR) and the National Journal Club

## Introduction

It has taken mental health nursing about a hundred years to reach the l professionalism that it has today (although whether or not it is a 'profe or indeed should aspire to being one is a matter for debate). In that t has had to deal with social prejudice, poor resources, segregation absence of a substantial body of specific clinical skills which would cl separate it from other nursing specialities, a lack of clear role definit inter-disciplinary tribalism associated with professional hierarchies a more recently, the recognition that sometimes it lacks evidence to supp its actions. Add to that any number of organisational, legal and structu changes and it is hardly any wonder that at times its identity as a acknowledged entity has been called into question. Yet survive and flouris it has, and currently it is recognised as an essential partner in the cor disciples of psychiatric care, along with medicine and psychology. Increasingly, its responsibilities have expanded to accommodate innovation and development and it has had to accept roles that allow it to function effectively with social, as well as healthcare agencies. In the UK alone, there are 56,000 mental health nurses registered with the United Kingdom Central Council for Nurses and their work activities are as diverse as the geography of the country in which they work.

However, life has changed around them and it is no coincidence that mental healthcare services themselves now face a series of questions about their credibility in a world that is fast becoming driven by evidence and the need to generate it. Psychiatry has been accused of lagging behind medicine generally in its attempts to establish its evidence base (Kennedy, 2000) and mental health nursing has not fared much better (Ward, 1994; Kempster, 1998). Even where there is sufficient evidence to influence practice, some authors have argued that there is not enough dissemination and practitioners are reluctant to use it even when it is made available to them (Waddell, 2001).

Nonetheless, mental health nursing has not achieved its success by default, nor has it relied upon the resources of psychiatry to provide it with its existing evidence base. This is all the more remarkable when one considers that, prior to 1989 and the introduction of a completely new approach to providing pre-registration nurse education (ENB, 1989), the only exposure to research and research findings that the vast majority of

of this work and even less chance of it coming together to form a substantial body of knowledge for use by the profession as a whole (Ward, 1994).

Following publication of the review, a meeting was organised by one of the authors for principal UK mental health academics and opinion leaders that took place in Oxford in May of 1994. Several options were open to this group. With no previous resource available there was a blank canvas but it was important that a network was not developed simply for the sake of it. What was needed was an organisation that would have meaning and purpose and plug a needed hole, not just any hole.

It was agreed that research had to form the basis of any new group. In the light of growing interest at that time in evidence-based practice it was seen as necessary that something was available which would promote the culture of research among mental health nursing and offer a forum for its dissemination. It would need to be a resource for those wishing to undertake research of their own, linking those who knew how to undertake the work with those wishing to learn. It needed to offer those who wanted to benefit from the work of others the opportunity to read about, and have access to, good practice activities while providing a method of linking people together, and not just their work.

Though the network did not fully materialise from this meeting certain fundamentals were agreed. The network would need to be:

- specific to mental health nursing, though it was hoped that other disciplines involved in psychiatric care and the social sciences would use or belong to it
- based upon research and its application into practice, ie. practice development (these terms were used as defined in the report of the task force of the strategy for research in nursing, midwifery and health visiting, Department of Health, 1993)
- consisted of two separate components. A database holding current, intended and completed projects plus a contact directory putting people in touch with each other for specific projects, interests, support and information
- for submitted research work from network members and not simply a trawl of existing research published in journals or held on other databases
- by postal access. (At that time the cost of technology for putting the network on to the Internet was prohibitive and e-mailing, as we know it today, was still only available to a minority)
- organised around a specific pre-formatted menu of mental health topics enabling access to the directories
- serviced by its own publication, a quarterly newsletter, which would be distributed to all network members
- supported by an annual conference
- expandable, so that in the event of new technologies becoming available or future demand changing it could remain active and

relevant. Good examples of this was the necessity for Internet access and an international directory

- used for providing live information about the state of mental health nursing research and practice developments through a review of the work of its members. It was envisaged that much of what was submitted to the network would not otherwise be published so such a review would provide data that was not available elsewhere
- use review material to comment on mental health nursing research strategies
- publish innovative work within its own publication
- regularly evaluated to ensure that it was meeting the needs of the research and development community and respond to any changes identified.

One of the less obvious roles of the network was seen as providing a passive voice co-ordinating the intended work of researchers and attempting to establish some sense of focus for the body of work being undertaken. At that time it was unclear how this was to be accomplished, but later it became obvious that, while it was virtually impossible to achieve, some influence could be maintained through the newsletter and the annual conference.

**Initial development**

A steering group was set up from those attending the initial meeting. Discussions were held with various network providers, including the Bath Information and Dissemination Service (BIDS) who provide electronic support to all UK universities but it became clear that if the network was to go that route it would need a substantial injection of funds. A paper was published (Ward, 1994) asking mental health nurses to identify topics that would inform the construction of the nursing index. It had to contain terms that were both contemporary and had meaning for nurses, not just a list of items that were considered to be current. This would aid both storage and retrieval functions. Contact was also maintained with the Speciality Assurance Team of the mental health topics for the READ code project, who were at that time developing a similar thesaurus for the NHS, and the NHS Centre for Reviews and Dissemination.

The Network had to be fully compatible with existing and intended NHS-wide networking systems to enable free flow and exchange of both projects and material. A 57-item index was developed over a six-month period which took into consideration the medical subject heading (MeSH) used by the NHS to register projects within their burgeoning Project Registration System database (PRS). In theory, this would have enabled an exchange of information between the two databases, but the reality was that the two systems were developed for different purposes (the NPNR for individual practitioners, PRS to enable large funders of research programmes to log their work) and this was never to take place. Documentation was developed around the index, and the operational mechanism designed so that the whole package would work. It was agreed that membership of the network would be via a small annual fee, both to cover individual administrative costs and to engender a sense of belonging among the members themselves. Finally, the name of the network was agreed. This was not as simple a task as you might imagine. When asked, half the nurses who responded to the original call for items in the index referred to themselves as mental health nurses, the other half as psychiatric nurses. The same split appeared on the steering committee. The term 'psychiatric' was eventually used because it was felt that this better reflected the wider aspirations of the intended network. Publicity material was constructed and funding sought.

**Funding the NPNR**

Funding options for the NPNR were limited by the availability of sponsors interested in mental health nursing and who would be in a position to extend their support over a period of years. It was never going to be possible to maintain the network from membership subscriptions alone and set-up costs in themselves were considerable. The network also had to be seen as independent of large companies and other professional agencies with mental health nursing being both the focus and the beneficiary of its activities. Initial difficulties were that many potential sponsors could neither see the necessity for a separate research network for mental health nurses, nor could some understand why nurses did not simply use existing resources or wait for those that were intended for coming on stream within the next few years. There was a perception that nurses did not undertake the quantity of research that would warrant an independent network. Moreover, mental health nurses were not seen as a priority group and, indeed, were not seen as making a real contribution to psychiatric or mental health research. In effect, there was a chicken and egg situation. Without a network to show the collective body of work, both completed and intended, or its application into practice, there was no clear way to identify the need to establish the network in the first place.

This situation was eventually overcome by undertaking a small review of relevant published material, relating it to the findings of the mental health nursing review and linking both these to the developing strategies for mental health care in the UK. The key potential sponsor was the Department of Health. They initially suggested that nurses use the PRS but as this was still being developed and the NPNR indexing system was completed and far more relevant to mental health nursing (the intended primary user of the system) they eventually agreed to support the work. Eventually, in March 1995, the DoH awarded the NPNR a fifty thousand pound pump-priming grant. This would at least enable the network to become operational and so increase the possibility of further maintenance funding in the future.

A full-time administrator was appointed, hardware purchased, database development undertaken and the NPNR became active from July 1995 onwards.

## Growth of the NPNR

One of the first tasks to be undertaken following the initial launch was to set up a system to evaluate the effectiveness and operational values of the network. In the case of the NPNR this was difficult. In the first place its primary function was to establish a network of contacts, assemble a bank of research abstracts relating to projects and disseminate these two elements to anyone within the membership who requested them. This was achieved by virtue of the network being live and its members using it. Simply counting the numbers of members and the amount of time they used the service was deemed to be very limited evaluation because it did not tell of the effectiveness of the process. For example, if only ten people had joined the NPNR and half of them lodged a project this could be seen as a failure. However, if they kept in regular communication with each other, used each other's work to inform their own and developed a research and development programme which combined their individual talents this could be seen to be a success of the NPNR. Similarly, if the network had 20,000 members, 10,000 projects it would be seen as a major success, especially for a potential sponsor. Yet, if these members never communicated with each other or contributed to the newsletter the NPNR would effectively be failing in its primary intention — networking. To evaluate the effectiveness of the NPNR it was necessary to set up a series of secondary functions upon which its performance over time could be reviewed.

This was achieved by considering the main purpose of the dissemination process, namely:

1.  The transfer and interchange of information between members.
2.  The reduction of academic or research duplication.
3.  The use of research to inform practice.

A series of dissemination sharing options were considered, put to the steering group for ratification and a functional strategy developed. Benchmarking of the NPNR was made and the first review undertaken in 2000.

The review showed that the exchange of information was the main concern of its members, with lodging projects of secondary interest. Interestingly enough, members wanted to find out about the work of others but often considered their own work to be of no value to the wider membership and were reluctant to make it available. The membership is not a constant value with a core body of approximately 800, changing over time and a total of nearly 2,000 who have been a member at one time or another. Three hundred projects contained within the database reflect a wide range of research interests but, to this day, there are still areas of the original indexing system that have no entries. The projects themselves show that nurses have taken service developments and the organisational structures of mental health services as key areas for research, with individual interventions coming a very close second. Low on the list of priorities is research into psychiatry itself, and this is a definite shift away from what used to be the case some fifteen years ago. Then nurses tended to explore areas of concern that could loosely be described as the domain of psychiatrists and possibly psychologists. It would seem that while there is still a perceived need for nurses to undertake some of this work, much of their research energy has been relocated to explore the work of nurses. As such, the time when a real body of research evidence exits to support the work activities of mental health nurses is at last becoming a reality.

The international membership has grown over the years without the necessity to introduce a separate international contact section. Seventeen countries are represented in the membership and the NPNR itself is organisationally linked to professional groups in Scandinavia, Australia Canada and the USA. It has two websites, one based in the UK and a Nordic group based in Norway and most contact with the network is now via e-mail. It publishes a quarterly newsletter, NetLink, which has been separately funded from sponsors and has established a base for its annual conference within Oxford University.

However, very early on in the life of the NPNR it became clear that one of the operational objectives of its work was not properly covered, either by its regular review or by the more substantial evaluation process. Dissemination is not just about the exchange of information. For it to be effective recipients have to understand the meaning of what they receive. At no time have the abstracts held by the NPNR been subjected to a quality assurance assessment, nor is any judgement made about the quality of the research processes used to gather the data. Equally, the NPNR was never intended to replace the traditional methods of gathering information from professional journals. It was always intended that the NPNR would extend members' knowledge and/or skills rather than short cut the system and do the work for them. A mechanism did not exist within the NPNR framework for ensuring that members were using the information they received in a constructive manner, nor was there any way of knowing whether members could independently review or critique literature. The NPNR recognised this deficiency in its workings and while accepting that it was not its responsibility to kite mark everything for its members, it was its responsibility to give them the skills that would enable them to make best use of the data contained on its databases. During late 1996 and most of 1997 work progressed on establishing a unique addition to the NPNR; a forum that would facilitate members' best use of the data, the development of its national journal club. Before describing the NPNR's National Journal Club, it is necessary to explore the nature of journal clubs.

## Journal clubs as a forum for promoting critique of research

According to Bury and Jerosch-Herold (1998), journal clubs normally involve a group of people who meet regularly to review and discuss one or several journal articles. These may or may not follow a chosen topic or theme. There is a limited literature which indicates the educational value of journal clubs. Linzer (1987) discovered that the critical skills of the members improves with journal club participation. Furthermore, Burnstein *et al* (1996) found that journal clubs that utilise a certain structure (eg. the use of a particular approach/model, a structured review instrument), appear to experience additional educational value. Bury and Jerosch-Herold (1998) point out that additional benefits to participating in journal clubs include: shared decision making about changes in practice; consideration of different perspectives and methods; learning from one's peers, and less sense of making judgements about work in an isolated position.

Since it needs to be acknowledged that our medical colleagues have made significant progress within the domain of evidence-based practice, it is perhaps not surprising that journal clubs are widely used by medics. Such clubs are increasingly being utilised by nurses, in a variety of settings, including formal education settings. These clubs are organised using a variety of formats, they do not need to have a fixed number of members, but do need to occur on a regular basis in order to get the maximum benefit (Morton, 1996). Clearly, clubs need an identified person (or persons) to organise the club, and sessions may derive additional benefit from having someone experienced in critiquing research take the lead in the initial meetings. The material to be critiqued needs to be distributed in advance of the club, as this allows members to read and be prepared for the ensuing discussion.

The authors of this text would suggest that there is no singular correct way to run a journal club and that members will find a method that suits them best. Bury and Jerosch-Herold (1998), for example, construct the case for multi-disciplinary journal clubs, whereas other clubs have been organised on a uni-disciplinary basis. Selection of papers for review is clearly a decision that appears to be bound up with the composition (and discipline) of the members and clubs should decide what, if anything, they are going to do with the 'conclusions' produced by the club.

## The NPNR National Journal Club

In September 1997, the NPNR National Journal Club was launched (uniquely for that year alone) at two annual conferences held in both Oxford and Edinburgh. This journal club has several aims and purposes:

❖ It serves as a forum where current issues in psychiatric/mental health nursing and research can be debated, explored and discussed.

❖ It serves as a means of education and personal development in that each of the National Journal Club members will have the opportunity to make a contribution. The NPNR wanted to create a forum where mental health nurses, nursing managers, and educationalists/researchers and students could create links with one another, comment on academic developments, and have the opportunity to collate feeling and feedback about national issues in mental health nursing.

❖ This would create a situation where nurses of all grades and specialities were able to exchange thoughts and feelings, network with one another and create a national dialogue, review academic manuscripts and contribute to four publications a year.

❖ This feedback could then be used to inform national strategic developments, research initiatives and both central and local policies concerning research implementation.

**How does the National Journal Club work?**

The National Journal Club meetings are held four times a year. In order to gain a national perspective it was first necessary to involve practitioners based in each of the regional health authorities. Initially, fifteen groups were established. Each of these smaller groups have an appointed regional co-ordinator (and usually some assistants) who act as a contact point for journal club members and prospective members. These individuals facilitate their regional journal club meetings, distribute manuscripts for reviews, feed back to the national co-ordinator any suggestions for improvement and development.

At each meeting, all the clubs systematically review the same manuscript dealing with an issue in psychiatric/mental health nursing or research, with an opportunity for each member to contribute. Group comments are then collected at the NPNR headquarters in Oxford and condensed into a single review paper. This produces a collective national response, from both NPNR and National Journal Club members, to the issues raised in the chosen manuscripts. This review is then published, four times a year, in the *British Journal of Mental Health Nursing* and the NPNR publication, *Netlink*. Additionally, since part of the 'core business' of the National Journal Club is critiquing research papers, all the clubs engaged in developing an approach or method that was suitable to their needs. Rather than 'wholesale' of an existing approach, the NPNR National Journal Club members wanted an approach that they felt comfortable with; that addresses the questions they want asking; and that facilitates them in their efforts to embrace evidence-based mental health care.

## Choice of publications

For the first year, manuscripts were chosen by key people within the NPNR, usually in response to national issues raised by the Department of Health, UKCC, (now the NMC [Nursing and Midwifery Council]), ENB, RCN or other nursing organisation. As the National Journal Club evolved, members of the club who had a clearer sense of what the current issues were for clinicians and clients, and what changes would make the most difference to these people, made suggestions for manuscripts to be reviewed. This resulted in the choice of particular papers for review and, indeed, certain 'themes' were followed, eg. violence and aggression. Additionally, these first sixteen reviews are then used as the examples of critiques in this book. One outcome of this process of the National Journal Club members selecting the papers for review, was that practitioners involved in working 'at the coal face' were able to respond (and influence) national agendas, on which issues should be raised and debated.

## What happens to the discussion notes produced?

Each appointed regional co-ordinator (and their assistant) collects and collates the feedback comments from the journal club meetings. These are then sent to the National Journal Club co-ordinator who, together with personnel from the NPNR, sums these up in a review paper. This review, reflecting the national perspective on the issue identified, is then published in the *British Journal of Mental Health Nursing* and the NPNR publication, *Netlink*. Also, if the manuscript addresses a specific issue raised by one of the national nursing organisations, then that organisation will be provided with a copy of the review. Comment will be fed back directly to the Department of Health, the UKCC (now the NMC), the ENB and the RCN. Comments may also be sent on to the author(s) concerned.

## Attending the National Journal Club

All NPNR members are encouraged to attend and contribute to the National Journal Club meetings. Members are asked to 'spread the word' and inform their colleagues of this important and exciting development. You do not have to be an NPNR member in order to attend the National Journal Club. Currently, the National Journal Club has over forty centres around the UK and it is hoped over the next few years that this will be extended to include feedback from international groups and members.

# Conclusion

The NPNR has filled a gap for mental health nurses. It provides resources and a method of networking that were previously unavailable to them, and it gives the opportunity for mental health nursing research and practice developments to impact upon the delivery of mental health care. In addition, it provides a mechanism to link people together so that their work has more meaning, can be better informed and provides them with peer support that would otherwise be absent from their personal development. Through its unique National Journal Club it offers a forum for discussion and debate around issues affecting mental health nursing, its research and evolution. National Journal Club reviews, published in a national professional journal as well as the NPNR publication, *NetLink*, have the opportunity to influence the quality and increase the accessibility of the work of future writers and researchers. The NPNR continues to be the only mental health nursing speciality network concentrating on the research activities of the profession and there are already plans in the pipeline to increase its support of members and future members. The remainder of this book would not have been possible without the existence of the NPNR. We hope you find it useful and informative, but most of all we hope that you use it to inform your understanding of research and take your place as an active member of your mental health nursing community.

Details about NPNR membership and events can be obtained by contacting the Network for Psychiatric Nursing Research, Royal College of Nursing Institute, Radcliffe Infirmary, Woodstock Road, Oxford OX2 6HE or e-mailing: mental.health.network@rcn.org.uk.

Having described the context and background to critiquing nursing research, explained the purpose and value of critiquing research and having detailed the evolution of the NPNR National Journal Club, the remainder of the book is concerned with the practice of critiquing nursing research. Accordingly, the next section is comprised of a range of approaches used to critique nursing research and each chapter identifies the strengths and limitations of these approaches. Each approach is also accompanied by two examples of critiques, which are based on critiques undertaken by the NPNR National Journal Club.

Section three describes the NPNR National Journal Club's approach to critiquing nursing research. Since this is a developmental approach, we provide two additional examples for each of the four stages identified.

# References

Barker PJ (1999) *The Philosophy and Practice of Psychiatric Nursing.* Churchill Livingstone, London

Bury T, Jerosch-Herold C (1998) Reading and critical appraisal of the literature. In: Bury T, Mead M, eds. *Evidence-based health care: A practical guide for therapists.* Butterworth Heinemann, Oxford:136–61

Burnstein JL, Hollander JE, Barlas D (1996) Enhancing the value of the Journal Club: use of a structured review instrument. *Am J Emerg Med* **14**(6): 45–50

Chung MC, Nolan P (1994) The influence of positivist thought on nineteenth century asylum nursing. *J Adv Nurs* **19**(2): 226–32

Clarke L (1999) *Challenging Ideas in Psychiatric Nursing.* Routledge, London

Department of Health (1993) *Report of the Task Force on the Strategy for Research in Nursing, Midwifery and Health Visiting.* HMSO, London

Department of Health (1994) *Working in Partnership: a collaborative approach to care. Report of the mental health nursing review team.* HMSO, London

English National Board for Nursing, Midwifery and Health Visiting (1989) *Project 2000: A new Preparation for Practice.* (Pre-registration Learning Outcomes. Item 1.2.3. The use of relevant literature and research to inform the practice of nursing). ENB, London

Hunt M, Hicks J (1983) Promoting research awareness in post-basic nursing courses. Nursing Times Occasional Papers. *Nurs Times* **79**(6)

Kempster M (1998) Evidence-based medicine in mental health. *Evidence-Based Nurs* **1**(40)

Kennedy P (2000) Is psychiatry losing ground with the rest of medicine? *Adv Psychiatric Treatment* **6**: 16–21

Linzer M (1987) The Journal Club and medical education: over one hundred years of unrecorded history. *Postgrad Med* **63**: 475–8

Morton SA (1996) Setting up a journal club. *Health Visitor* **69**(11): 465–6

Waddell C (2001) So much research evidence, so little dissemination and uptake: mixing the useful with the pleasing. *Evidence Based Mental Health* **4**: 3–5

Ward MF (1994) In search of a purpose. Nursing Times Mental Health Supplement. *Nurs Times* **90**(8): 69

Ward MF (2000a) Developing a mental health nursing network to support research. *Nurse Researcher* **7**: 24–31

Ward MF (2000b) Campaign fails to tackle mental health staff crisis. *Nurs Times* **96**(15)

Ward MF, Gournay K, Thornicroft G, Wright S (1999) *The 1998 Census: A review of acute in-patient mental health services within inner London.* Royal College of Nursing, London

# Section two: Examples of a range of approaches used to critique nursing research

**3**

# An introduction, and Duffy's (1985) research appraisal checklist approach to critiquing nursing research

## Introduction

This chapter builds on the introduction to the background and context of critiquing nursing research, which was outlined in chapter one. It is accepted as axiomatic that there is no such thing as the 'perfect' study. Consequently, one might postulate that there may, similarly, be no such thing as the 'perfect' approach to or model of critiquing research. Accepting this premise, and the need for nurses to be able to engage in critiquing research under the auspices of evidence-based practice, there are several key issues which need to be considered.

Firstly, nurses should be aware that a range of approaches to critiquing research exist, as a result, it is one of the aims of this book to introduce the reader to the variety of approaches.

Secondly, accepting that there appears to be range in the quality of the approaches to critiquing research, we have attempted to include a diverse selection and we offer our own views of the strengths and limitations of these approaches. We include two well known and two lesser well known examples of such approaches.

Thirdly, nursing research has a history of being strongly influenced by the medical profession (Pearson, 1992; Cutcliffe, 1998).The philosophical, epistemological and methodological beliefs of the biomedical model have been adopted by some (many) nurse researchers. As a result, positivistic philosophies, quantitative methods and the hegemony of the RCT can be seen throughout the history of nursing research. Given nursing research's historical emphasis with quantitative methods, we suggest that this emphasis can be seen in the range of approaches for critiquing nursing research. Wherein, the bulk of these approaches reflect this emphasis on quantitative methods, and appear to be designed to critique the research according to certain positivistic/quantitative criteria.

Fourthly, this historical emphasis on approaches that are designed to critique a study according to quantitative criteria indicates that models of critiquing need to evolve and develop in parallel with the development of research methods and methodologies.

Fifthly, accepting the argument that approaches to critiquing need to evolve, we include a range of approaches, which when ordered chronologically, familiarise the reader with evolution of approaches to critiquing. Importantly, this issue also highlights that scope exists for additional development work in the area of approaches to critiquing, leading logically into the third section of the book, the NPNR National Journal Club's approach to critiquing research.

The remainder of this chapter focuses on Duffy's (1985) 'Research appraisal checklist' approach to critiquing nursing research. It identifies the fifty-one criteria, ordered under eight major research categories, which Duffy uses as the basis for his checklist, and provides some brief instructions on how to use the checklist when critiquing research. Following this, we provide two detailed examples (drawing from the reviews carried out by the NPNR National Journal Club). Having described the approach and provided examples, we highlight some of the advantages and disadvantages of this approach.

## Duffy's (1985) research appraisal checklist approach to critiquing research

Duffy (1985) suggests that in order to use his approach, the reviewer should examine each of the fifty-one criteria. Each of these should then be given an individual rating which best describes the degree to which the criterion is met (or not) within the research report. His rating scale ranges from one to six, with one indicating that the criterion was not met and six indicating that the criterion was completely met. Duffy adds that reviewers should add brief comments to criteria that score less than five, in order to explain the decision. Additionally, if the reviewer thinks the criterion is not applicable, then this should be marked as NA. The scores for each criterion are added together in order to give; a) a score for each separate category (eg. a score for the abstract) and, b) a total score for the paper. Following this, the reviewer is encouraged to produce a brief summary which indicates the major strengths and limitations of the report, and this summary should reflect the scores indicated for the categories. The fifty-one criteria are outlined below.

| 1. | The title is readily understood | 123456 NA | |
|----|---------------------------------|-----------|--|
| 2. | The title is clear | 123456 NA | |
| 3. | The title is clearly related to content | 123456 NA | |
| 4. | The abstract states the problem, and where appropriate, hypotheses clearly and concisely | 123456 NA | |
| 5. | The methodology is identified and described briefly | 123456 NA | |
| 6. | The results are summarised | 123456 NA | |
| 7. | The findings and/or conclusions are stated | 123456 NA | |
| **Category score =** | | | |
| 8. | The general problem of the study is introduced early in the report | 123456 NA | |
| 9. | Questions to be answered are stated precisely | 123456 NA | |
| 10. | Problem statement is clear | 123456 NA | |
| 11. | Hypotheses to be tested are stated precisely in a form that permits them to be tested | 123456 MA | |
| 12. | Limitations of the study can be identified | 123456 NA | |
| 13. | Assumptions of the study can be identified | 123456 NA | |
| 14. | Pertinent terms are/can be operationally defined | 123456 NA | |
| 15. | Significance of the problem is discussed | 123456 NA | |
| 16. | The research is justified | 123456 NA | |
| **Category score =** | | | |
| **4.** | **Review of the literature** | | |
| 17. | Cited literature is pertinent to the research topic | 123456 NA | |
| 18. | Cited literature provides rationale for the research | 123456 NA | |
| 19. | Studies are critically examined | 123456 NA | |
| 20. | Relationships of the problem to previous research is made clear | 123456 NA | |
| 21. | A conceptual framework/theoretical rationale is clearly stated | 123456 NA | |
| 22. | The review concludes with a brief summary of relevant literature and its implications to the research problem under study | 123456 NA | |
| **Category score =** | | | |
| 23. | Subject population (sampling frame) is described | 123456 NA | |
| 24. | Sampling method is described | 123456 NA | |
| 25. | Sampling method is justified (especially for non-probability sampling) | 123456 NA | |
| 26. | Sample size is sufficient to reduce Type II error | 123456 NA | |
| 27. | Possible sources of sampling error can be identified | 123456 NA | |
| 28. | Standards for the protection of subjects are discussed | 123456 NA | |
| **Category score =** | | | |
| 29. | Relevant reliability data from previous research are presented | 123456 NA | |
| 30. | Reliability data pertinent to the present study are reported | 123456 NA | |

| | | | |
|---|---|---|---|
| 31. | Relevant previous validity data from previous research are presented | 123456 NA | |
| 32. | Validity data pertinent to present study are reported | 123456 NA | |
| 33. | Methods of data collection are sufficiently described to permit judgement of their appropriateness to the present study | 123456 NA | |
| **Category score =** | | | |
| 34. | The design is appropriate to the study question and/or hypotheses | 123456 NA | |
| 35. | Proper controls are included where appropriate | 123456 NA | |
| 36. | Confounding/moderating variable are/can be identified | 123456 NA | |
| 37. | The description of the design is explicit enough to permit replication | 123456 NA | |
| **Category score =** | | | |
| **6. Data analysis** | | | |
| 38. | Information presented is sufficient to answer research questions | 123456 NA | |
| 39. | The statistical tests used are identified and obtained values are reported | 123456 NA | |
| 40. | Reported statistics are appropriate for hypotheses/research questions | 123456 NA | |
| 41. | Tables and figures are presented in an easy to understand, informative way | 123456 NA | |
| **Category score =** | | | |
| **7. Discussion** | | | |
| 42. | The conclusions are clearly stated | 123456 NA | |
| 43. | The conclusions are substantiated by the evidence presented | 123456 NA | |
| 44. | Methodological problems in the study are identified and discussed | 123456 NA | |
| 45. | Findings of the study are specifically related to the conceptual/theoretical basis of the study | 123456 NA | |
| 46. | Implications of the findings are discussed | 123456 NA | |
| 47. | The results are generalised only to the population on which the study is based | 123456 NA | |
| 48. | Recommendations are made for further research | 123456 NA | |
| **Category score =** | | | |
| **8. Form and style** | | | |
| 49. | The report is clearly written | 123456 NA | |
| 50. | The report is logically organised | 123456 NA | |
| 51. | The tone of the report displays an unbiased, impartial, scientific attitude | 123456 NA | |
| **Category score =** | | | |

**Grand total =**

Strengths (based on the 51 criteria) are...
Limitations (based on the 51 criteria) are...

> Grand total score corresponding to overall
> categorisation of the research.
> Score between 205–306 = superior paper
> Score between 103–204 = average paper
> Score between 0–102 = below average paper

# Example one: The Network for Psychiatric Nursing Research National Journal Club, review from the seventeenth meeting

> The paper reviewed first appeared in 1999, in the *Journal of Psychiatric and Mental Health Nursing* (**6**: 125–35), 'Research utilisation and attitudes towards research among psychiatric nurses in Northern Ireland' (Parahoo K).

## Abstract/overview

This paper reports on a survey which attempted to determine psychiatric nurses' attitudes towards research, and their perceptions of their use of research and other research-related activities. The author obtained a convenience sample of 236 nurses, from the six main psychiatric hospitals in Northern Ireland and from the psychiatric wards within the general hospitals. The author states that the results of the survey show that, while the nurses report positive attitudes towards research, their perception of their use of research in practice indicates that evidence-based practice is far from being realised. The author then discusses the implications of these findings.

Note: Duffy's original maximum score is 306 (51 x 6) and consequently the overall quality of the paper is calculated according to comparison of the total score with the maximum total score. However, since Duffy includes a 'not applicable' score for each of the criteria, it might be considered as inaccurate to consider the overall quality of the papers reviewed without taking any 'not applicable's into account. Therefore, we include two scores for each category and for each paper; one which does not take account of the 'not applicables' and one which does. We have termed this way of scoring; pro rata scoring.

Criteria/appraisal rating                                    Comments

| 1. Title | Comments |
|---|---|
| 1. 123456 NA | Could have clarified what the term 'research utlization' means |
| 2. 123456 NA | Perhaps the title could have identified that the study was conducted on only qualified psychiatric nurses. |
| 3. 123456 NA | Members felt that it may have been useful for the title to identify that the study was conducted only on hospital-based psychiatric nurses, and not on a sample that included hospital and community-based psychiatric nurses. |
| Category score = | 13/18 Pro rata score 13/18 |
| 2. Abstract | |
| 4. 123456 NA | Yes — clear |
| 5. 123456 NA | Further details of the survey (eg. that it used a questionnaire) may have been useful |
| 6. 123456 NA | The results are summarised in the main, but there appears to be some confusion regarding the nature of evidence-based practice and research-based practice (see McKenna *et al*, 2000), in that one can have evidence-based practice (at least in part) without the presence and application of research evidence. |
| 7. 123456 NA | The abstract does not state any conclusions, it states only that the implications of the findings are discussed. |
| Category score | 16/24 Pro rata score 16/24 |
| 3. Problem | |
| 8. 123456 NA | The general problem is introduced in the second paragraph of the introduction. |
| 9. 123456 NA | The questions are stated clearly, although the members felt they had to work through a substantial section of the paper before they reached the questions. |
| 10. 123456 NA | The research question is posed as a question, not as a problem statement |
| 11. 123456 NA | No hypothesis included |
| 12. 123456 NA | The limitations can be identified and the author makes some attempt to identify the limitations himself. |
| 13. 123456 NA | There is an assumption in the paper that remains implicit, and that is the hegemony of the Randomised Control Trial (RCT). There is a significant debate surrounding this issue (Leininger, 1992; Pearson, 1992; McKibben and Walker, 1994; McKenna *et al*, 2000). Since certain research questions can only be answered using certain research methods/paradigms (Leininger, 1992), and since different research methods/paradigms produce different types of knowledge (Dickoff and James, 1968; Carper, 1978; Benner and Wrubel, 1989; Chinn and Kramer, 1995), what is clearly indicated is that it is inaccurate to proclaim the hegemony of one method/paradigm over another. Different methods will have inherent value depending on the research question asked and the nature of the knowledge required. Furthermore, within the context of mental health nursing, the hegemony of RCTs and the evidence they produce has received additional challenge and these challenges are grounded in the notion that much of mental health nursing can be regarded as invisible and unmeasurable, and thus not accessible to quantitative methods (Micheal, 1994; Stevenson, 1996; Altschul, 1997; Chambers, 1998; Cutcliffe and McKenna, 2000). |

| 14. | 123456 NA | The pertinent terms are defined in part, for example, the author explores and defines the term 'research utilization', but the questionnaire that was distributed to the participants does not make such a distinction. |
|---|---|---|
| 15. | 123456 NA | |
| 16. | 123456 NA | Clearly, this is a much under-researched area and thus this study is entirely justified. |
| **Category score** | **34/54 Pro rata score 34/42** | |
| **Review of the literature** | | |
| 17. | 123456 NA | While much of the literature cited in the review appears to be either directly or indirectly related to the research question, members felt that large sections of the literature review did not appear to be particularly relevant to the study. Indeed, the extensive section of the author's paper that precedes the 'Methodology' reads much more akin to a discursive piece; exploring the relative merits/drawbacks of different methods/types of evidence for psychiatric/mental health (P/MH) nurses. There is little doubt that this is an issue that warrants discussion and debate, but the members felt that much of it fell outside the context of this study. |
| 18. | 123456 NA | See comments in response to question 17 |
| 19. | 123456 NA | Members felt that many of the studies that had been reviewed for this study had not been reviewed critically, particularly when one considers the cumulative nature of knowledge generation (McKenna, 1997), in that the author failed to show how the previous studies had subsequently built upon one another. |
| 20. | 123456 NA | The relationship of the research problem to the previous research is made clear. |
| 21. | 123456 NA | |
| 22. | 123456 NA | No such summary is included, however, members wondered if such a summary is warranted or indeed, common practice. |
| **Category score =** | **15/30 Pro rata score 15/24** | |
| **5. Methodology Part A: subjects** | | |
| 23. | 123456 NA | |
| 24. | 123456 NA | |
| 25. | 123456 NA | Members stated that they wanted more information about the author's remarks regarding the limited resources forcing the author into using a convenience sample. |
| 26. | 123456 NA | |
| 27. | 123456 NA | |
| 28. | 123456 NA | The subjects would be largely anonymous, however, the nursing managers would know which wards the nurses worked on and thus complete anonymity was not achieved. |
| **Category score =** | **19/30 Pro rata score 19/24** | |

| Methodology Part B: instruments | | |
|---|---|---|
| 29. | 123456 NA | The paper does not include reliability scores from the previous research. However, the members felt that to criticise automatically this paper on this matter would be inappropriate. Their concerns go to the use of reliability tests on surveys. Surveys, such as the instrument used in this study, used to determine attitudes and canvas opinion, both of which can and do, change over time. Given that reliability is concerned with consistency over repeated measures (Burns and Grove, 1993), it would be inappropriate to criticise a study on the grounds of reliability, when it demonstrates that opinions have changed over time. The researcher could have addressed this to some extent by repeating his survey within a short space of time of the initial survey. This may have provided the data to calculate reliability scores, but these scores would still be subject to the valid criticisms regarding opinions changing over time. |
| 30. | 123456 NA | There are no reliability scores mentioned for this current study, however, see comments in response to question number 29. |
| 31. | 123456 NA | There is no reference to the validity of the previous studies which are cited in this paper. |
| 32. | 123456 NA | The paper includes some references to validity, eg. how content validity was achieved, and he acknowledges the absence of current validity tests due to the paucity of previous empirical work in this area. |
| 33. | 123456 NA | |
| Category score = | | 11/30 Pro rata score 11/24 |
| Methodology Part C: design | | |
| 34. | 123456 NA | The design is appropriate to the study question, though scales more in keeping with measuring attitudes (Burns and Grove, 1993; Polit and Hungler, 1997) could have been used. |
| 35. | 123456 NA | |
| 36. | 123456 NA | |
| 37. | 123456 NA | There is sufficient information to allow replication. |
| Category score = | | 10/25 Pro rata score 10/12 |
| 6. Data analysis | | |
| 38. | 123456 NA | |
| 39. | 123456 NA | |
| 40. | 123456 NA | |
| 41. | 123456 NA | Tables and figures are very clear. |
| Category score = | | 12/24 Pro rata score 12/12 |

| 7. Discussion | | |
|---|---|---|
| 42. | 123456 NA | This whole section of the paper was regarded by the members as strong. The members pointed out that the only limitation was the author's inclusion of results from general nurses, when he had stated that he would use only the results from the P/MH nurses. |
| 43. | 123456 NA | |
| 44. | 123456 NA | |
| 45. | 123456 NA | |
| 46. | 123456 NA | |
| 47. | 123456 NA | |
| 48. | 123456 NA | |
| Category score = | | 35/42 Pro rata score 35/42 |
| 49. | 123456 NA | Written in a reasonable academic style. |
| 50. | 123456 NA | The logical sequence/organisation was disrupted, according to the members, due to the paper reading akin to a combination of a discursive paper and an empirical paper. |
| 51. | 123456 NA | Tone impartial. |
| Category score = | | 13/18 Pro rata score 13/18 |

**Grand total = 178**

*Strengths*

Clearly, this is an under-researched issue and therefore quality papers that attempt to provide such research are timely.

The development of the questionnaire indicates an evolution of the design and methods required to investigate certain issues in this area.

The discussion is particularly strong, and raises the relevant (and for some key) point regarding the potential reasons why P/MH nurses may not make use of research findings.

Written in a clear, concise style and is accessible, easy to read.

*Limitations*

Some of the article reads more akin to a discursive piece and the bulk of the paper reads more akin to an empirical piece of work, which perhaps causes a degree of confusion.

The author claims to report only on the data from the P/MH nurses, however, much of the results section and discussion (to a lesser extent) reports on findings from the general nurses.

Omits the size of the sample of P/MH nurses who were invited to participate, providing only the size of the sample who responded and the size of the overall sample (ie. general nurses, P/MH nurses, etc).

Perhaps contains an element of confusion between research-based and evidence-based practice.

> Grand total score corresponding to overall categorisation of the research.
> Score between 205–306 = superior paper
> Score between 103–204 = average paper
> Score between 0–102 = below average paper
> **Grand total score was 178, therefore, categorised as an average paper.**

> Grand total pro rata score corresponding to
> overall categorisation of the research.
> Score between 161–240 = superior paper
> Score between 81–160 = average paper
> Score between 0–80 = below average paper
> **Grand total score was 178, therefore, using
> the pro rata scoring method, the paper
> would be categorised as a superior paper.**

# References

Altschul A (1997) A personal view of psychiatric nursing. In: Tilley S, ed. *The Mental Health Nurse: Views of practice and education*. Blackwell Science, London

Benner P, Wrubel J (1989) *The Primacy of Caring: Stress and coping in Health and Illness*. Addison-Wesley, New York

Burns N, Grove stock (1993) *The Practice of Nursing Research: Conduct, critique and utilization*. 2nd edn. WB Saunders, Philadelphia

Carper BA (1978) Fundamental patterns of knowing in nursing. *Adv Nursing Science* 1(1): 13–23

Chambers M (1998) Interpersonal mental health nursing: research issues and challenges. *J Psychiatr Ment Health Nurs* 5: 203–11

Chinn P, Kramer MK (1995) *Theory and nursing: A Systematic approach*. CV Mosby, St Louis

Cutcliffe JR (1998) Is psychiatric nursing research barking up the wrong tree? *Nurse Educ Today* 18: 257–8

Cutcliffe JR, McKenna HP (2000) Generic nurses: the nemesis of psychiatric/mental health nursing? *Ment Health Practice* 3(9): 10–14

Dickoff J, James P (1968) A Theory of theories: A position paper. *Nurs Res* 17: 3

Duffy M (1985) A research appraisal checklist for evaluating nursing research reports. *Nurs Healthcare* 6(10): 539–47

Estabrooks CA, Field PA, Morse JA (1994) Aggregating qualitative findings: An approach to theory development. *Qualitative Health Research* 4(4): 503–11

Leininger M (1992) Current issues, problems and trends to advance qualitative paradigmatic research methods for the future. *Qualitative Health Research* 2(4): 392–415

McKenna HP (1997) *Nursing Theory and Models*. Routledge, London

McKenna HP, Cutcliffe JR, McKenna P (2000) Evidence-based practice: Demolishing some myths. *Nurs Standard* 14(16): 39–42

McKibbon KA, Walker CJ (1994) Beyond ACP journal club: How to harness Medline for therapy problems. *Ann Intern Med* 121(1): 125–7

Micheal S (1994) Invisible skills. *J Psychiatr Ment Health Nurs* 1: 56–7

Pearson A (1992) Knowing nursing. In: Robinson K, Vaughan B, eds. *Knowledge for Nursing Practice*. Heinemann, Oxford: 213–26

Polit DF, Hungler BP (1997) *Essentials of Nursing: Methods, appraisal and utilisation*. 4th edn. Lippincott, Philadelphia

Stevenson C (1996) Taking the pith out of reality: A reflexive approach for psychiatric nursing research. *J Psychiatr Ment Health Nurs* 3: 103–10

# Example number two: The NPNR National Journal Club, review from the fourteenth meeting

The paper reviewed first appeared in 1999, in the *Journal of Psychiatric and Mental Health Nursing* (**6**: 3–8), 'Spiritual high versus high on spirits: Is religiosity related to adolescent drug abuse?' (Pullen L, Modrcin-Talbot MA, West WR and Meunchen R).

## Abstract/overview

This paper attempted to investigate the relationship between alcohol/drug abuse and the frequency of religious service attendance in adolescents, within the south eastern United States of America. The authors collected data using a survey from a total sample of 217 adolescents (aged twelve to nineteen). This sample was comprised of both a non-clinical and a clinical group. Their results indicate that as attendance at religious services increased, alcohol and drug abuse decreased. They conclude that spirituality is a concept that warrants further study, in order to determine if its inclusion within treatment programmes could help enhance recovery or reduce recidivism.

Note: Duffy's original maximum score is 306 (51 x 6) and consequently the overall quality of the paper is calculated according to comparison of the total score with the maximum total score. However, since Duffy includes a 'not applicable' score for each of the criteria, it might be considered as inaccurate to consider the overall quality of the papers reviewed without taking any 'not applicables' into account. Therefore, we include two scores for each category and for each paper; one which does not take account of the 'not applicables' and one which does. We have termed this way of scoring; pro rata scoring.

Criteria/appraisal rating                                                 Comments

| 1. Title | Comments |
|---|---|
| 1. 123456 NA | The members felt the title was easily understood, although some wondered what the authors meant by the term 'religiosity'. |
| 2. 123456 NA | The members felt the title was clear. |
| 3. 123456 NA | Members felt the title and content of the paper were entirely congruent. |
| Category score = | 15/18 Pro rata score 15/18 |
| **2. Abstract** | |
| 4. 123456 NA | It was noted that, within the abstract, the relationship is stated, however there is no reference to a research problem. Members felt that the abstract was clear and concise. Indeed, some expressed the view that the authors could have included more relevant detail within the abstract without it becoming too long. |
| 5. 123456 NA | The abstract states that a survey was used, but perhaps it could also have provided some information on the type of survey; and whilst it does indicate that the data was analysed, it doesn't indicate how. |
| 6. 123456 NA | The results are summarised, albeit very briefly. |
| 7. 123456 NA | Members pointed out that the abstract could have contained more detail about the findings; the discussion and the conclusions. |
| Category score | 20/24 Pro rata score 20/24 |
| **3. Problem** | |
| 8. 123456 NA | The general problem is introduced in the first paragraph of the introduction. |
| 9. 123456 NA | The questions are stated clearly, although the members felt they had to work through a substantial section of the paper before they reached the questions. |
| 10. 123456 **NA** | The research question is posed as a question, not as a problem statement. |
| 11. 123456 NA | The hypotheses are included at the start of the 'Methods' section, and are stated clearly. However, some members did wonder if the 'Methods' section was the most appropriate place for the research hypotheses. |
| 12. 123456 NA | There did not appear to be a section that referred to the limitations of the study, and that in itself was regarded as a significant limitation of this study by the members. |
| 13. 123456 NA | There is an assumption in the paper that remains implicit, and that is the authors apparent belief that attendance and/or participation at religious activities (eg. church attendance) is inherently a 'healthy' activity. Members noted that all of the literature cited in the review indicated 'positive' outcomes. Additionally, the authors draw upon certain grand theories (eg. Roy's adaptation model, 1980) in order to illustrate the value of engaging in 'religious' activity. Consequently, members wondered if such a selection of literature provided a balanced and objective view of the substantive area, and felt that it indicated the possible presence of the authors' assumptions. Now while there is an abundance of literature that lends support to the argument of attending to one's 'spiritual' needs (Dyson *et al*, 1997; Walter, 1997; Brandon, 1999) and there is evidence that such needs can be met by engaging in 'religious' activities, it would be inaccurate to consider religious activities as the **only** way of meeting such needs. |
| 14. 123456 NA | The pertinent terms are defined. Indeed, this was regarded as one of the strengths of the paper. |

| | | |
|---|---|---|
| 15. | 123456 NA | Members noted that while the author draws attention to the body of literature regarding the inappropriate use of drugs/alcohol, it was felt that a summary of the key problems such behaviours provoke would have been useful. |
| 16. | 123456 NA | Within the literature review, the authors include a comprehensive precis of the research within this substantive area. The current extent of understanding revealed in this literature appears to indicate that the relationship between drug/alcohol abuse and 'religiosity' is very well established. Consequently, members were left wondering why it was necessary to undertake another study to confirm further what appeared to be already known? Particularly when many unanswered, yet relevant questions, within this substantive area remain. For example, why and how does increased 'religiosity' make a difference in drug/alcohol abuse? What intra and inter personal dynamics occur (if any!) within this complex process that helps prevent drug/alcohol abuse? |
| Category score | | **29/54 Pro rata score 29/48** |
| **4. Review of the literature** | | |
| 17. | 123456 NA | Members felt the literature cited was clearly relevant to the research. |
| 18. | 123456 NA | Members pointed out that the literature included in the review indicated that the relationship between drug/alcohol abuse and religiosity was already well established and well researched. Consequently, the literature did not appear to indicate a need for this research question, but perhaps was a strong indication of the need for other relevant questions. |
| 19. | 123456 NA | Members felt that many of the studies that had been reviewed for this study had not been reviewed critically, but had been reported. |
| 20. | 123456 NA | This was a difficult area to assess. The relationship of the research problem to the previous research is clear, in that this study appears to be very similar to the studies that have already been undertaken. However, how this study builds upon these earlier studies (and this is another aspect of the relationship between previous and current empirical work, see McKenna, 1997) is not made clear. |
| 21. | 123456 NA | The conceptual framework is included and described. |
| 22. | 123456 NA | No such summary is included, however, members wondered if such a summary is warranted or indeed, common practice. |
| Category score = | | **19/30 Pro rata score 19/24** |
| **5. Methodology Part A: subjects** | | |
| 23. | 123456 NA | The authors provide detailed information on the characteristics of the sample. |
| 24. | 123456 NA | The authors do not appear, however, to justify any of their choices in their sampling frame, and this may have enhanced the paper (Morse, 1991). For example, members wondered, was this a convenience sample? Why the differences in sample size for each group? Did all the non-clinical subjects attend the same church? |
| 25. | 123456 NA | Members stated that they felt the authors could have indicated more clearly their particular reasons for the sampling choices they made. |
| 26. | 123456 **NA** | |
| 27. | 123456 **NA** | |

| 28. | 123456 NA | It was noted that formal ethical approval was granted, and this is to the betterment of the paper. However, the paper contained no indication of the ethical issues or considerations, and such an inclusion may have enhanced the quality of the paper (Schrock, 1991). |
|---|---|---|
| **Category score =** | **11/36 Pro rata score 11/24** | |
| **Methodology Part B: instruments** | | |
| 29. | 123456 NA | |
| 30. | 123456 NA | Members pointed out that their paper did not appear to contain any information regarding reliability or validity of this study, or previous studies. As a result, this was regarded as a significant limitation. |
| 31. | 123456 NA | |
| 32. | 123456 NA | |
| 33. | 123456 NA | |
| **Category score =** | **5/3 Pro rata score 5/30** | |
| **Methodology Part C: design** | | |
| 34. | 123456 NA | The design was appropriate to the study question, and provided some data that would enable the hypotheses to be tested. However, given the wide range of confounding variables and interactions of variables that could impact on patterns of drug/alcohol use, and relationship with religiosity, it is debatable that the method used provided the clearest and most meaningful result. For example, there are arguments that posit drug/alcohol use as a symptom of a disease (ie. addiction as a disease, Gerace, 1993), arguments that indicate that the social, economic, political and cultural factors as the basis for explaining drug/alcohol abuse (see Williams and Harris-Reid, 1999). Given the possible interaction of these and other influences on drug/alcohol abuse, the members doubted that the design used in this study provided the clearest and most meaningful results. Therefore, as an alternative, the researchers may have considered a qualitative method. The choice of a qualitative method would have enabled the researchers to ask the clients: 'tell me about your experiences of/attitudes towards drug/alcohol use and how religiosity affects these? |
| 35. | 123456 NA | |
| 36. | 123456 NA | |
| 37. | 123456 NA | There is sufficient information to allow replication. |
| **Category score =** | **10/24 Pro rata score 10/12** | |
| **6. Data analysis** | | |
| 38. | 123456 NA | This whole section was felt to be very clear, relevant and appropriate, and was regarded as a strength of the paper |
| 39. | 123456 NA | |
| 40. | 123456 NA | |
| 41. | 123456 NA | |
| **Category score =** | **24/24 Pro rata score 24/24** | |

| 7. Discussion | | |
|---|---|---|
| 42. | 123456 NA | The conclusions are stated clearly. |
| 43. | 123456 NA | Members felt that, on first consideration, it appears as though the conclusions are substantiated by the evidence presented. However, as it indicated previously, it was also regarded as somewhat simplistic to posit a direct correlation between an increase in religiosity with a corresponding decrease in drug/alcohol abuse. Since the authors appeared to have made no attempt to isolate the dependent variable and control other influencing variables, the change in drug/alcohol use may be attributed to increased religiosity; but it may be attributed to any number of confounding variables (or a combination of these variables) (see Polit and Hungler, 1997; Burns and Grove, 1993). Consequently, whilst it would be appropriate to suggest the presence of a correlation, it may have been prudent for the authors not to make such an assertive claim. Particularly, given the limitations of the study. |
| 44. | 123456 NA | There did not appear to be any discussion of the methodological problems. |
| 45. | 123456 NA | The findings did appear to be linked to the conceptual framework used in the study. |
| 46. | 123456 NA | Members stated that the paper did discuss the implications of the findings to a degree. However, this discussion was limited and furthermore, perhaps provided further evidence of the authors' implicit assumption/belief that attendance and/or participation at religious activities (eg. church attendance) is inherently a 'healthy' activity. |
| 47. | 123456 NA | There did not appear to be any evidence of generalising outside of the study population. |
| 48. | 123456 NA | The authors do not indicate the need for some additional research, but members felt there were additional questions and issues that warrant investigation which do not appear to be indicated in this paper. For example, what is it about the process and interaction of engaging in religiosity that makes a difference to drug/alcohol use? |
| Category score = | **29/42 Pro rata score 29/42** | |
| 8. Form and style | | |
| 49. | 123456 NA | Written in a reasonable academic style. |
| 50. | 123456 NA | The paper has a logical sequence/organisation. |
| 51. | 123456 NA | Members felt that the tone of the paper was rather biased towards the view/belief that attendance and/or participation at religious activities (eg. church attendance) is inherently a 'healthy' activity, and therefore should be encouraged. |
| Category score = | **12/18 Pro rata score 12/18** | |

**Grand total = 174**

*Strengths*

Many of the terms used within the paper are clearly defined.
The paper is succinct and contains no unnecessary text.
The data analysis section was regarded as being particularly strong.
Written in a clear, concise style and is accessible, easy to read.

## Limitations

The omission of reliability and validity scores was regarded as a significant limitation. The study appears to posit a rather simplistic, linear relationship between alcohol/drug abuse and religiosity and there is a large body of evidence that suggests drug/alcohol use or abuse are very complex, multi-dimensional problems. The paper appeared to contain an implicit bias or assumption that attendance to, or participation in religious activities is a 'healthy' activity.

# References

Brandon D (1999) Mental health and spirituality: two survivors. *Mental Health Practice* **2**(6): 16–19

Burns N, Grove SK (1993) *The Practice of Nursing Research: Conduct, critique and utilization*. 2nd edn.WB Saunders, Philadelphia

Duffy M (1985) A research appraisal checklist for evaluating nursing research reports. *Nurs Healthcare* **6**(10): 539–47

Dyson J, Cobb M, Forman D (1997) The meaning of spirituality: a literature review. *J Adv Nurs* **26**: 1183–88

Gerace LM (1993) Addictive Behaviour. In: Rawlins RP, Williams SR, Beck CK *Mental Health – Psychiatric Nursing: A Holistic life-cycle approach*. 3rd edn. Mosby, St Louis: 357–81

McKenna HP (1997) *Nursing Theory and Models*. Routledge, London

Morse JM (1991) Strategies for sampling. In: Morse JM, ed. *Qualitative Nursing Research: A contemporary dialogue*. Sage, London: 127–45

Polit DF, Hungler BP (1997) *Essentials of Nursing Research: Methods, Appraisal and utilisation*. 4th edn. Lippincott, Philadelphia

Schrock R (1991) Moral issues in nursing research. In: Cormack DFS, ed. *The Research Process in Nursing*. 2nd edn. Blackwell Science, London: 30–9

Roy C (1980) The Roy adaptation model. In: Riehl JP, Roy C, eds. *Conceptual Models for Nursing Practice*. 2nd edn. Appleton-Century-Crofts, New York: 179–89

Walter T (1997) The ideology and organisation of spiritual care: three approaches. *Palliative Med* **11**: 21–30

Williams DR, Harris-Reid M (1999) Race and mental health: Emerging patterns and promising approaches. In: Horwitz AV, Scheid TL *A Handbook for the Study of Mental Health: Social contexts, theories and systems*. Cambridge University Press, Cambridge: 295–314

# Critique and summary: Strengths and limitations of Duffy's (1985) research appraisal checklist approach to critiquing nursing research

## Strengths

❖ The approach follows a logical sequence; one which often mirrors that of the paper reviewed (particularly if the paper uses a quantitative method), and this makes it straightforward to follow.

❖ The approach produces a numerical value, which Duffy argues is representative of the overall quality of the paper, and this 'numerical' approach may be favoured by some, eg. for many years educationalists within nursing have ascribed a numerical value to provide an indication of the quality of work.

❖ It is possible that the author of the research paper reviewed may learn from a critique using Duffy's approach, particularly if the reviewers include extensive comments rather than focusing on the score.

❖ The approach does enable both strengths and limitations of a study to be identified.

❖ The approach allows room for data and/or argument to be introduced to support the reviewer's criticisms/observations and suggestions for improvement. However, again, this relies on the reviewer making extensive use of the 'comments' section and not relying on the 'score'.

❖ The approach does lead the reviewer towards considering the implications of the study, but perhaps greater emphasis could have been placed on this.

## Limitations

❖ Tends to ascribe high scores, indicating that papers are of high quality, whereas the views of the members of the papers would not indicate such a result.

❖ Clearly orientated towards evaluating quantitative studies and may not be appropriate (or have only limited application) for evaluating qualitative studies.

❖ The approach ascribes an equal weighting to each of the criteria and this may not be appropriate. For example, there may be certain criteria that are more important than others.

❖ The lack of guidance on whether or not the total score should or should not include the items regarded as 'not applicable' is rather confusing.

❖ There are significant problems with (and a concomitant debate surrounding) the practice of assigning a numerical value to a judgement of quality. While it has to be acknowledged that educationalists have been doing exactly that for many years, when they ascribe a numerical value to a student's assignment, the process is still problematic. For example, the approach has unequal distribution of Duffy's fifty-one separate criteria within his categories. The section on 'Analysis' contains four criteria, whereas the section on 'Method' contain a total of fifteen criterion. This begs questions such as, does Duffy indicate that the methods section is nearly four times as valuable than the analysis, to the overall quality of the study?

❖ Further problems with the scoring system include: where bands of scoring exist, eg. 204 = average research and 205 = superior research, the addition or subtraction of one or two points can make the difference between superior and average research. Such simplistic margins suggest that explicit demarcations exist between average and superior research, and the authors of this book would argue that this is not the case. The approach does not indicate how the scores and demarcations were derived.

❖ The approach might be regarded as a form of simplistic reductionism, where a crude attempt is made to reduce the research to its simplest constituent parts, and then the reviewer attempts to 'measure' these parts.

# 4

# Burns and Grove's (1987) critical appraisal approach to critiquing nursing research

This chapter focuses on Burns and Grove's (1987) approach to critiquing nursing research. Burns and Grove posit that there are different academic 'levels' of research critiquing which correspond to the academic levels of the nurse qualification. Accordingly, each of these different levels of critiquing involves different processes. The guidelines are applicable whatever the level of critiquing the reviewer is aiming for. This chapter outlines their guidelines for conducting a research critique and then paraphrases the key questions the reviewer should ask, under key headings/areas identified by Burns and Grove. Following this we provide two detailed examples (drawing from the reviews carried out by the NPNR National Journal Club). Having described the approach and provided examples, we highlight some of the advantages and disadvantages of this approach.

Burns and Grove argue that there are eight guidelines which a reviewer should remain mindful of when conducting a critique.They describe these as:

1  Read and critique the entire study.
2  Examine the research and clinical expertise of the authors.
3  Examine the organisation and presentation of the research report.
4  Identify strengths and weaknesses.
5  Provide specific examples of strengths and weaknesses.
6  Be objective and realistic in identifying the study's strengths and weaknesses.
7  Suggest modifications for future studies.
8  Evaluate the study.

Burns and Grove also identify five different levels of critiquing research and they link these with specific levels of academic qualification:

| | | |
|---|---|---|
| 1 | Comprehension | } Baccalaureate level |
| 2 | Comparison | |
| 3 | Analysis | Masters level |
| 4 | Evaluation | } Doctorate/experienced |
| 5 | Conceptual clustering | researcher |

*Footnote:* It is interesting to note that within Burns and Grove's description of the levels of critiquing research/academic level of qualification, there is no reference to diploma level studies. This may be a reflection of the different patterns of nurse education between Britain and the United States of America. If we accept Burns and Grove's description then the implicit implication is that the large majority óf nurses within Britain would not need any comprehension of or skills in critiquing nursing research. (Since the large majority of nurses in Britain have either undertaken a diploma level or certificate level pre-registration qualification.) Clearly, this is at odds with the emphasis on evidence-based practice (*Chapter 1*). We argue that it is incumbent on all practising nurses to have some understanding of approaches to critiquing nursing research, irrespective of the level of their academic preparation.

**Paraphrased questions the reviewer should ask, under key headings/ areas identified by Burns and Grove**

*Research problems and hypothesis*

❖ Is the problem clearly stated?
❖ Are the key variables identified?
❖ Are the hypotheses clearly stated?

*Review of the literature*

❖ Were Investigators suitably qualified?
❖ Are classic/other studies cited?
❖ Is the review logical and organised?
❖ Has related literature been explored?

*Variables*

❖ What variables are defined?
❖ Are there any undefined variables?
❖ Are independent and dependent variables clearly delineated?

*Research design*

❖ Is the design clearly indicated?
❖ Is it appropriate?
❖ How does the design control threaten validity?
❖ Could others replicate the study?

*Research instruments*

❖ Are data collecting instruments clearly defined?
❖ Are instruments appropriate?
❖ Are they valid and reliable?
❖ Are limitations addressed?

## Measurement

❖ Is the level of measurement described?
❖ Are there data to support reliability and validity measures?

## Sampling

❖ Is the sampling procedure clearly described?
❖ Is the sample random or non-random?
❖ Is the sample size adequate?

## Analysis of data

❖ Are statistical values reported?
❖ Was the most effective statistic chosen?
❖ Was the level of significance reported?

## Interpretation of results

❖ Are the results grounded in the data?
❖ Are weaknesses in the data honestly addressed?
❖ Are conclusions justified?

## Report of the results

❖ Does the title of the study reflect the key variable?
❖ Is there a clear abstract?
❖ Has the investigator been honest?
❖ Is non-sexist language used?
❖ Is the report interesting?

## Protection of human rights

❖ Are procedures ethical?
❖ Is informed consent obtained?
❖ Are privacy and anonymity safeguarded?

# Example number three: The NPNR National Journal Club, review number thirteen

The paper reviewed first appeared in 1999, in the *Journal of Psychiatric and Mental Health Nursing* (**6**:137–145), 'Education for community psychiatric nurses: content, structure and trends in recruitment' (Hannigan B).

## Abstract/overview

This paper reported on a survey which was designed to measure aspects of community psychiatric nursing (CPN) education in the UK. It indicates that thirty-two of the thirty-nine course leaders who ran post-qualifying programmes for CPNs responded to a nine-page postal questionnaire. Findings indicated that the majority of courses are now run at degree level; most courses appeared to include education in key areas of specialist content pertinent to contemporary CPN practice (eg. collaborative working with service users). Overall however, the paper reported that courses for CPNs appeared to be characterised by considerable variation in specialist content. The paper concludes by offering possible explanations for this variation and some suggestions for future research.

1A    Within the 'Introduction' of the paper, the author describes the primary aim of the study: to investigate the specialist content of CPN courses currently available in the UK. However, the aim of the study is not phrased as a 'problem'. Members wondered if this was because the focus of the research was not an actual problem. Consequently, questions were raised concerning whether or not the study was required, particularly given that a similar study (with similar aims) had been carried out each year for most of the previous ten years. Alternative views were raised which indicated the value in monitoring the trends in nurse education, including CPN education, since educational curricula should, at least in part, reflect the needs of the local population and current national policies and agendas (Parkes, 1997; Norman, 1998).

1B    As the study uses a survey design, and was not concerned with measuring causal relationships between variables, no key variables are mentioned in the study, and this was regarded as appropriate by the members.

1C    The paper did not posit a hypothesis or a null hypothesis. Again, given that the research used a straightforward survey design, it was appropriate for the researcher not to include a hypothesis (Polit and Hungler, 1997.)

2A    The reported piece of research was carried out as the dissertation for a masters degree. Given that the author had a bachelors degree, and had access to supervision from senior researchers, and that the research used a straightforward survey design, and minimal use of statistics in the analysis, members felt that the investigator was suitably qualified to undertake the study.

2B    The study appropriately describes, and subsequently draws upon, the previous studies carried out to determine the extent of, and trends in, CPN education.

2C    Members stated that the literature review was well organised and logical.

2D    In addition to drawing on the literature mentioned in 2B, the author also includes some of the discursive texts which consider positions and arguments regarding the developments in CPN education. Members wondered if the author had considered drawing upon a slightly wider literature, which may have been relevant to this issue. For example, White and Brooker (1998) CPN surveys, or literature that has examined alternative developments in CPN education, eg. 'Thorn' training (Gamble, 1995).

3A/B/C   As this study used a straightforward survey design, and was not attempting to test or measure the relationship between variables, no variables were highlighted.

4A   The author stated that he used a postal questionnaire, which was distributed to each education centre that provided CPN courses. Members felt that the design was clearly stated.

4B   In order to obtain information, which can be expressed in numerical form from a wide population, a survey design is appropriate (Parahoo, 1997). Consequently, the members felt that the design used by the author was appropriate.

4C   The paper does not make any reference to threats to validity. However, members constructed an argument that indicated that to criticise automatically this paper on this matter might be inappropriate. Their concerns were the use of reliability tests on surveys. Surveys, such as the instrument used in this study, used to determine 'concrete' matters that are not 'open to debate' (eg. the number of nurses on a course, whether or not the nurses are studying for a degree or a diploma), but which also aim to compare the changes of these figures over time, may not be best considered in terms of reliability. Given that reliability is concerned with consistency over repeated measures (Behi and Nolan, 1995), it might be inappropriate to criticise a study on the grounds of reliability, when it demonstrates that numbers of nurses on courses fluctuates from year to year.

Where surveys are attempting to measure less 'concrete' variables or phenomenon, then it may be prudent for authors to address this by repeating the survey within a short space of time of the initial survey. This would then provide the data to calculate reliability scores. However, members felt that there were no such fluctuating variables within this paper.

4D   Given the precise nature of the detail included in this paper (eg. sample composition, design), and the fact that this study is, in the main, a replication of a study that has been conducted almost every year for the last ten years, members stated that it would be relatively easy and entirely plausible for others to replicate the study.

5A/B   Members stated that the description of the survey gave them a clear indication of the nature and type of questions asked. The question was raised why the instrument did not include any questions about the clinical component of the courses. Since these courses appear to have been designed purposefully, blending theoretical and clinical input, one could argue that the nature of the clinical input to CPN education and training is relevant and important. Consequently, any study that intends to gain a more complete understanding of the content, structure and trends in CPN education may benefit from investigating the clinical input in addition to the theoretical input.

5C    The paper does not make any reference to the validity of the instrument. Again, given that the instrument was based on an instrument which was used in previous studies, members felt that the author could have used data from the previous studies to indicate/determine the validity. Furthermore, the additional work carried out to extend the instrument may have benefited from some consideration of content or face validity (Polit and Hungler, 1997).

5D    The author did make reference to the limitations regarding the absence of any questions in the survey pertaining to the clinical input on a course.

6A    The report states that 'measurements' used in the survey were 'self-reported' measures, for example, self-reports of the number of hours in the course, self-reports on the number of the students.

6B    The arguments regarding validity and reliability have been made earlier in this chapter.

7A    Members stated that the sampling strategy could be regarded as one of the strengths of the paper since it sampled the total population (ie. each education centre that provided the CPN course). Furthermore, it achieved a response rate of 82%, which is high for a postal return survey. The members felt that such results could be taken to be indicative or representative of the total population.

7B    The sample was not random, but since the study sampled the entire population, a randomised sample was not required.

7C    As stated above, the sample size was considered to be highly adequate.

8A    The paper utilised statistics in only a very limited way, in that percentages were used. Members felt that this was appropriate given the design of the study, and the inclusion of any unnecessary statistics may indicate an attempt to gain 'pseudo-scientific credibility' for the paper, without adding anything of real substance.

8BC    There were no statistical tests carried out and correspondingly, no mention of levels of significance.

9AB    Members felt that this section could be regarded as another strength of the paper as the author appears to 'ground' his results in the data and does not appear to have 'conjured' or manufactured results. Furthermore, the author is honest, open and clear about the weaknesses of the results (eg. the absence of a response from seven education centres and how this may have effected the results/conclusions).

9C    Members stated that the author could have made the conclusion clearer. The author does allude to some interesting discussion points (although a thorough critique of the discussion points falls outside of the headings of Burns and Grove's approach). However, members felt that the discussion points would have benefited from further development. Of particular interest was the variation in the course content between sites. The author offers limited explanation for this variation, however, members felt that the author had perhaps missed an opportunity to explore this issue in more detail. It was the hope of the members that future research in this area might follow up these points and ask questions, such as: how is current mental health policy and the current research agenda reflected in your course content? Does your course content reflect the specific mental health care needs of your local population and local mental healthcare workforce? How does the course content reflect the theoretical orientation of the individual course leaders?

10A    Members felt the title reflected the focus of the study and identified the key variables, such as they were.

10B    The paper contained an abstract which provided an accurate synopsis of the paper.

10C    Members felt that the apparent honesty of the author, both with regard to the limitations and reporting of the study could be regarded as one of the strengths of the paper, as this honesty was evident throughout the paper.

10D    There was no evidence of sexist language.

10E    It is reasonable to say that opinion was divided on this matter. Clearly, papers that focus on 'specialist' rather than generic issues will be directly applicable to a more narrow audience and perhaps less interesting to the wider audience. As stated previously, members also felt that perhaps the author had missed the opportunity to explore some of the 'big' questions and this omission maybe made the paper less interesting. Nevertheless, opinion was offered that suggested this paper did add something to the knowledge base in this area.

11ABC    There is no mention of ethical issues in the paper. Members felt this was not a significant limitation given the focus and design of the study. Additionally, the guidelines on the practice of ethics committees in medical research involving human subjects, produced in 1990 and 1996 by the Royal College of Physicians, specify that ethical approval is required for a study when:

- the research involves any NHS clients (past or present)
- the research involves the use of client notes
- the study was undertaken on NHS premises.

Given that the study did not meet these criteria, members felt formal ethical approval was not required.

# References

Behi R, Nolan M (1995) Reliability: Consistency and accuracy in measurement. *Br J Nurs* 4(8): 472–5

Gamble C (1995) The Thorn nurse training initiative. *Nurs Standard* 9: 31–4

Norman I (1998) The Changing emphasis of mental health and learning disability nurse education in the UK and the ideal models of its future development. *J Psychiatr Ment Health Nurs* 5: 41–51

Parahoo K (1997) *Nursing Research: Principles, process and issues*. Macmillan Press, London

Parkes T (1997) Reflections from outside in: My journey into, through and beyond psychiatric nursing. In: Tilley S, ed. *The Mental Health Nurse: Views of Practice and Education*. Blackwell Science, Oxford: 58–72

Polit DF, Hungler BP (1997) *Essentials of Nursing Research: Methods, appraisal and utilization*. 4th edn. JB Lippincott, Philadelphia

Royal College of Physicians (1990) *Guidelines on the practice of ethics committees in medical research involving human subjects*. The Royal College of Physicians, London

Royal College of Physicians (1996) *Guidelines on the practice of ethics committees in medical research involving human subjects*. The Royal College of Physicians London

White E, Brooker C (1998) Community Mental Health Nursing: National Surveys. *Ment Health Practice* 2(2): 8–16

# Example number four: The NPNR National Journal Club, review from the eleventh meeting

The paper reviewed first appeared in 1999, in the *Journal of Psychiatric and Mental Health Nursing* (**6**: 9–14), 'The process of constant observation: perspectives of staff and suicidal patients' (Fletcher RE).

## Abstract/overview

This paper reports on a study which attempted to explore the perceptions of staff regarding the nursing activity of 'constant observations' of suicidal clients in mental health settings. The paper also attempts to elicit the perceptions of clients and then compare the two. The two categories of nursing interventions; therapeutic and controlling, were identified by both groups. Inconsistencies of the perceptions between the two groups were also noted. The author then discusses and explores the implications of these findings.

1A      Feedback comments from the members indicated that the author initially listed three objectives which appeared to be clear. Further on in the paper, the author changes the stated objectives from, identifying nurses'/ clients' perceptions of the purpose, nature and meaning of constant observations, to identifying the perceived purposes, nursing actions and feelings of clients and staff. Such disparity was felt to confuse matters.

1B    As the study used a qualitative design, and was not concerned with measuring causal relationships between variables, no key variables are mentioned in the study. This was regarded as appropriate by the members.

1C    Given that the paper claimed to utilise a qualitative, ethnographic research method, it was not necessary to include a formal hypothesis and the omission of a hypothesis need not be regarded as a flaw.

2A    Members stated that the author appeared to be suitably qualified for a study of this type.

2B    Comments from the members regarding the literature review were less encouraging with some members expressing a sense of puzzlement. Much of the literature cited by the author appeared to be out-of-date, which was curious given that a wealth of important and more contemporary material on suicide prevention, and the nursing care of suicidal people is available (Busteed and Johnstone, 1983; Mental Health Act Commission and Sainsbury Centre for Mental Health, 1997; Moore, 1998 ).

2C/D  Members raised further questions with respect to the logical sequence, the organisation and content of the literature review. For example, there was a question raised about why the review commenced with a reference to risk assessment, when this was perhaps outside of the scope or remit of the review. Other members noted that the bulk of the literature reviewed was from the United States of America (USA) which appeared somewhat inappropriate given that the study was undertaken in the United Kingdom (UK). Other members felt that the review perhaps lacked critical reading of the literature and failed to provide a clear picture of how each subsequent study had built upon the findings of the previous work in that substantive area. The literature review did include evidence that indicated the alleged benefits and drawbacks of the experience of being placed on 'constant observations', and offering such a balanced view within the review was thought to be a strength of the paper. Although some members stated that the claims that 'constant observations' promote the freedom of the individual needed greater substantiation and evidence.

4A/B  Members raised several questions concerning the research design and method. The author described the study as 'ethnography', however, members could not agree with this description. Ethnographic studies are commonly associated with 'thick description' (Atkinson and Hammersley, 1994) yet such description did not appear to be present in the study. Since, according to Morse and Field (1995), ethnography is always informed by the concept of culture, and thus ethnographers ask; 'In what ways do members of a community actively construct their world?' it would appear reasonable to use an ethnographic method to examine the culture of constant observations on mental health wards. However, qualitative studies that are more concerned with uncovering the meaning of being in the world in certain experiences, would perhaps benefit from using a phenomenological method (Heidegger, 1962; Benner and Wrubel, 1989; Walters, 1995). Since the author proposed to explore the 'meaning of constant observation' (Fletcher, 1999: 10), a phenomenological method may have been more appropriate.

4C    Members noted that attempts to determine the 'validity' of a qualitative study have been strongly criticised. For example, according to Leininger (1994: 97), this would indicate attempting to judge the credibility of a qualitative design by using criteria designed for quantitative studies. However, the author clearly made some attempt to establish the credibility of his findings. Firstly, by drawing on a colleague to sort responses according to operational definitions (although the members pointed out that these definitions were not described). Secondly, by attempting to triangulate the data by obtaining data from the clients. While these endeavours to establish the credibility of the findings should be applauded, it should be noted that there are fundamental epistemological, philosophical and methodological flaws with the methods used by the author.

Firstly, the philosophical underpinnings of quantitative research approaches and qualitative research approaches are very different and such differences have been highlighted many times within the methodological literature (Denzin and Lincoln, 1994; McKenna, 1997; Cutcliffe and McKenna, 1999). Consequently, key authorities on qualitative research point out that it is inappropriate to attempt to apply positivistic and empiricist views of the world to qualitative research (Benner and Wrubel, 1989; Morse, 1991a; Denzin and Lincoln, 1994; Ashworth, 1997). For the author to strive for 'objectivity' within a qualitative study can be regarded as inappropriate.

Members wondered why the author had drawn upon qualitative research texts with a noted 'vintage' and had not made use of the more contemporary qualitative research texts. Perhaps the use of these texts, at least in part, explains the author's inappropriate use of terms developed for establishing the authenticity of quantitative findings. A more current examination of these issues may have highlighted that qualitative research findings should be tested for credibility or accuracy using terms and criteria that have been developed exclusively for this very approach (Hammersley, 1992; Cutcliffe and McKenna, 1999). Indeed, Leininger (1994) makes this point most clearly when she states:

> *We must develop and use criteria that fit the qualitative paradigm, rather than use quantitative criteria for qualitative studies. It is awkward and inappropriate to re-language quantitative terms.*

4D    On a similar note to 4C, given that the author claimed to be using a qualitative design, it would have been inappropriate to criticise the paper on the grounds of replicability, since this is a criteria developed specifically for use within the quantitative paradigm.

5A/B/C/D Members noted that each of the questions raised in this section appear to be more appropriate for quantitative studies, and should not be criteria for judging the quality of a qualitative piece of research. With regard to the congruency between the research design and the data collection method, the use of participant observation within an ethnographic study would have been entirely appropriate (Atkinson and Hammersley, 1994). This can be regarded as a sound methodological decision within the paper. Perhaps the author could have improved this section of the paper by adding further detail and substantiation to the methodological, data collection decisions he made. For example, what is gained by combining participant observation with interviews? Did the interview schedule evolve or remain static? Were there any questions asked by the participants regarding elements that they felt may have been overlooked?

6A/B    Just as in section 5, members noted that each of the questions raised in this section appear to be more appropriate for quantitative studies, and should not be criteria for judging the quality of a qualitative piece of research.

7A    Members raised several issues regarding the sampling procedures and felt that they could have been described more clearly. For example, while the composition of the sample was described, unfortunately, the author provided no explanation of the sampling procedure. Given the relatively small sample size, and the qualitative nature of the study, members assumed that the author had used purposeful sampling, which would be in keeping with the method (Morse, 1991b). Yet this was not indicated in the paper. The author included one criterion for inclusion for the sample of clients, though did not include any inclusion criteria for the sample of staff. Members felt that the author should have included an indication of the minimum criteria for inclusion in the sample, pointing out what constituted a 'good informant' for this study (Morse, 1991b).

7B/C    Given that the author claimed to be using a qualitative design, it would have been inappropriate to criticise the paper on the grounds of the lack of random sampling or the size of the sample. Sampling within qualitative studies is purposefully biased, a point made by Morse (1998: 734). She states:

> ... that means that we seek informants who have experience, **the most experience** *[original emphasis]* in the topic of interest. Yes, the sample is biased; **it must be biased** *[original emphasis]*.

8A/B/C    Given that the author claimed to be using a qualitative design, it would have been inappropriate to criticise the paper on the grounds of the lack of statistical analysis, or the choice of inappropriate statistical tests, or the absence of levels of significance.

9A Members felt that the results did appear to be grounded in the data, and the author substantiated his findings by using text from the interviews; adding to the sense that the results were grounded in the data provided by the interviewees.

9B/C Some members stated that the results resonated very clearly with their own experiences and supported themes in this substantive area; namely, the perception of 'constant observations' as a controlling or therapeutic activity (Briggs, 1974; Barker and Walker, 1999; Conway, 1999; Barker and Cutcliffe, 1999). Other members felt the results and conclusions could have been explained more clearly.

10A Members felt the title was concise and reflected the area under study.

10B Both the title and the abstract aroused the interest of the members and they stated that the substantive area warranted investigation and study.

10C/E Members found the paper to be interesting and it was particularly refreshing to see such 'honest' data regarding the use and purpose of 'constant observations'. An example of such honesty is the author's finding that acknowledges that, despite the rhetoric of 'supportive observation' (Barker and Cutcliffe, 1999), the use of 'constant observations' clearly has an element of serving the needs of the organisation rather than the needs of the individual. A further strength of the paper, according to the members, was the author's attempt to obtain data from, and subsequently induce a theory from the clients' perspectives. Emotionally charged and sensitive topics within psychiatric/mental health nursing, such as; the use of 'constant observations', physical restraint, being detained under the mental health act, or considering a client's sexual needs, each appear to be under researched. Furthermore, examination of the empirical literature in this area appears to indicate that there is a distinct paucity of research that seeks to elicit the client's perspectives, feelings and experiences of emotionally charged topics. A study such as this, despite its limitations, might be regarded as a useful combination to this under-researched substantive area.

10D There was no evidence of sexist language used.

11A/B/C Members stated that there appeared to be no mention of ethical concerns within the study, and such an oversight was regarded as a significant limitation of the study. The members' difficulty can perhaps be located in the concerns regarding research and vulnerable groups. and Childress (1994) reasoned that vulnerable groups are those captive populations. Examples of such populations include; the mentally ill, the acutely ill and the terminally ill. Usher and Holmes (1997) argue that vulnerable research participants are those that are considered to be unable, or less able, to make autonomous decisions regarding their participation in the research. According to Watson (1992), when considering whether or not people from these populations should be asked to participate in research studies, there are several key factors to consider. The most frequently cited being the seriousness and probability of risk to the client, whether or not the subject or society receives any benefits, and the capability of the subject to give informed consent. While it should be noted that, given the emergent nature of the design of some (most) qualitative studies, it may not always be possible for researchers to balance the benefit to risk ratio of such studies in advance (Raudonis, 1992; Lacey, 1998). However, *ex post facto* consideration of ethical issues or the use of the ethics as process approach (Ramcharan and Cutcliffe, 2000) is more common in social science research, and would have been entirely appropriate for this study.

# References

Ashworth P (1997) The variety of qualitative research: Introduction to the problem. *Nurse Educ Today* **17**: 215–18

Atkinson P, Hammersley M (1994) Ethnography and participant observation. In Denzin NK, Lincoln YS, eds. *Handbook of Qualitative Research*. Sage, London: 248–61

Barker P, Walker L (1999) *A survey of care practices in acute admission wards*. Report submitted to the Northern and Yorkshire Regional Research and Development Committee, Newcastle

Barker P, Cutcliffe JR (1999) Clinical risk: A need for engagement not observation. *Ment Health Practice* **2**(8): 8-12

Beauchamp TL, Childress JF (1994) *Principles of Biomedical Ethics*. 4th edn. Oxford University Press, Oxford

Benner P, Wrubel J (1989) *The Primacy of Caring: Stress and coping in health and illness*. Addison-Wesley, New York

Briggs PF (1974) Specialising in psychiatry: therapeutic or custodial? *Nurs Outlook* **22**: 632–5

Busteed EL, Johnstone C (1983) The Development of suicide precautions for in-patient psychiatric units. *J Psychosoc Nurs Ment Services* **21**: 15–19

Conway E (1999) *A multidimensional audit of observation policy*. Report to Newcastle City Health Trust, Newcastle

Cutcliffe JR, McKenna HP (1999) Establishing the credibility of qualitative research findings: The plot thickens. *J Adv Nurs* **30**(2): 374–80

Denzin N, Lincoln YS (1994) Introduction: Entering the field of qualitative enquiry. In: Denzin N, Lincoln YS, eds. *Handbook of Qualitative Research*. Sage London

Hammersley M (1992) *What's wrong with Ethnography?* Routledge London

Heideggar M (1962) *Being and Time*. Harper Row, New York

Lacey EA (1998) Social and medical research ethics: Is there a difference? *Soc Sciences in Health* **4**(4), 211–7

Leininger M (1994) Evaluation criteria and critique of qualitative research studies. In: Morse JM, ed. *Critical Issues in Qualitative Research Methods*. Sage, London: 95–115

McKenna HP (1997) *Nursing Theories and Models*. Routledge, London

Mental Health Act Commission and Sainsbury Centre for Mental Health (1997) *The National Visit*. Sainsbury Centre, London

Moore C (1998) Acute in-patient care could do better, says survey. *Nurs Times* **94**(3): 54–6

Morse JM (1991a) Qualitative nursing research: A free for all? In: Morse JM, ed. *Qualitative Nursing Research: A contemporary dialogue.* Sage London: 14–22

Morse JM (1991b) Strategies for sampling. In: Morse JM, ed. *Qualitative Nursing Research: A contemporary dialogue.* Sage, London: 127–45

Morse JM (1998) What's wrong with random selection? *Qualitative Health Res* **8**(6): 733–5

Morse JM, Field PA (1995) *Qualitative Research Methods for Health Professionals.* 2nd edn. Sage, London

Ramcharan P, Cutcliffe JR (2000) Judging the ethics of qualitative research proposals: The ethics as process approach. *Health Social Science* **9**(6): 358–66

Raudonis BM (1992) Ethical considerations in qualitative research with hospice patients *Qualitative Health Res* **2**(2): 238–49

Usher L, Homles C (1997) Ethical aspects of phenomenological research with mentally ill people. *Nurs Ethics* **4**(1): 49–56

Walters AJ (1995) The phenomenological movement: implications for nursing research. *J Adv Nurs* **22**: 791–9

Watson AB (1992) Informed consent of special subjects. *Nurs Res* **31**: 43–7

# Summary: Strengths and limitations of Burns and Grove's (1987) approach to critiquing nursing research

## Strengths

❖ The approach is easy to follow.

❖ It does not contain unnecessary jargon and is, accordingly, accessible.

❖ The approach leads the reviewer to most of the key components of quantitative studies.

❖ It is possible that the author of the research paper reviewed may learn from a critique using Burns and Grove's approach, particularly, if the reviewers include extensive comments.

❖ The approach does enable both strengths and limitations to be identified.

❖ The approach allows room for the data and/or argument to be introduced to support the reviewer's criticisms/observations and suggestions for improvement. However, this relies on the rigour and thoroughness of the reviewer(s), in that the questions asked within the key areas are 'closed questions' ie. questions that can be adequately answered using single word responses.

## Limitations

❖ Specifying the need to consider variables (see key area/question 3) shows a limitation of the approach to critiquing. Since the absence of variables might not necessarily be indicative of an absence of quality.

❖ The approach does not tell the reviewer all they need to consider in the study. For example, the 'ethics' key area (area 11) asks specific questions about anonymity, confidentiality and informed consent. However, it does not include specific questions about equally important ethic issues, eg. the balance of risk to benefit ratio.

❖ A criticism of the Burns and Grove approach is the lack of emphasis on the 'discussion' section and the implications of the results. This is another important example of the approach not informing the reviewer to consider key aspects of a study. In addition to being methodologically sound, and having accurate results, studies should explore, in detail, the implications of these findings. Practitioners need to see the results examined and discussed within the context of current knowledge, conflicting findings and supporting evidence. The absence of a 'discussion' key area within Burns and Grove's approach might be regarded as a significant omission.

❖ A further important criticism is the clear emphasis of this approach for critiquing quantitative studies and using quantitative criteria. In fact, we would argue that this approach is unsuitable for critiquing qualitative studies given the focus of the key areas and questions.

❖ Burns and Grove do not indicate why there are three questions within most of their eleven key areas, four questions in some key areas and two questions in one key area. Thus, reviewers might be left wondering if this indicated implicitly the relative importance that Burns and Grove ascribe to each of the key areas.

❖ This approach, like Duffy's (1985) approach, might be regarded as a form of simplistic reductionism, where an attempt is made to reduce the research to its simplest constituent parts, and then the reviewer attempts to 'measure' these parts.

Footnote: It should be noted that Burns and Grove perhaps recognised the limitations of their 1987 approach, and subsequently, in their later editions of the same book (1993; 1997) they provide more comprehensive approaches suggesting that quantitative and qualitative studies should be critiqued according to different criteria. However, it is only within the 3rd edition (1997) that they include a separate and comprehensive approach for critiquing qualitative studies.

# 5

# Morrison's (1991) approach to critiquing nursing research

This chapter focuses on Morrison's (1991) approach to critiquing nursing research. Morrison argues that each of us needs to be critical of the research we read in order to discriminate between the high and lower quality papers. He provides a series of reasons for the need to critique research, including the need to 'de-mystify' research. Morrison then describes what he claims are the five essential features of a critique. He acknowledges that while there any many ways that a reader can critique a study, each of these appears to involve a questioning approach; asking key and/or relevant questions at certain stages of the report. Included in Morrison's approach are questions that he feels need to be asked of the reviewer; questions regarding the reviewer's knowledge base and depth of background reading. The remainder of his approach is concerned with key questions about the different aspects of the study. This chapter lists Morrison's key questions under each of the headings he identifies. Following this, we provide two detailed examples (drawing from the reviews carried out by the NPNR Journal Club). Having described the approach and provided examples, some of the strengths and limitations of this approach are highlighted.

Morrison (1991) argues that the central features of a good critique are that the critique should be:

- objective
- constructive
- unbiased
- a penetrating analysis
- a decisive analysis of the quality of the research.

The key questions that need to be asked are grouped under these headings.

*Questions about the researcher*

❖ Who is the researcher and what is his or her background?

*Questions to ask about the research problem*

❖ Is the problem clearly stated?
❖ Can it be easily researched?
❖ Has it been researched already or is the researcher providing a new and creative slant?
❖ Does the question relate to nursing practice?

## Questions to ask about the literature review

❖ Is it relevant to the topic?

❖ Is it comprehensive or have key references been ignored or missed out?

❖ Are the sources current and up-to-date or has the author relied solely on well known but out-of-date references?

❖ Is it laid out logically and coherently?

❖ Is a summary provided at the end of the review which accurately captures the crucial aspects of the relevant literature and spells out the relevance of this literature for the study?

## Questions to ask about the design of the study

❖ Is there a statement about the overall design of the study, such as 'case study', 'experiment' or 'survey', which conveys immediately the type of report which is being discussed?

❖ Are the relevant theoretical frameworks discussed?

❖ If hypotheses are offered, are they stated clearly?

❖ Is there a straightforward description of what the researcher planned to do and why, and how was it done (ie. aims and methods)?

❖ Could we repeat the procedure on the basis of the information provided?

❖ Are the technical terms clearly defined or does the author assume that these are understood?

## Questions to ask about the data collection

❖ Is the method used discussed in sufficient detail?

❖ Is the rationale provided for the choice of method?

❖ Does the method stand up to criticism?

❖ What details are provided about the sample used in the study?

❖ Was the sample appropriate?

❖ Are details given about the special instruments used in the study (eg. questionnaires, interview schedules, measuring techniques)?

❖ Is the reliability and validity of the findings discussed?

## Questions to ask about the data analysis

❖ Are the analyses appropriate for the type of data collected?

❖ Is the method of analysis clearly described, step-by-step, and easy to follow?

❖ Are the findings presented clearly with the help of graphs, tables or highlighted themes?

❖ Are the results discussed adequately?

❖ Does the discussion emphasise some aspects of the results and ignore others, and is such emphasis justified?

*Questions to ask about the conclusions and recommendations*

❖ Are the conclusions justified on the strength of the findings?

❖ Are the conclusions linked closely to the original purpose of the research?

❖ Have any new insights been uncovered during the research?

❖ Have new research questions emerged unexpectedly from the study?

❖ Are the recommendations made by the researcher feasible and are they excessive and costly?

❖ Is a change in nursing practice justified on the strength of these findings or is more research needed before embarking on a programme of major change?

❖ What are the implications of the study for further research in the field?

❖ Does the researcher evaluate the study and point out possible limitations?

# Example number five: The NPNR National Journal Club, review from the fifteenth meeting

The paper reviewed first appeared in 1998, in the *Journal of Psychiatric and Mental Health Nursing* (**5**: 451–62), 'A survey of psychiatric nurses' opinions of advanced practice roles in psychiatric nursing' (Allen J).

## Abstract/overview

In this paper, the author attempted to survey established psychiatric nurses' opinions of the content of advanced practitioner nursing roles by sending a questionnaire to a random sample of 100 members of the NPNR network, and received a response rate of 78%. The results identified elements of the 'normal' nursing roles (eg. basic psychotherapeutic practices), and elements of the 'advanced' nursing role (eg. enhanced autonomy in admission and discharge). The study concluded that an advanced psychiatric nursing role was supported by psychiatric nurses and recommended that pilot sites, to test the acceptability and effectiveness of the role, should be established.

1     The author is a RMN, with a background and current interest in acute psychiatry. He appears to have limited experience of research (assuming that the MSc qualification involved the production of a research dissertation).

2A     The author alludes to the research problem early in the paper (2nd paragraph, introduction), but members felt that the problem could have been stated more clearly. Later in the paper, the author does indicate a research question, however this occurs at the end of a somewhat discursive section. Members stated that as a consequence, it was difficult to locate the research question as it was somewhat obscured by the discursive text. While acknowledging the need to set the background to the study, members felt that, perhaps, this section of the paper did not add to the overall clarity of the paper. Furthermore, they added that this section rather confused matters since it gave the paper a 'discursive' appearance rather than an 'empirical' appearance. Perhaps there may have been merit in condensing this section.

2B    The problem can be researched, but members noted that since opinions change over time, any results obtained would need to be acknowledged as a cross-sectional, 'snap shot' in time.

2C    The author points out that there is a distinct paucity of empirical work in this area. The author makes reference to some of the theoretical and policy literature in this substantive area, but given the paucity of empirical work, particularly exploration of psychiatric nurses' views of advanced practice, the research has the potential to be contributing new knowledge.

2D    Members felt that the research question clearly relates directly to nursing practice and, potentially, could relate to psychiatric nursing education, policy and further research.

3A    Members noted that the paper does not include an identified literature review. There appeared to be no systematic or logical review of the previous studies undertaken in this substantive area.

3B    The author does include a review of some of the theoretical literature (eg. the arguments regarding specialist or advanced, extended or expanded practice) and draws upon additional literature which may be related to this substantive area (eg. nurse prescribing). However, as mentioned previously, members stated that while this did allude to the background of the study in part, it retained a discursive feel and did not appear to provide a comprehensive review of all the research in this area. Having said that, it may be that such texts do not currently exist within the British literature. Given that the author drew upon North American theoretical texts, it may have been prudent for the author to review the empirical work that also originated from America.

3C    The sources used are current but, as stated previously, they are primarily from theoretical and policy literature, not from empirical work.

3D    Members felt that this section of the paper was perhaps somewhat confusing as they wished to see a review of the empirical work carried out in this area, in order that they could see the current extent of the knowledge base in this substantive area.

3E    There did not appear to be a summary at the end of the review which accurately captured the crucial aspects of the relevant literature.

4A      The paper does include a statement that suggests the research design used a postal survey. However, members pointed out that this statement was misleading. Further into the paper (p. 455), the author points out that the study included a qualitative analysis. Therefore, to describe the research design as using only a survey could be regarded as inaccurate, and it may have been more accurate to describe the study as using a triangulated design (Nolan and Behi, 1995; Fu-Jin, 1998)

4B      The author includes some information on the survey design, but members still raised some questions over this matter. Firstly, they felt that some justification for the use of a survey may have enhanced the quality of the paper, particularly when arguments about the longitudinal and cumulative nature of knowledge generation are considered (May, 1994). Additionally, the members recognise the inclusion of some operationally defined terms regarding 'normal, generalist, and specialist' practice, and they felt that such definitions were a strength of the paper. However, they did wonder if the respondents had been provided with these terms, since their own understanding of these terms may have been different to the author's. Such differences may not necessarily invalidate the results, but members felt it may have been useful to know if all the respondents were responding to the same conceptualisations of different 'levels' of practice.

4C      No hypotheses were used.

4D      The paper included some information regarding the description of the study, but as stated previously, perhaps could have included more. Members suggested, for example, some rationale for using what the author refers to as 'qualitative data', and how this would address the aims of the study.

4E      Members felt there was enough information to enable a repeat of the study, although they added that they would clarify and enhance the 'qualitative' component before repeating this study.

4F      The feedback from the members indicated that they felt that, on the whole, the technical terms had been clearly defined.

5A      The method used was described.

5B      As stated previously, the author could have explained his justification for using a survey in more detail.

5C      Members noted that the author claimed to have undertaken a qualitative analysis of the comments written in response to the questions, and they went on to level strong criticisms of this section of the paper. Firstly, the members noted that there is no description later in the paper of the 'themes' the author claimed he would induce. Perhaps more importantly, members questioned whether or not the author had undertaken what could accurately be described as qualitative research at all.

While acknowledging the many forms of qualitative research, both Morse (1991) and Cutcliffe (1997) point out that many studies that purport to be using a qualitative method, are arguably not doing so. In this paper, there does not appear to be any evidence of analysis, or evidence of the analytical processes required in qualitative research. Counting the same word or phrase, contained in the additional 'comments' in response to deductive questions, such as the author has in this paper, does not constitute qualitative data analysis. Qualitative researchers need repeated and in-depth contact with their data. This is often expressed in terms of 'immersing oneself in the data' (Streubert and Carpenter, 1999), and it is this repeated contact which enables them to witness re-occurring patterns and themes in the data: qualitative researchers are not concerned with searching for the same word or phrase. Indeed, awkward attempts to count the frequency of the same word in qualitative data analysis have been strongly criticised as inappropriate. Morse (1995: 148) makes this point most clearly when she states:

> *I repeat: The* **quantity** *[original emphasis] of data in a category is not theoretically important to the process of saturation. Richness of data derived from detailed description, not the number of times something is stated. Frequency counts are out.*

Additionally,

> *Frequency of occurrence of any specific incident must be ignored. Saturation involves eliciting all forms of types of occurrences, valuing variation over quantity.*

> (p. 147)

5D     Members felt that the size of the sample appeared to be adequate for a preliminary study, although they noted the absence of power calculations (Cohen, 1977). Power calculations or 'power analysis' can be carried out in order to determine how large the sample needs to be (by using an estimation of the size of the difference expected between two groups). Questions were raised about the representativeness of the sample, as it was taken from the NPNR members. The author did acknowledge this as a limitation of the study.

5E     Parts of the questionnaire were described in detail, including some operational definitions.

5F     Unfortunately, the paper contains no reference to reliability or validity; this was thought to be a significant omission. It may have been particularly valuable and prudent to use a 'test/re-test' design in order to establish the reliability of the instrument (Behi and Nolan, 1995; Parahoo, 1997), particularly as the study was concerned with measuring opinion, and it is well accepted that opinions change over time.

6A     The members raised several issues with regard to the choice and the use of the statistical tests of the author. According to Watson and McFaden (1997) paper on non-parametric tests (note: one of these authors is a senior lecturer in statistics), it would have been more appropriate to use the

Wilcoxon signed rank test to determine statistical significance differences within the single sample, rather than the Mann Whitney U test which is most often associated with testing for significant differences between two independent samples. Perhaps it could be argued that the author achieved two independent samples (ie. practice-based and academic staff). The author states that he selected a random sample of 100 NPNR members and does not appear to have purposefully selected independent samples. Furthermore, given that Chi-square tests are usually undertaken to determine statistical significance associations between two categorical scales (Watson and McFaden, 1997), it was unclear which two categorical scales the author was referring to in his paper.

6B    There was mixed opinion in response to this question; some members felt the methods of analysis were adequately described, whereas other members thought they were confusing. For example, members wondered if it was legitimate to manipulate/remove the results and how this manipulation may effect the results?

6C    Opinion was mixed on this matter. Some members felt the methods of analysis were adequately described, others thought that they were confusing and could have been made clearer. Maybe the use of percentages would have helped. Furthermore, the jumps in the item question numbers (eg. 1.1 then 12.4, then 14.1) was rather confusing.

6D    Again, opinion was mixed on this matter, but on the whole, the members felt that the results could have been described more clearly. They raised a particular concern over the use of the term 'a high level of comments' (p. 459), as this indicated evidence of confusion of and combining qualitative and quantitative methods in an inappropriate manner (Cutcliffe and McKenna, 1999).

6E    The discussion appears to offer a balanced argument, and an argument that arises out of the findings. However, given the paucity of the research in this area, and the disparity on the nature of advanced practice evident within the results, perhaps a more appropriate study to undertake would have been to ask: what activities should 'normal, advanced and specialist' psychiatric nursing practice be composed of?

7A    Members felt that the conclusions were partially justified by the results. However, given the methodological limitations, the possible unrepresentative nature of the sample; the absence of any reliability or validity measures; and the cross-sectional nature of the study, it may have been more appropriate for the author to phrase his conclusion in a tentative manner, rather than the 'assertive' manner used in the paper.

7B    Members stated that the conclusions are linked closely to the original purpose of the research.

7C    Members stated that while the research did not uncover any new insights with this research, the findings did reiterate theoretical (and valuable) positions, in particular, the importance in ensuring that advanced nursing roles do not become a 'dumping ground' for practices no longer desired by medics.

7D     The author mentions the need for future additional surveys, with different and wider professions, however, no new research questions were identified and the members felt that this was a notable omission.

7E     Members felt that the practice and educational recommendations posited by the author were feasible, but as with any new training initiative, would have an additional cost attached.

7F     Members felt that far more research was required before it would be reasonable to justify major changes in nursing practice/service delivery.

7G     Members felt that the paper highlighted additional lines of enquiry and the need for further research. Perhaps studies could be conducted with psychiatric nurses who work in different clinical areas. Additional surveys with larger and more representative samples might be worthwhile. But perhaps more importantly, this study would lead to studies that ask related questions, but questions more appropriate to the current extent of knowledge in this substantive area (see 6E).

7H     The author does point out some of the limitations of the study, but perhaps it would have been prudent to acknowledge more (eg. absence of reliability/validity measures, methodological limitations).

# References

Behi R, Nolan M (1995) Reliability: Consistency and accuracy in measurement. *Br J Nurs* **4**(8): 472–5

Cohen J (1977) *Statistical Power Analysis for the Behavioural Sciences*. Revised edn. Academic Press, New York

Cutcliffe JR (1997) Qualitative research in nursing: A quest for quality. *Br J Nurs* **6**(17): 969

Cutcliffe JR, McKenna HP (1999) Establishing the credibility of qualitative research findings: The plot thickens. *J Adv Nurs* **30**(2): 374–80

Fu-Jin S (1998) Triangulation in nursing research: Issues of conceptual clarity and purpose. *J Adv Nurs* **28**(3): 631–41

May KA (1994) Abstract knowing: The case for magic in the method. In: Morse JM, ed. *Critical Issues in Qualitative Research Methods*. Sage London: 10–21

Morrison P (1991) *Critiquing research. Surgical Nurse* **6**(1):20–22

Morse JM (1991) Qualitative Nursing research: A free-for-all? In: Morse JM, ed. *Qualitative Nursing Research: A Contemporary Dialogue*. Sage London: 14–22

Morse JM (1995) The significance of saturation. *Qualitative Health Research* **5**(2): 147–9

Nolan M, Behi R (1995) Triangulation: The best of all worlds? *Br J Nurs* **4**(14): 829–32

Parahoo K (1997) *Nursing Research: Principles, process and issues*. Macmillan Press, London

Streubert HJ, Carpenter DR (1999) *Qualitative Research in Nursing: Advancing the Humanistic Imperative*. 2nd edn. Lippincott, Philadelphia

Watson H, McFaden A (1997) Non-parametric analysis. *Nurse Researcher* 4(4): 28–40

# Example number six: The NPNR National Journal Club, review from the eighth meeting

The paper reviewed first appeared in 1998, in the *Journal of Psychiatric and Mental Health Nursing* (**5**: 255–64), 'The meaning of caring for patients on a long-term psychiatric ward as narrated by formal care providers' (Pejlert A, Asplund K, Gilje F and Norberg A).

## Abstract/overview

This paper reports on a study that interviewed seventeen care providers about their caring experiences on a hospital psychiatric ward, and attempted to illicit the meaning of this work. The study used Ricoeur's (1976) phenomenological hermeneutic method, and induced three themes which illuminated the meaning of care provided. These were described as; being in the midst of human storage, moving towards a human care of relations, and struggling with the old and the new. The authors then interpreted and discussed these findings in the light of a previously published interview study, one which obtained the experiences of the patients who lived on a long-term psychiatric ward. The authors conclude that attending to ingrained attitudes of the past and their influence on the new approaches to care is essential to understanding, not only changes in ways of doing nursing tasks, but also ways of relating.

1      From the qualifications of the authors, it appeared as though the authors represented a collection of nurse educators from several academic centres, some of whom appeared to have a clinical background. It was unclear from these qualifications precisely what the nature of this clinical background may have been.

2A      Members felt that the research question was not clearly stated. They added that while the title appears to be clear, it does not accurately reflect the content of the paper. It should be noted that the introduction creates more confusion around the nature of the study. While the title indicates that the study is concerned with eliciting the meaning of caring for long-term psychiatric patients, the introduction claims that the study aims to elicit the narratives of patients as well as carers. Consequently, members thought that the paper could have made the research question clearer.

2B    Members stated that they had difficulty in answering this point, since they were unclear what 'easily researched' means. However, exploring or attempting to understand the meanings people ascribe to their lived experiences or basic social processes is entirely appropriate (and plausible) for a qualitative study (Streubert and Carpenter, 1999). Therefore, it is reasonable to argue that the problem can be researched (although whether or not this is 'easy' is another matter).

2C    It was noted that the introduction consists largely of a detailed account of a previous but linked study conducted by the same authors, and a review of some other studies that appear to be linked to this substantive area. While there appears to exist a limited body of work in this (or related) substantive area, members posited that there appeared to be a paucity of empirical work focused on this research issue with this particular client population. Consequently, the paper had the potential to add something new to the formal area of 'caring'.

2D    The problem clearly relates to nursing practice. Indeed, it claimed to be a study concerned with understanding the very nature of nursing practice for a specific population.

3A    Members stated that it appeared that the introduction and literature review were blurred. Additionally, that it might be regarded as inappropriate to have such a detailed account of the previous study at this point in the paper. However, it would seem appropriate and relevant to cite the previous studies of the authors and thereby highlight an ongoing theme or context to their research.

3B/C   The literature review appeared to contain few references. However, given that the authors claimed to be using a qualitative method, it could be argued as inappropriate to carry out a comprehensive literature review at this point (Glaser and Strauss, 1967). If this limited reviewing of the literature was a purposeful and necessary component of the method, the authors do not make this clear. Furthermore, they appear to allude (briefly) to the theoretical literature and limited empirical literature in this substantive area (ie. experiences of 'caring' for mental health clients). Members were unsure if this was a purposeful and necessary component of the method or evidence of an incomplete literature review.

3D    As stated above, the sequence and layout were regarded as rather confusing, since the author appeared to have combined the introduction and the literature review, and the members questioned the inclusion of so much detail of the author's previous study.

3E    There was no evidence of a summary of the main points of the literature review.

4A    There did not appear to be a statement about the overall design of the study. The methods section was subdivided into four sub-sections; participants and setting, interviews, interpretation and results, and naïve reading. Questions raised by the members included the inquiry if each of these sub-sections was appropriate to the methods section of the study. The first sub-section, participants and setting, says very little about the methods but does include detailed information on the participants.

4B     There did not appear to be a discussion of the relevant theoretical frameworks.

4C     The paper did not appear to contain any stated hypotheses. However, given that the authors claimed to be using a qualitative method, it could be argued that a formal hypothesis was not required (Glaser, 1978). Bearing in mind that a hypothesis refers to a proposed relationship between variables, and this study was concerned with examining the 'meanings' of caring for a certain client group, the absence of a formal hypothesis was not felt to be a limitation of the study; rather it was a methodological choice that was congruent with the design.

4D     Members felt that while the paper contained one sentence which described the aims of the study (within the introduction, p. 257), the methods and sub-sections were rather confusing. Members noted how the authors claim they asked three questions in the interview. Yet in this section alone, there are at least five questions. Unfortunately, there is no indication of the actual nature of these questions, but if this is an example of the multiplicity of the questions used, members felt it raised doubts about the ability of the authors to identify appropriately matched responses. Members wondered, if the questions and responses do not link, how could the data be coded correctly?

4E     Once again, given that the study claimed to be using a qualitative method, and that qualitative approaches are not concerned with establishing reliability by the use of replication (Morse and Field, 1995), members felt it would have been inappropriate to criticise this study on the grounds of it lacking the necessary information to make replication possible.

4F     The members did not raise the over use of technical 'jargon' as an issue for this text; they were, however, of the opinion that the structure and the arrangement of the information contained in the paper was somewhat equivocal and confusing. Furthermore, they felt that the paper contained too much tautological and unnecessary text and, as a result, this text may detract from the overall message of the paper.

5A     As stated above (in 4D), the section titled 'interviews' appeared to include sufficient detail, yet further reading of the paper indicated contra-dictions and inconsistencies with this information.

5B     The paper does not appear to contain a rationale for the method chosen.

5C     The method of data collection (ie. interviews) was felt to be congruent with the research design (Morse and Field, 1995).

5D    The paper contained a wealth of information regarding the characteristics of the sample. However, members pointed out that there did not appear to be any indication of the sampling strategy. At the very least, it would have strengthened the paper if the authors stated that they had used a sampling strategy that is in keeping with the research design, ie. purposeful sampling.

5E    Given that all seventeen care providers from the particular hospital ward were interviewed, members felt that this was an appropriate and adequate sample for this study.

5F    As stated above (in 4D/5A), the section titled 'interviews' appeared to include sufficient detail, yet further reading of the paper indicated contradictions and inconsistencies with this information.

5G    Given that this claimed to be a qualitative study, members noted that the absence of validity and reliability measures need not be construed as a limitation. But what would be expected to be present is some attempt or attention to establishing the credibility or authenticity of the findings, and this would be in keeping with qualitative methods (Leininger, 1992). In response to this, members raised some questions concerning the authors' attempts to establish the credibility of their findings by 'checking with a colleague'. There are benefits to this process, in that it provides the opportunity for challenging the robustness of the emerging themes. For instance, there may be issues or patterns that the researcher has missed which the colleague may highlight. It should also be noted that this approach has several philosophical and epistemological difficulties (Cutcliffe and McKenna, 1999). Firstly, since the process of theory induction and the subsequent generation of themes depends upon the unique creative processes between the researcher and the data, it is unlikely that two people will interpret the data in the same way. Secondly, enlisting the help of a colleague to 'check' or verify the induced themes, somehow suggests that if more than one person thinks or agrees with the induced themes, then this must be more accurate than one person's induction. If this argument is expanded, it begins to support the positivistic philosophy that there is only one accurate inter-pretation, only one reality, and the accuracy of an interpretation is increased as the number of people agreeing increases.

6A/B  Members described the method of data analysis as being congruent with a qualitative design. However, it is reasonable to suggest that they also identified some problems. Members indicated that the third sub-section, 'Interpretation and results' did include the description of the method of data analysis used, but unfortunately, did not adequately illustrate how the analysis or interpretation occurred. It did contain a brief explanation of the stages involved in the analysis, but perhaps this section could have been strengthened considerably by providing an example of how a particular theme was induced from the three-stage process described. This may have enhanced the understanding and explanation of the process and added some credibility to the theory, in that the reader would be able to see the evolution of the theory from the transcripts of the lived experiences of the interviews. The authors state that the interviewees' texts were read with the pre-understanding of the results of their previous study (p. 257). Arguments exist in the qualitative research literature that would appear to support such disclosure. Lincoln and Guba (1985) wrote of neutrality, where researchers can minimise their subjectivity and increase the credibility of their findings. This position is based upon the notion that the researcher's previous 'theoretical baggage' would influence unduly the interpretations of the findings. Other authors (eg. Husserl, 1964; Rose *et al*, 1995; Jasper, 1994) describe this process as 'bracketing'. They argue that one's experience, judgement and beliefs can be bracketed to avoid these perceptions effecting the findings. Similarly, Ashworth (1993; 1997) holds the view that the credibility of the findings is increased if researchers first make explicit their pre-suppositions and acknowledge their subjective judgement.

A vigorous counter argument to this position exists. Morse (1994) contends that qualitative methods have been plagued with conflicting advice concerning the application of prior knowledge. Many qualitative authors (Benner, 1984; Benner and Wrubel, 1989; Schutz, 1994; Walters, 1995) describe the creativity and interpretation that researchers bring to the study, and that this interpretation can be made richer by immersing all of themselves in the subject's world. Turner (1981) and Stern (1994) posit that it is the reflexivity and researcher's creativity that make qualitative methods so valuable and Cutcliffe (2000) argues that to deny a qualitative researcher's access to their prior knowledge and restrict the creativity necessary to utilise it, is likely to limit the depth of understanding of the phenomenon and impose unnecessary, rigid structures. However, the authors of the reviewed paper decided to disclose one particular pre-understanding and this led the members to ask the question: why disclose only this pre-understanding and not any other pre-understandings that they have? Are the authors suggesting this is the only pre-understanding they have?

6C    The paper appears to report and explain its findings under the headings: structural analysis, content, form, interpreted whole and reflection. Members stated that this section contains some limited explanation of the process of analysis, and this improves the overall quality of the paper. Additionally, this section does explain each of the induced themes and the members stated that they could see how the lived experiences and subsequent data had been analysed to form the themes. This section was also felt to be rather repetitive.

6D/E    The paper states that the results of the analysis of the data from the care givers (new data) will be presented with the results of the patients' analysis (old data). Members declared that the end product was, realistically, more about the old data than the new. Subsequently, this was felt to be somewhat deceptive and detracted from the overall quality of the paper as it confused rather than enlightened members. This was felt to be unfortunate, since the group members thought that there were some interesting points and findings in this section, but that they were often obscured and difficult to 'dig out'. There was a great deal of material presented by the authors, and members felt that this was perhaps too much. For example, the paper included a table which took up a whole page of the journal. Perhaps the authors could have condensed this to reflect the key points, or provide examples, and consequently maybe make the paper more 'punchy'. A significant point raised by the members was that, once again, a study that sought to uncover the opinions or experiences of recipients of mental healthcare, found that nurses who were 'kind' and understanding, were equated with providing 'good' care.

7A/B   Members pointed out that it was difficult to answer this question as the authors had not included or identified a specific 'Conclusions' section within the manuscript.

7C/D   Feedback from the group members suggested that they felt this was an interesting paper, which at times, raised some important questions about the nature of care-giver relationships with clients. In particular, it highlighted the shift in emphasis in nursing from the role of 'care-giver' to a 'partner in a therapeutic alliance'. These findings reflect a re-occurring theme within current psychiatric and mental health nursing literature; that of the centrality and value of forming relationships with clients, engaging in human care (Barker, 1999). While for some mental health nurses there appears to be a current emphasis on cure, neuroscience and biological interventions, it is important to note that for many others, this is regarded as entirely inappropriate. This paper can be seen as adding to the argument that many psychiatric and mental health nurses are becoming increasingly aware of the need to remind themselves of several key questions, such as: what do people need psychiatric or mental health nurses for? How can these nurses establish the genuinely, collaborative forms of care or partnerships, described in the 1994 Report of the Mental Health Review Team? How can we develop a technology of human care which is undeniably about mental health nursing? (Barker, 1999).

7E   The paper did not appear to contain any recommendations.

7F   Members felt it would be unwise to instigate a change in practice on the grounds of the findings of one study. However, this is not necessarily a reflection on the quality of this paper, but is more indicative of applying an appropriate level of caution when interpreting and subsequently implementing any research findings.

7G   As stated above (7C/D), the findings in this study perhaps indicate the need to undertake empirical work in order to address certain key questions. Such as: what do people need psychiatric or mental health nurses for? How can these nurses establish the genuinely, collaborative forms of care or partnerships, described in the 1994 Report of the Mental Health Review Team? How can we develop a technology of human care which is undeniably about mental health nursing? (Barker, 1999).

7H    The authors do not appear to have included a 'Limitations of the study' section, or indicated the possible limitations in the study. The members thought this was a significant oversight.

# References

Ashworth PD (1993) Participant agreement in the justification of qualitative findings. *J Phenomenological Psychology* **25**: 3–16

Ashworth PD (1997) The Variety of qualitative research: Non-positivist approaches. *Nurse Educ Today* **17**: 219–24

Barker P (1999) *The Philosophy and Practice of Psychiatric Nursing.* Churchill Livingstone, Edinburgh

Benner P (1984) *From Novice to Expert: Excellence and power in clinical practice.* Addison-Wesley, New York

Benner P, Wrubel J (1989) *The Primacy of Caring: Stress and coping in health and illness.* Addison-Wesley, New York

Cutcliffe JR, McKenna HP (1999) Establishing the credibility of qualitative research findings: The plot thickens. *J Adv Nurs* **30**(2): 374–80

Cutcliffe JR (2000) Methodological issues in grounded theory. *J Adv Nurs* **31**(6): 1476–84

Department of Health (1994) *Working in Partnership: A collaborative approach to care. Report of the Mental Health Nursing Review Team.* HMSO, London

Glaser BG, Strauss AL (1967) *The Discovery of Grounded Theory: Strategies for qualitative research.* Aldine, Chicago

Glaser BG (1978) *Theoretical Sensitivity.* The Sociology Press, Mill Valley, California

Husserl E (1964) *The Idea of Phenomenology* (W Alston, G Nakhikan). Nijhoff, The Hague

Jasper MA (1994) Issues in phenomenology for researchers in nursing. *J Adv Nurs* **19**: 30–14

Leininger M (1992) Current issues, problems and trends to advanced qualitative paradigmatic research methods for the future. *Qualitative Health Res* **2**(4): 392–415

Lincoln YS, Guba EG (1985) Naturalistic Inquiry. Sage, Newbury Park

Morrison P (1991) Critiquing research. *Surgical Nurse* **3**(1): 20–22

Morse JM (1994) Emerging from the data: The cognitive processes of analysis in qualitative enquiry In: Morse JM, ed. *Critical Issues in Qualitative Research Methods.* Sage, London: 23–43

Morse JM, Field PA (1995) *Qualitative Research Methods for Health Professionals.* 2nd edn. Sage, London

Ricoeur P (1976) *Interpretation Theory: Discourse and the surplus of meaning.* Christian University Press, Fort Worth

Rose P, Beeby J, Parker D (1995) Academic rigour in the lived experience of researchers using phenomenological methods in nursing. *J Adv Nurs* **21**: 1123–9

Schutz SE (1994) Exploring the benefits of a subjective approach in qualitative nursing. *J Adv Nurs* **20**: 412–17

Stern P (1994) Eroding grounded theory. In: Morse JM, ed. *Critical Issues in Qualitative Research.* Sage, London: 210–23

Streubert HJ, Carpenter DR (1999) *Qualitative Research in Nursing: Advancing the humanistic imperative.* Lippincott, Philadelphia

Turner B (1981) Some practical aspects of qualitative data analysis: One way of organising the cognitive processes associated with the generation of grounded theory. *Qual Control* **15**: 225–45

Walters AJ (1995) The phenomenological movement: implications for nursing research. *J Adv Nurs* **22**: 791–9

## Summary: Strengths and limitations of Morrison's approach to critiquing nursing research

*Strengths*

❖ The approach is easy to follow and apply.

❖ It follows a logical sequence that usually matches that of the reviewed paper.

❖ It appears to give consideration to most of the fundamental components to which each research report should make reference.

❖ It does not contain an overuse of terminology or jargon, but requires the reviewer to have some understanding of basic concepts and practices within research.

❖ It is possible that the author of the research paper reviewed may learn from a critique using Morrison's approach, particularly, if the reviewers include extensive comments.

❖ The approach does enable both strengths and limitations to be identified.

❖ The approach clearly encourages the reviewer(s) to think about how the findings in the reviewed paper(s) may impact on nursing practice. Indeed, the reviewers are encouraged to place the findings in the overall context of the substantive/formal area researched and that is a notable strength of the approach.

❖ The approach does include some useful and thought-provoking questions within the headings. For example, question 6E, 'does the discussion emphasise some aspects of the results and ignore others, and is this emphasis justified?'

❖ The approach allows room for the data and/or argument to be introduced to support the reviewer's criticisms/observations and suggestions for improvement. Furthermore, this is perhaps facilitated more easily using Morrison's approach, than with the two previous approaches (Duffy 1985; Burns and Grove, 1987). This is because some of the questions used in Morrison's approach use 'open ended' rather than closed questions, and thus stimulate more than comments/debate.

*Limitations*

❖ Some of the terminology used in Morrison's questions, or the meaning of the questions, is unclear and difficult to assess. For example, what does the author mean by the expression 'easily researched?' How should a reviewer determine whether or not something is 'easily researched?' Just because something may be difficult to research, does that make a study any less valuable or appropriate?

❖ This approach appears to be more focused on critiquing quantitative studies (eg. questions about hypotheses, questions about replication of the study, the question about graphs and tables). Consequently, the usefulness of this approach in critiquing qualitative studies may be limited.

❖ There are several questions that need to be asked of each reviewed paper which this approach does not indicate or facilitate the reviewer in asking (eg. the approach makes no reference to ethical issues or ethical considerations).

❖ The approach suggests the reviewer should consider if a change in practice is required as a result of the findings. However, since it would be unwise to instigate a change in practice on the grounds of the findings of one study, this seams like a superfluous question.

❖ One of Morrison's questions (3C) asks, 'are the sources (of literature) current and up-to-date or has the author relied solely on well known but out-of-date references?' There are several limitations arising out of this question (even ignoring the tautology). Firstly, Morrison does not indicate when a paper would become 'out-of-date'. Secondly, and this issue is of greater importance, what reviewers should be considering is the quality of the references included, not necessarily the age. Age, as the sole criteria, does not always indicate poor quality. Indeed, prudent researchers usually make reference to seminal or key works. It is difficult to imagine a physics researcher being criticised for including the work of Newton, Faraday or Einstein. Similarly, it would be inappropriate to criticise the work of a researcher examining issues within psycho-dynamic therapy for including the work of Freud, Klein or Jung.

❖ As with Burns and Grove's approach, Morrison does not appear to indicate why there are different numbers of questions within the key areas he identifies. Indeed, the range of the number of questions is wider than in Burns and Grove's approach. Morrison's approach has a key area with one question, some key areas with four questions and even one key area with eight questions! Reviewers were left wondering if this indicated, implicitly, the relative importance that Morrison ascribes to each of the key areas.

❖ This approach, like Duffy's (1985) approach and Burns and Grove's (1987) approach might be regarded as a form of simplistic reductionism, where an attempt is made to reduce the research to its simplest constituent parts, and then the reviewer attempts to 'measure' these parts.

# 6

## Polit and Hungler's (1997) approach to critiquing nursing research

This chapter focuses on Polit and Hungler's (1997) approach to critiquing nursing research. It describes their guidelines (*Box 6.1*) and the five key areas that the reviewer needs to consider. In order to facilitate the application of this approach, we have summarised the key issues in each of these areas into lists of questions. Following this we provide two detailed examples (drawing on the reviews carried out by the NPNR National Journal Club). Having described the approach and provided examples, we then highlight some of the strengths and limitations of this approach.

Polit and Hungler (1997, p. 410) declare that a research critique is:

*... not just a review or summary of a study but rather a careful, critical appraisal of the strengths and limitations of a piece of research.*

They argue that each research report has a number of important dimensions and that a thorough critique of the paper would include consideration of each of these dimensions. They describe these dimensions as: substantive and theoretical, methodologic, ethical, interpretive and presentational/ stylistic. In addition to these five areas, Polit and Hungler (1997) provide a set of overall guidelines for critiquing research reports (*Box 6.1*) and guidelines for considering the interpretive dimensions of the study and the presentational dimensions of the study (*Boxes 6.2* and *6.3*).

### Substantive and theoretical dimensions

1.  Was the study important in terms of:
    *   the significance of the problem
    *   the soundness of the conceptualisations
    *   the appropriateness of the theoretical framework
    *   the creativity and insightfulness of the analysis.
2.  Is the research problem relevant to nursing? Would it have been more appropriate for the study to have been conducted by a discipline other than nursing?
3.  The researcher should ask; given what we know about this topic, is this research the right next step? (As knowledge development is often incremental and sequential, it is wise to avoid unnecessary repetition.

However, the reviewer should consider; has the researcher taken several 'leaps ahead?')
4.  Is the study question congruent with the methods used to address it?
5.  Has the researcher appropriately placed the research problem into a larger theoretical context?

---

**Box 6.1: Guidelines for the conduct of a written research critique**

❖ Be sure to comment on the study's strengths as well as its limitations. The critique should be a balanced consideration of the worth of the research. Each research report has **some** (original emphasis) positive features. Be sure to find them and note them.

❖ Give specific examples of the study's strengths and limitations. Avoid vague generalisations of praise and fault finding.

❖ Try and justify your criticisms. Offer a rationale for how a different approach would have solved a problem that the researcher failed to address.

❖ Be as objective as possible. Try to avoid being overly critical because you are not particularly interested in a topic or because you have a world view that is inconsistent with the underlying paradigm.

❖ Be sensitive in handling negative comments. Try to put yourself in the shoes of the researcher receiving the critical appraisal. Do not be condescending or sarcastic.

❖ Suggest realistic alternatives that the researcher (or future researchers) might want to consider. Don't just identify problems — offer some recommended solutions, making sure that the recommendations are practical ones.

❖ Evaluate all aspects of the study — its substantive, theoretical, methodologic, ethical, interpretive and presentational dimensions.

---

(From Polit and Hungler, 1997)

## Methodologic dimensions

**Four main design decisions in quantitative studies:**

1   Design: Was the most appropriate design for the study used? Which design would provide the clearest and most meaningful results regarding the hypothesis/null-hypothesis?

2   Participants: What was the composition of the sample? How large was the sample, was this adequate? How were they recruited, was this appropriate?

3   Measures: Which measuring instruments/tools were used? Consider, how can the variable under study be operationalised (isolated) and reliably/validly measured for each participant?

> ❖ Does the report suggest overt biases?
> ❖ Is the report written using tentative language as befits the nature of the disciplined enquiry, or does the author talk about what the study did or did not prove?
> ❖ Is sexist language avoided?
> ❖ Does the title of the report adequately capture the key concepts of the population under investigation? Does the abstract (if any) adequately summarise the research problem, study method, and important findings?

(from Polit and Hungler, 1997)

# Example number seven: The NPNR National Journal Club, review from the first meeting

The paper reviewed first appeared in 1995, in the *Journal of Advanced Nursing* (**22**: 855–861), 'A study to identify the attitudes and needs of qualified staff concerning the use of research findings in clinical practice within mental health care settings' (Veeramah V).

## Abstract/overview

This paper reported on a small scale exploratory survey which attempted to assess the attitudes and needs of qualified nurses working within mental health settings. A total of 150 questionnaires were sent to trained nurses working in the south east of England and 118 questionnaires were returned, which indicates a response rate of 78%. The researcher claimed that the main findings were that although the vast majority of nurses in the study have a positive attitude to research, very few actually make significant use of research findings to enhance their practice. The author then lists some of the variables that seem to contribute to this state of affairs and points out that most of the nurses said they would be involved in research activities if the time was provided for them to do so.

## Substantive and theoretical dimension

1A    The identified research problem certainly warrants investigation, in that it appears to be 'covering new ground' or, at the very least, investigating an area that appears to be distinctly under researched. Therefore, the study can be regarded as important.

1B    It appears that the paper did contain concepts that lacked definition or perhaps suffered from a lack of clarity. This was particularly noticeable in the introduction and the literature review. Some of the members wondered even if the author fully understood what was meant by research as there appeared to be a confusion between evidence-based practice and research-based practice (McKenna *et al*, 2000). It may have been useful to include some definitions of what constitutes 'research-based practice' and the author could have included some extra detail in order to 'demystify' research. Furthermore, the crucial issue that nursing research should inform practice, not dictate practice, was absent.

1C    There is little evidence of a theoretical framework within the study.

1D    The members felt that there were many opportunities in this paper where the researcher could have been more creative and insightful and in a sense, had not 'extended him/herself' fully. These are explored in the 'Interpretive dimension' section in more detail.

2    The research problem is highly relevant to nursing and this can be viewed as one of the strengths of the paper. The emphasis on evidence-based practice has clearly increased over recent years and it is not surprising that new journals (eg. *Evidence-Based Nursing*), a growing body of literature (eg. Muir-Gray, 1997) and centres for disseminating research evidence (eg. the Cochraine centre) have also emerged. Consequently, few (if any) credible healthcare professionals would deny that sound evidence should be an integral part of clinical decision making. Therefore, while recognising that research-based practice is but one of the four components of evidence-based practice (McKenna *et al*, 2000), it is still appropriate and necessary to investigate issues involved in the use of research- (and evidence-) based practice.

3    Opinion was divided among the members as to whether or not this research was the right 'next step'. The author ends the literature section by listing seven propositions. It should be noted that the researcher points out that these propositions are based mainly on literature reviews and are not well supported empirically. Nevertheless, it is evident that the researcher includes questions in the questionnaire that appear to be in response to the issues highlighted by these seven propositions (but not all of them). It could be argued that the researcher is trying to build upon existing knowledge.

Several questions were begged by the National Journal Club members: Why did the author not construct a questionnaire to address each of the seven propositions? If the researcher acknowledges that several of the propositions are not based on empirical study, does that not indicate a direction for study that the researcher could follow? Does the absence of any empirically-based theory in these areas indicate the need for a qualitative study?

4    This was another question where opinion was mixed. It would appear to be entirely appropriate, once having decided that the study

question is concerned with determining the 'research needs' of qualif. staff, that a survey design is used to measure the extent and nature of the needs (Parahoo, 1997). The researcher did not limit himself/herself to measuring the needs, indeed, the principal objective of the study was to assess the attitudes of the staff towards nursing research. Consequently, there may have been merit in exploring the different ways that attitudes may be measured and it was perhaps remiss of the researcher not to mention the significant difficulty and wide debate that surrounds the practice of measuring attitudes. This is explored in more detail in the 'Methodological dimension' section.

5    The researcher appears to have located the research problem within a larger theoretical context; namely, the need for nursing to move towards being an evidence- (research-) based discipline.

## Methodological dimension

Since the study purports to be using a quantitative method, the key questions relating to design, sample, measures and procedures are considered in this section.

1    The study uses a simple survey design and while surveys have been used previously to investigate this phenomenon (Hunt, 1981; Lacey, 1994), it may not have been the most appropriate method. Attempts to measure attitudes present a range of methodological difficulties (Parahoo, 1997), and it was felt by some members of the National Journal Club, that the paper may have benefited from some attention to this matter. The members' difficulty resides not in the ultimate choice of a survey, but rather the absence of any consideration of methodological options or consideration of the methodological difficulties in attempting to measure attitudes. It may have been worthwhile for the author to have explored alternative scoring systems, for example, using questions with visual analogue scales or semantic differential scales, which have particular value in measuring subjective experiences, and this would have been more in keeping with measuring attitudes (Parahoo, 1997).

Alternatively, perhaps the use of focus groups could have been considered since according to Roberts (1999), focus groups as a means of gathering (qualitative) data offers several advantages, particularly when trying to understand the behaviour, attitudes and perception of a group. These advantages include synergism, stimulation from other group members, security and speed. Additionally, the semi-structured nature of focus groups would have allowed the researchers to:

- let the focus group participants respond to one another as they discuss their attitudes towards research (adding to the richness and depth of the data)
- pick up on and subsequently follow any key issues or particular themes that emerged during the focus group.

*second* alternative method that was suggested by the members was to use triangulated design and combine the qualitative component with a *subsequent* quantitative survey. Using this design, the researcher would perhaps have first induced a theory of P/MH nurses' attitudes to research, and could then have measured the extent to which this theory was accurate for a wider population of P/MH nurses.

2      It is difficult to comment on the composition of the sample, as the precise details of the sample are not included in the paper. This can be regarded as an oversight and limitation of the paper. The researcher stated that he/she attempted to sample as many qualified mental health nurses from specific clinical areas (both in-patient and community areas). Unfortunately, their paper contains no breakdown of how many questionnaires were distributed to each clinical area, or a breakdown of community/hospital distribution. Consequently, members were left guessing how the questionnaires were distributed and who they were distributed to.

3      It appeared that the author had largely attempted to replicate a previous study undertaken in this area, and had augmented the questionnaire used in that study with two further questions. Members stated that the additional questions added something extra to the original questionnaire, but felt that the tool could have withstood further refinement. For example:

• had the tool undergone any tests for validity?
• were the terms used in the questionnaire operationally defined?
• some of the questions appear to have an element of ambiguity and thus may cause confusion. In question one, for example, are the respondents being asked to agree/disagree with the 'research-based' aspect, the 'professional' aspect or both? In question 2, what does, 'research activity' refer to? Conducting research, implementing research or reading research?

4      There is no mention in the paper of when the measurements occurred and the members were left assuming that the results refer to a 'single time point' measurement.

## Ethical dimension

The researcher does state that the necessary permissions were gained from all the appropriate managers, however, there appears to be no mention of ethical considerations. Given that the research appeared to take place (at least in part) on NHS premises, and Department of Health's (1991) guidelines on research and Local Research Ethics Committees (LRECs), it would have been prudent for the researcher to submit the research proposal to the LREC for approval.

## Interpretive dimension

1    The view of the members was that the discussion section did not offer conclusions or interpretations of all the important results. The discussion appeared to be largely a reiteration of the findings and some comparison of the results to the studies cited in the literature review. Suggestions regarding what the researcher may have included in the discussion are listed in question 7.

2    The limited interpretations appear to be congruent with the results and are considered within the context of the limitations.

3    The researcher draws upon the evidence of the previous findings of the studies cited in the literature review.

4    It does not appear that alternative explanations are offered. One such alternative explanation might have been an argument that suggested that those nurses who feel more positive towards research are more likely to complete and return a questionnaire of this nature. Indeed, perhaps the absence of such consideration may even cast doubt on the validity of the findings, and this led members to wonder if the most appropriate question had been asked. Some members felt that a more appropriate question to ask was: 'What do nurses understand by the term research?' Perhaps an important question that the researcher could have asked of the data was: 'How easy would it have been for nurses to say they have a negative attitude towards research?' Particularly, when nurses are frequently told in policy documents, published papers and in their pre- and post-registration education, that research is 'good' and should be embraced.

5    There does not appear to be any mention of statistical significance, but the researcher did state that he/she intended to avoid 'jargon' and keep the analysis simple in order that the majority of nurses might understand it.

6    There does not appear to be any evidence of unwarranted generalisations within the discussion.

7    There is evidence of only limited discussion of the implications for nursing practice/theory/research. Members highlighted that there are so many relevant issues relating to this matter and the findings of the research, and felt that the researcher rather 'sold himself/herself short'. For example, the researcher could have considered; is research-based practice always something to strive for (McKenna *et al*, 2000) and if not, how might this consideration have effected the results? Is there the body of research in mental health nursing for the nurses to be using in their practice? (Ward *et al*, 2000). Has the most valuable/useful or most appropriate type of knowledge been uncovered in the research that has been conducted for nursing, and if not, how might this effect the nurses attitudes towards and utilisation of research findings? Several authors have alluded to the different types of knowledge that nurses need (see Benner, 1984; Pearson, 1992; McKenna, 1997) and if nursing research is producing knowledge that has

only limited relevance or application to clinical practice, this may have an impact on the nurses' attitudes towards those research findings (Cutcliffe, 1998). There is another question that warrants consideration: would it always be in the best interests of nurses to be aware of the latest research findings? That is, would the nurses be placed in a dichotomous position if the research evidence indicated one way of practice and the organisation or medical colleagues advocate another? A crucial issue which the members felt was a particularly significant omission was that research should inform practice — not dictate it (McKenna *et al*, 2000).

8      The paper does make specific recommendations and these were felt to have sense and value. While they appear to have some resonance with the results, they do not appear to have been uncovered through the research process. That is, many of the recommendations do not appear to have evolved directly from the results and consequently, the members felt that some of these had an element of impracticability.

**Presentational and stylistic dimension**

1      The report contains most of the detail required, but some important details appear to be missing. For example, the paper contains no (null) hypothesis or research question (however, it does contain a series of study objectives), there is a distinct absence of detailed consideration of any ethical issues, and members felt that a thorough discussion of the implications of the results was absent.

2      Members described the paper as reasonably well written and noted that it appears to have been written purposefully to enable the reader's understanding. (Indeed, the author makes such claims within the paper.) Consequently, one of the strengths of the paper can be considered to be the absence of unnecessary jargon or tautology. However, in attempting to be, as the researcher states, 'as simple as possible' (p. 858), the paper perhaps loses rigour.

3      In the main, the paper had a logical flow and conformed to the standard format of; introduction, literature review, methods, results, discussion, conclusion (Tierney, 1991). However, as stated above, the collection of recommendations at the end of the paper appear to be based on a review of the literature, and not necessarily based on the findings. The inclusion of these recommendations at this point in the paper might be regarded as inappropriate.

4      Members described the paper as being reasonably well organised and there was no evidence of irrelevant detail. The author acknowledges the omission of an important detail; the total number of the sample. The lack of information concerning the distribution of the questionnaire was thought to be an oversight. The paper left the members assuming that each participant

only filled in one questionnaire each, yet this is not made clear in the pap and importantly, this might be because the researcher could not be sure th. was the case. Some more detail of the distribution and subsequent collectior of the questionnaires may have helped.

5      The paper does not appear to contain any evidence of overt biases.

6      The researcher uses tentative language throughout the report, although it should be noted that members felt that, in places, the report had almost an apologetic feel with expressions such as; 'unfortunately, although the study was small scale... despite the sample size'.

7      The was no evidence of sexist language within the report.

8      The title and abstract both appear to be clear and concise.


## References

Benner P (1984) *From Novice to Expert: Excellence and power in clinical nursing.* Addison-Wesley, Menlo Park

Cutcliffe JR (1998) Is psychiatric nursing research barking up the wrong tree? *Nurse Educ Today* **18**: 257–8

Department of Health (1991) *Local Research Ethics Committees.* DoH, London

Hunt J (1981) Implications for nursing practice: The use of research findings. *J Adv Nurs* **6**: 1898–194

Lacey EA (1994) Research utilization in nursing practice – a pilot study. *J Adv Nurs* **19**: 987–95

McKenna HP (1997) *Nursing Theories and Models.* Routledge London

McKenna HP, Cutcliffe JR, McKenna P (2000) Evidence-based practice: Demolishing some myths. *Nurs Standard* **14**(16): 39–42

Muir-Gray JA (1997) *Evidence-based health Care.* Churchill Livingstone, Edinburgh

Parahoo K (1997) *Nursing Research: Principles, process and issues.* Macmillan Press, London

Pearson A (1992) Knowing nursing: emerging paradigms in nursing. In: Robinson K, Vaughan B, eds. *Knowledge for Nursing.* Butterworth Heinemann, Oxford

Polit DF, Hungler BP (1997) *Essentials of Nursing Research: Methods, appraisal and utlisation.* 4th edn. Lippincott, Philadelphia

Roberts P (1999) Planning and running a focus group. *Nurse Researcher* **4**: 78–82

Tierney AJ (1991) Reporting and disseminating research. In Cormack D, ed. *The Research Process in Nursing.* 2nd edn. Blackwell Scientific, Oxford: 318–28

Ward M, Cutcliffe JR, Gournay K (2000) *The Nursing, midwifery and health visiting contribution to the continuing care of people with mental health problems: A review and UKCC action plan.* UKCC, London

# ample number eight: The NPNR National Journal Club, eview from the twelfth meeting

> The paper reviewed first appeared in 1994, in the *Journal of Psychiatric and Mental Health Nursing* (1, 85–92), 'An observational study of associations between nurses behaviour and violence in psychiatric hospitals' (Whittington R and Wykes T).

## Abstract/overview

This paper described a cyclic model of violence to psychiatric nurses and then reports on a partial test of the model. The paper argued that stress induced by exposure to violence leads to impaired staff performance and adoption of behaviours which make the re-occurrence of violence more likely. The paper then reports how the researchers tested part of this model by proposing that certain staff behaviours (eg. expressing verbal hostility) would be associated with an increased risk of assault. The paper reports that there was some evidence of the proposed association and the researchers then claim they discuss the implications of these findings for psychiatric nursing.

## Substantive and theoretical dimension

1A    The research area certainly warrants investigation. Violence continues to be a cause for concern within the National Health Service (NHS). Recent evidence indicates that the problem of violence towards nurses is increasing (Health Services Advisory Committee, 1987; Crichton, 1995). Consequently, any study that potentially contributes to a greater understanding of the dynamics and processes involved and helps to reduce the incidence of violence, can be regarded as a significant study.

1B    Opinion was divided on this matter. The paper posits an interesting model and few would doubt that the nurses' feelings and resulting behaviour could have an effect on client violence. However, the paper presents a rather simplistic and linear model, and importantly, omits many additional variables that could be similarly involved or contribute to the exacerbation of violence, eg. experiential learning, clinical supervision (Cutcliffe, 1999), cultural or organisational factors (Morrison, 1990)

1C    Members again reported some concerns about the theoretical framework, given the concerns outlined in response to 1B. There was also the feeling that the model may contain an element of disciplinary prejudice. Examination of the approach to understanding and exploring that appears to be preferred within the discipline of psychology appears to emphasise the following process. Psychologists, in the main, look to individual behaviour to explain outcomes and decontextualise the material. Then they attempt to generalise to the wider population. Members wondered if this paper (given that one of the authors was a psychologist) might be one example of that process.

1D    Opinion was varied concerning the insightfulness and creativity of the analysis. Some members felt that the model represented an attempt to translate theories/ideas of stress and coping, into simplistic and unlikely scenarios in avoidant and confrontative coping. Other members felt that only limited empirical work has been undertaken which considers the possible effects of the nurse's feelings and behaviours on client violence, and this paper maybe offers insight into such dynamics.

2    The research is clearly appropriate to nursing and one of the strengths of the paper was the researchers' willingness to address potentially awkward and yet highly relevant questions.

3    Opinion was divided with regard to this question. Some members felt that given the relative lack of empirical work in this area, a qualitative method was indicated. Such a position is supported by the well-documented argument that a qualitative method is indicated when little or nothing is known about the phenomenon (Dickoff and James, 1968; Munhall, 1993; Morse and Field, 1995). Other members felt that perhaps by positing and subsequently testing, simplistic hypotheses (ie. there is a relationship between client violence, the nurse's feelings and the nurse's behaviour) was an appropriate choice. While it may have been appropriate to posit hypotheses, it should be noted that the members felt the model was too simplistic and failed to take account of the many confounding variables.

4    Given the question posed by the researchers, that certain types of nurse behaviour are more associated with violence by psychiatric clients than other types of behaviour, it was appropriate to use a quantitative, deductive method; in that the question is concerned with measurement and testing (Parahoo, 1997).

5    The researchers alluded to the larger theoretical context, in terms of the ramifications of violence within the NHS, but only to a limited extent. They have attempted to locate the study, or at least link the study, to the wider formal area of 'stress and coping'.


**Methodological dimension**

Since the study purports to be using a quantitative method, the key questions relating to design, sample, measures and procedures are now considered.

1    The design was appropriate to the study question and provided some data that would enable the hypotheses to be tested. However, given the wide

ange of confounding variables and interactions of variables that could impact on client violence, it is debatable that the method used provided the clearest and most meaningful results. For example, there are arguments that posit violence as having a biological basis (Kreuz and Rose, 1972), arguments that indicate the 'organisation's' role or/and culture in perpetuating violence (Morrison, 1990) and 'social learning' theories as the basis for explaining violence (Bandura, 1973). Given the possible interaction of these and other influences on client violence, the members doubted that the design used in this study provided the clearest and most meaningful results.

As an alternative, the researchers might have considered either a qualitative method or a different quantitative method. The choice of a qualitative method would have enabled the researchers to ask the clients: 'tell me about your experiences of the nursing staff and if/how their behaviour contributes to client violent behaviour?' An alternative quantitative method would have involved the use of a survey; and could have asked the clients to indicate from a range of nursing responses/behaviours, which of these would contribute to client violent behaviour?

2    The sample had two 'tiers' and consisted of certain wards and certain individuals on the wards. The nurses were selected by chance in that they happened to be on duty when the observations were made. The researchers state that the sample of nurses was representative of the overall population on the wards in terms of grade and sex.

With regard to the sample of wards, there are significant problems with designating wards as violent or non-violent, not least because of the ambiguity around defining an incident as violent (Cutcliffe, 1999; Turnbull, 1999). Indeed, the researchers made reference to this difficulty themselves. In the absence of any previous empirical work on which to base sampling decisions (ie. previous studies could have determined that certain wards could be designated as violent and non-violent as a result of the wards meeting certain evidence-based criteria), the researchers have made some attempt to differentiate between such wards. Perhaps it would have been prudent for the researchers to acknowledge the limitations of their attempts to differentiate between violent and non-violent wards. Other members wondered, given the hypothesis and the bulk of the results, why such differentiations had been made at all?

3    The detail provided by the authors concerning the measures used was thought to be a strength of the paper. One minor point was raised with regard to the 'availability' measure. It was pointed out that nurses could well be unavailable to clients because they were engaged in therapeutic activity and not necessarily distancing themselves as a result of the stress they were feeling (as the researchers allude to).

4    The procedure used for measurement was also thought to be a strength of the paper. Although, the reviewed paper made no reference to the Hawthorne effect (Polit and Hungler, 1997) which was thought to be an oversight.

## Ethical dimension

The paper contains no mention of consideration of ethical issues or ethical approval. This was felt to be a major limitation of the paper. For example, members wondered about how the researcher may have responded if he witnessed any purposeful provocation of a client.

## Interpretive dimension

1/2     Members stated that the discussion contained some interpretation of what appear to be important results, yet, it also contained some contradictions. For example, the researchers suggest that charge nurses were the least 'available' grade of nurse, yet tended to speak to clients more and were also at high risk of assault. On the other hand, enrolled nurses were a highly 'available' grade of nurse, made more rejecting statements, used touch more often, yet were less at risk of assault. Perhaps what this discussion could have mentioned, given the confounding and often conflicting relationships between variables, is that simplistic, proposed causal relationships do not offer a complete understanding of the processes, dynamics and interactions involved in violence between clients and staff.

3     The researchers draw upon previous empirical work in this substantive area. However, it may be worth noting that of the six references used in the discussion, four of the papers referenced were written by the author(s) of the current paper.

4     The researchers make reference to some of the contradictions in their findings, but instead of positing these as evidence to reject their model and hypotheses (and thus consider alternative explanations), they attempt to justify why these findings may have occurred, resulting in much unsupported casual hypothesising.

5     The study includes 'P' values and distinguishes between practical and statistical significance.

6     The study does not make any unwarranted generalisations.

7     Members felt that the paper contained important implications for psychiatric/mental health nursing practice, yet these were largely implicit in the paper. Only the final paragraph of the discussion section contained any explicit indication of the implications and further attention to the implications may have been advisable. If, as the researchers posit, there appear to be some staff who use certain behaviours which provoke (or contribute to) client violence, then this has clear education and training implications. For example, self-awareness or awareness raising is often regarded as an integral component of P/MH nurse preparation (Burnard, 1995) and many approaches exist to facilitate an increase in awareness (Heron, 1990; Duck, 1992). It is possible that the nurses who engage in behaviour that provokes client

violence may do so unknowingly. (Indeed, if such behaviour is engaged in knowingly, then that raises a whole series of additional training/education issues!) If one accepts that the nurses are acting unknowingly, then the need for further self-awareness training becomes very clear. Furthermore, while there is little consensus in the literature on the practice of de-escalation (Patterson *et al*, 1997), few authors in this substantive area would disagree that an awareness of the nurse's feelings and resultant behaviour is inextricably linked to the practice of de-escalation. The argument goes like this: if a nurse is unaware of their own behaviour (eg. use of touch, eye contact, body posture, verbal behaviours), then how can they engage competently in de-escalation techniques, since much of this practice involves monitoring oneself and adjusting potentially provocative actions.

Additionally, if we accept the researchers' argument that nurses who feel stressed may be more likely to engage in distancing behaviours and inadvertently provoke further violent actions, then there is a clear indication that nurses require support systems and methods of dealing with stress. The need for formal support systems for nurses who deal with violent incidents has been highlighted many times in the literature. Arguments proposing the introduction of post incident counselling or de-briefing services (Ryan and Poster, 1993; Turnbull, 1993; Wykes and Mezey, 1994; Thomas, 1995 ) and the continuing need for clinical supervision (Cutcliffe, 1999) are perhaps the most common, and it may have benefited the reviewed paper if further attention had been given to these particular service/education implications.

8       The paper contains limited recommendations for practice and for further study; stating only that further research is required to evaluate the importance of interpersonal behaviours in this significant problem. Additional implications that perhaps warranted discussion have been outlined in response to question 7. Supplementary areas or issues for further study that the authors could have considered include: research aimed at understanding how nurses feel following client violence; how they deal with any resultant stress and how any residual stress effects their subsequent interactions; how clients feel when they perceive nurses behaving in avoidant or provocative ways; how the culture of the ward/unit may contribute to violence; how prepared or trained nurses feel in engaging with potentially violent clients.

**Presentational dimension**

1       On the whole, members felt that the paper contained enough information to allow a thorough critique of the study's purpose, conceptual framework, design, methods, analysis and interpretations. There was a distinct absence of information regarding ethical issues and ethical considerations.

2       The report was written in a good academic style.

3       The report is, in the main, well organised and has a logical structure. The addition of a clearer conclusion section was suggested by some members.

4    The report is concise and does not include irrelevant detail.

5    Members felt that the paper did appear to contain some evidence of overt bias, and that was a bias towards the validity and accuracy of the proposed model. Evidence of this bias was in the form of the researcher's apparent unwillingness to: consider alternative explanations; or consider using the evidence obtained as the basis for rejecting their model, and their apparent attempts to justify why these anomalous findings may have occurred.

6    The report uses tentative language as befitting of the nature of disciplined enquiry.

7    Sexist language is avoided.

8    Members felt the title was an accurate reflection of the content of the paper. The abstract did not appear to provide a description of the methods employed.

# References

Bandura A (1973) *Aggression: A social learning analysis*. Prentice Hall, New Jersey

Burnard P (1995) *Counselling skills for healthcare professionals*. 2nd edn. Chapman Hall, London

Crichton J (1995) A review of psychiatric inpatient violence. In: Crichton J, ed. *Psychiatric Patient Violence: Risk and response*. Duckworth, London

Cutcliffe JR (1999) Qualified nurses' lived experiences of violence perpetrated by individuals suffering from enduring mental health problems: a hermeneutic study. *Int J Nurs Stud* **36**: 105–16

Dickoff J, James P (1968) A theory of theories: a position paper. *Nurs Res* **17**(3): 197–203

Duck S (1992) *Human Relationships*. 2nd edn. Sage, London

Health Services Advisory Committee (1987) *Violence to Staff in the Health Service*. HMSO, London

Heron J (1990) *Helping the Client: A creative practical guide*. Sage, London

Kreuz LE, Rose RM (1972) Assessment of aggressive behaviour and plasma testosterone in a young population. *Psychometric Med* **34**: 321–2

Morrison EF (1990) The tradition of toughness: a study of non-professional nursing care in psychiatric nursing settings. *Image: J Nurs Scholarship* **22**(1): 32–8

Munhall PL (1993) Language and nursing research. In: Munhall PL, Boyd CO, eds. *Nursing Research: A qualitative perspective*. National League for Nursing Press, New York

Morse JM, Field PA (1995) *Qualitative Research Methods for Health Professionals*. 2nd . Sage, London

Parahoo K (1997) *Nursing Research: Principles, process and issues*. Macmillan Press, London

Patterson B, Leadbetter D, McComish A (1997) De-escalation in the management of aggression and violence. *Nurs Times* **93**(36): 58–61

Polit DF, Hungler BP (1997) *Essentials of Nursing Research: Methods Appraisal and utlisation*. 4th edn. Lippincott, Philadelphia

Ryan J, Poster E (1993) Workplace violence. *Nurs Times* **89**(48): 38–41

Thomas B (1995) Risky business. *Nurs Times* **91**(7): 52–4

Turnbull J (1993) Victim support. *Nurs Times* **89**(23): 30–2

Turnbull J (1999) Violence to staff: Who is at risk? In: Turnbull J, Patterson B, eds. *Aggression and Violence: Approaches to effective management*. Macmillan Press, London

Wykes T, Mezey G (1994) Counselling for victims of violence. In: Whittington R, Wykes T, eds. *Violence and Healthcare Professionals*. Chapman Hall, London: 180–98

## Summary: Strengths and limitations of Polit and Hungler's approach to critiquing nursing research

### *Strengths*

❖ This is a very thorough and comprehensive approach. Furthermore, as this is the most recent of the four approaches we have included, it perhaps indicates the evolutionary or developmental nature of approaches to critiquing research; wherein this approach has built upon the earlier approaches and has managed to address some of the limitations of the earlier approaches.

❖ The dimensions that have the detailed guidelines are thorough.

❖ It appears to give consideration to most of the fundamental components that each research report should make reference to.

❖ The approach does not have a 'sequential' 'step-by-step' method that could mirror the reading of the article. For example, questions asked of the title and abstract occur at the very end of the guidelines. Consequently, the reviewer is likely to need to read all the paper before any comment can be made and this may necessitate re-reading several sections. This may add to the rigour of the critique (while others may regard this as a limitation).

❖ It does contain some research terminology, but this is not excessive or inappropriate. However, this does necessitate the reviewer to have some understanding of basic concepts and practices within research.

❖ If a reviewer follows and subsequently addresses each of the questions contained within each of the five dimensions, then it is very likely that the author of the research paper reviewed may learn from a critique using Polit and Hungler's critique.

❖ As with Morrison's approach, Polit and Hungler's approach encourages the reviewer(s) to think about how the findings in the reviewed paper(s) may impact on nursing practice.

❖ The approach includes many useful and thought-provoking questions within the headings.

❖ The approach allows room for the data and/or argument to be introduced to support the reviewer's criticisms/observations and suggestions for improvement.

## *Limitations*

❖ The approach provides lists of questions/guidelines for the interpretive and presentational dimensions, and yet does not provide lists/guidelines for the other three dimensions, yet it does not explain why this is the case. This leaves reviewers wondering if Polit and Hungler are suggesting a greater 'weighting' for these dimensions? Yet they do not appear to make this case explicitly.

❖ As with the other approaches, this appears to be quantitatively orientated, in that the reviewer is encouraged to ask specific questions of quantitative studies, eg. in quantitative studies, does the interpretation distinguish between practical and statistical significance? And, are generalisations made that are not warranted on the basis of the sample used? However, the reviewer is not encouraged to ask questions specific to qualitative studies. Unlike the three previous approaches, this approach does ask specific (and separate) methodological questions for both qualitative and quantitative studies.

❖ Some of the specific guidelines might be considered to be repetitive.

❖ As Polit and Hungler themselves point out, a critique should highlight the positive elements of a study in addition to the limitations. However, the lists of questions in the guidelines appears to usher the reviewer into considering the limitations more than the strengths.

# Section three: The development of the NPNR National Journal Club's approach to critiquing nursing research

# 7

# The NPNR National Journal Club's approach to critiquing research: First phase of the National Journal Club development

The previous chapters have highlighted that there exist a wide range of approaches to critiquing nursing research, and we have focused on four such approaches. These represent only a sample of the different models or approaches that exist within the nursing research literature. The previous chapters have also indicated some of the strengths and limitations of these approaches.

The authors would argue that there is no one, singular 'best' way to critique nursing research and we would also argue that no one, singular model or approach will suit every nurse. Perhaps there would be merit in nurses trying out a variety of models or approaches until they find one with which they feel comfortable. Alternatively, maybe there is merit in nurses developing approaches for themselves and consequently feeling empowered by such a development. With such a possibility in mind, members of the NPNR National Journal Club sampled and subsequently tried out the approaches highlighted in this book and came to the following conclusions.

1.   Each of the approaches appears to have strengths and limitations. The following criticisms could be levelled at each of the approaches (to a greater or lesser extent).

2.   The approaches appeared to be orientated towards (or influenced by) quantitative methods rather than qualitative methods, and appeared to be critiquing the study according to quantitative criteria rather than qualitative criteria. As indicated previously, nursing research has a history of being influenced by the medical profession (Pearson, 1992), and consequently, the philosophical, epistemological and methodological beliefs of the biomedical model have been adopted by some nurse researchers. Consequently, positivistic philosophies, quantitative methods and the hegemony of the Randomised Control Trial (RCT) can be seen throughout many nursing research reports. Given such an influence, it is maybe no surprise that approaches to critiquing nursing research also reflect this 'quantitative' favouritism or leaning.

3.   There is a growing recognition of the need to embrace qualitative research methods within nursing research (Leininger, 1992), hence the movement towards a more pluralistic approach, and concurrently, a need for approaches to critiquing nursing research to mirror this

movement towards qualitative studies. Approaches should be able to facilitate an adequate critique of a qualitative research study.

4.  The approaches appear to judge the studies according to the degree which the results are generalisable. While this may be entirely appropriate for some studies, it may not be appropriate for all studies.

5.  Perhaps the approaches do not emphasise enough the need for the reviewer to consider the key practice issues that arise out of the study. That is, given that nursing is a practice-orientated discipline, ultimately the research should have some implications (or potential impact) on practice.

The authors of this book would argue that for a model of critiquing nursing research to be comprehensive and useful, it needs to consider the theoretical, methodological, ethical substantive and presentational issues. Additionally, we would wholeheartedly agree with the view that critiques must emphasise both the strengths and limitations of the research. However, because nursing is a 'practice-led' discipline, we would argue that additional criteria for judging models or approaches for critiquing nursing research might include the following questions:

❖ Is it easily understandable by and accessible to nurses? Or does the extent of excessive jargon or terminology discourage the review from reading the paper? (We acknowledge that there is a need for methodological clarity and precision and, accordingly, the use of some terminology. Nevertheless, too much jargon/terminology within research reports is often cited as a reason for nurses not utilising the study in clinical practice.)

❖ Does the model/approach to critiquing help nurses decide whether or not the research makes a difference to their practice?

❖ Does the model/approach to critiquing help nurses decide whether or not the research has potential to make a difference to practice?

❖ What are the key points that arise from the study; in particular, the key points for practice?

❖ Does the model/approach to critiquing necessitate the need for a PhD, MSc or a BSc degree in order to be able to make sense of the critique and subsequently the research?

We would argue that the approach developed by the NPNR National Journal Club perhaps addresses some of these issues, and furthermore, is an approach developed by nurses, for nurses out of a need to do so. The approach attempts to comment not only on the reviewed paper but locates arguments, issues and questions within broader contexts. Be they larger 'policy' contexts (see increased use of evidence-based practice, *Chapter 6, p. 88*), or practice context (see experiences of violence, *Chapter 10, p. 151*), or methodological contexts (see methodological issues in measuring attitudes, *Chapter 9, p. 139*). Consequently, an individual reading one of the NPNR

Journal Club style critiques, not only hopefully gains a sense of the pape strengths and limitations, but additionally, is directed to relevant, linke material that supports the critique and leads the reviewer in the direction o. some of the associated literature. This enables the reviewer (and the author of the paper reviewed) to become better informed on the matters raised.

Some of the emerging strengths/features of the NPNR National Journal Club approach to critiquing might include the following:

⌘ It asks: how does the reviewed piece of work effect/help/benefit you as a clinician, educationalist, researcher or manager?
⌘ The inclusion of three key points for each reviewed paper.
⌘ The approach can be used for both qualitative and quantitative research.
⌘ It urges the reviewer to consider; what meaning or worth does the study have for the practice and knowledge base of P/MH nursing?
⌘ It urges the reviewers to reference their criticisms/points raised and this hopefully, raises the level of academic debate.
⌘ It urges the reviewers to consider the paper in a 'holistic' rather than 'reductionalist' manner. It urges reviewers to consider each of these identified sections separately and as part of the 'whole'.
⌘ It embraces the notion of evolutionary/developmental approaches to critiquing research. The approach is not static and can evolve over time; aggregating reviewers' confidence in the approach as it is used.

As with the introduction of any new practice (Ward *et al*, 1998), it takes time for the practitioners to feel 'at ease' and familiar with the introduction of a new approach to critiquing research. In the early stages of such an introduction, practitioners perhaps lack confidence in the new approach/ new practice, until they can experience the benefits for themselves. Importantly, in the early days of the National Journal Club, we adopted the empowering philosophy of practice development described by Ward *et al* (1998) to facilitate the uptake of the National Journal Club's approach to critiquing research. Consequently, it was emphasised to each Journal Club, that the approach was developmental. It could and indeed, should, evolve over time, in direct response to the members' feedback, derived from their experience of using the approach. Reviews produced during the 'early days' of the National Journal Club perhaps are less comprehensive, less extensive and less expansive than later reviews. Concomitantly, the members' confidence in the critiques they produced, also increased over time, as they became more familiar with the approach, felt more involved with its development, and saw their reviews published.

---

**Box 7.1: Guidelines of the NPNR National Journal Club approach to critiquing nursing research**

❖ Follow the sequence of the paper as laid out by the author(s).

❖ Consider each of the theoretical, substantive, methodological, ethical and presentational dimensions of the for each of the sections (headings) identified by the paper's author.

❖ Consider each of these identified sections separately and as part of the 'whole', since individually well written sections may not necessarily add up to become a cumulative whole. Thus, minimising the sense of reductionalism present in most critiquing approaches.

❖ Ask methodological questions in keeping with the design/paradigm identified by the author.

❖ Draw upon any existing approach to critiquing for specific questions if you feel these add to your critique.

❖ Locate the questions/issues you raise in your critique within the broader practice, education, research and policy literature.

❖ Reflect on and identify, how does the reviewed piece of work effect/ help/benefit you as a clinician, educationalist, researcher or manager?

❖ Reflect on and identify, what meaning or worth does the study have for the practice and knowledge base of P/MH nursing?

❖ Identify three key points, of which at least one is positive and one negative.

❖ Do ensure that you look for, and highlight at least one strength of the paper. It is all too easy to over emphasise the negative.

❖ Provide references to substantiate your critique.

---

# References

Leininger M (1992) Current issues, problems and trends to advance qualitative paradigmatic research methods for the future. *Qualitative Health Res* **2**(4): 392–415

Pearson A (1992) Knowing nursing: emerging paradigms in nursing. In: Robinson K, Vaughan B, eds. *Knowledge for Nursing Practice*. Butterworth Heinemann, Oxford: 213–26

Ward M, Titchen A, Morell C, McCormack B, Kitson A (1998) Using a supervisory framework to support and evaluate a multi-project practice development programme. *J Clinical Nurs* **7**: 29–36

# The first phase of the NPNR National Journal Clu◄ development: Early attempts

## Example number nine: The NPNR National Journal Club, review from the second meeting

The paper reviewed first appeared in 1997, in the *Journal of Advanced Nursing* (**26**: 295–303), 'Learning from Practice: Mental Health Nurses' Perceptions and Experiences of Clinical Supervision' (Scanlon C and Wier WS ).

## Abstract/overview

This paper reports on a small scale qualitative study which attempted to explore mental health nurses' perceptions and experiences of clinical supervision. The authors conducted a series of semi-structured interviews, analysed the data and found encouraging early indicators that mental health nurses are becoming better able to reflect upon their formative learning needs, and so take seriously their need for professional support, as they strive towards therapeutic relationships with clients. The authors discovered evidence that suggests 'good enough supervision' was the exception rather than the rule.

## Introduction

Feedback comments indicated that members felt each of the three questions identified within the introduction were worthy of investigation in their own right. Furthermore, comments indicated that members felt the purposes of the study were indicated in the research questions; however, it was not clear if the study was intended to induce a theory where no current theory existed, and/or add to knowledge and understanding that already exists.

## Literature review

Feedback comments indicated that members felt that this paper, like many papers on clinical supervision, lacked a complete representation of all that supervision can be. Additionally, while it is appropriate to discuss parallel processes within supervision, certainly if one uses a psychodynamic model (Hawkins and Shohet, 1996), members felt it was not appropriate to describe all clinical supervisor/supervisee relationships in terms of parallel processes.

## esearch design: sample

While some reservations were raised concerning the size of the sample, it was acknowledged that relatively small sized samples can still provide rich data for qualitative studies (see, for example, Cutcliffe, 1995). However, concerns were raised concerning the composition of the sample. While purposeful sampling is entirely appropriate with the qualitative method advocated (Morse, 1991), it was felt that a little more effort could have gone into obtaining the sample rather than the convenience sample used. Reed *et al* (1996), for example, argue that the research question and methods used dictate the need for a sample that is relevant to the theoretical development within the study. To limit this sample to nurses who were known to the researchers perhaps imposes unnecessary limitations and may well have had an impact on the richness of the data gathered.

## Research design: data collection

Comments indicated that members felt that the method of data collection was appropriate. Another point of view argued that since the researchers were concerned with obtaining the 'lived experiences' of mental health nurses who receive clinical supervision, it may have been more appropriate to have used a phenomenological approach (Heidegger, 1962; Walters, 1995). More detail was necessary, for example, about what type of qualitative approach was used and why? Were other approaches considered? The paper may have been better for having more detail in some areas.

## Ethical considerations

The paper appeared to lack information on ethical issues, eg. did anyone not consent to take part.

## Data analysis

Feedback comments indicated that members felt that while the methods appeared to be appropriate, it was not clear how the development of the emergent themes was achieved. Consequently, members were left wondering if there had been some slurring of the methodology (Baker *et al*, 1992) and what influence this might have had on the results. The use of interviewees' statements was felt to be particularly useful not only in terms of establishing the credibility of the findings, but also adding to the understanding of the emerging theory. Efforts appear to have been made to ensure the rigour of the data analysis. However, importing such terms and methods that were developed for quantitative methods such as 'inter-rater reliability' was felt to be inappropriate for this study (Cutcliffe and McKenna, 1999).

## Results, discussion and conclusions

The results section contained some valuable themes, and these themes are supported by previous studies (Bishop, 1994; Fowler, 1995; Severinsson, 1995; Butterworth *et al*, 1997). While in response to the results, the authors make some useful comments in the discussion section, it might have been worthwhile to expand the implications for their findings to include issues such as training/education in clinical supervision.

## Final comments: what meaning does this have for psychiatric and mental health nurses?

The key points raised from the review of this paper are listed in *Table 7.1*. Few would dispute that the practice and evaluation of clinical supervision continues to be an important issue for nurses, and the continued interest in the subject is reflected in the number of articles in the nursing literature that feature supervision. It is also reasonable to suggest that there remain many unanswered questions. Any attempt to examine these issues and address these questions appears to have merit. Since, within the substantive area there remain epistemological questions; questions concerning the process and questions concerning the outcomes and efficacy, there is a clear need to conduct both qualitative and quantitative enquiries. The contribution of qualitative studies should not be ignored even though there is growing pressure from some managers to discover a direct correlation between receiving clinical supervision and improved client care.

However, while this paper does add evidence to certain current arguments, eg. the problems and difficulties of having a direct line manager as your supervisor, and the distinct lack of specific supervision training that individuals have had, it does not appear to be saying a great deal that is new. Perhaps it may have been more worthwhile to focus on these identified problems and either investigate them qualitatively, more fully, eg. how do the problems of having a direct line manager as a supervisor affect the process of supervision? Or, investigate quantitatively how many individuals have encountered the problems, eg. how many of the nurses receive supervision from their direct line manager? Such studies may then provide a deeper, more complete understanding of the extent of the problem.

The last issue, that of sampling strategies, is relevant to all nursing research studies. The results presented in this study, as with any research study, are only as credible as the methodology allows (Polit and Hungler, 1997). Practitioners concerned with conducting studies that would either support or refute the practice of clinical supervision need to consider methodological and sampling issues. In this instance there may have been merit in sampling all psychiatric nurses from one clinical area, or one particular grade. While any theory induced would only be pertinent to that clinical area studied or group of individuals, each microcosm of nursing *rs* a resemblance to nursing as a whole. As Denzin and Lincoln (1994: *1*) state:

*Every instance of a case or process bears the general class of phenomena it belongs to. However, any given instance is likely to be particular and unique.*

While the authors are cautious about generalising the experiences of clinical supervision described, there may well be elements of the theory that all nurses recognise as having meaning for themselves and which can be related to their own practice and experience of clinical supervision.

**Table 7.1: Key points arising from the second review**

| | |
|---|---|
| 1 | The article reflected a current and important theme within mental health nursing: clinical supervision as a vehicle for improving practice, and attempts to explore and evaluate clinical supervision should be supported. |
| 2 | Members were not convinced that the paper was saying anything new, while it did add weight to certain arguments, eg. not having a manager as your supervisor. |
| 3 | The limitations of the sampling strategy may have had an impact on the results. |

# References

Baker C, Weust J, Stern PN (1992) Method slurring: The grounded theory/phenomenology example. *J Adv Nurs* **17**: 1355–60

Bishop V (1994) Clinical Supervision Questionnaire. *Nurs Times* **90**(48): 40–42

Butterworth T, Carson J, White E, Jeacock J, Clements A, Bishop V (1997) *It is good to talk. Clinical supervision and Mentorship. An evaluation study in England and Scotland.* The School of Nursing, Midwifery and Health Visiting, The University of Manchester

Cutcliffe JR (1995) How do nurses inspire and instil hope in terminally ill HIV patients? *J Adv Nurs* **22**: 888–95

Cutcliffe JR, McKenna H (1999) Establishing the credibility of qualitative research findings: the plot thickens. *J Adv Nurs* **30**(2): 374–80

Denzin NK and Lincoln YS (1994) Entering the field of qualitative research. In: Denzin NK, Lincoln YS, eds. *Handbook of Qualitative Research.* Sage, London: 1–17

Fowler J (1995) Nurses' perceptions of the elements of good supervision. *Nurs Times* **91**(22): 33–7

Hawkins P, Shohet, R (1996) *Supervision in the Helping Professions.* Open University Press, Milton Keynes

Heidegger M (1962) *Being and Time.* Harper Row, New York

Morse JM (1991) Stategies for sampling. In: Morse JM, ed. *Qualitative Nursing Research: A contemporary dialogue.* Sage, London: 127–45

Polit DF, Hungler BP (1997) *Essentials of Nursing Research: Methods, Appraisal and utilization.* 4th edn. Lippincott, Philadelphia

Reed J, Procter S, Murray S (1996) A sampling strategy for qualitative research. *Nurse Researcher* 3(4): 52–69

Severinsson EI (1995) The phenomenon of clinical supervision within psychiatric health care. *J Psychiatr Ment Health Nurs* 2: 301–9

Walters AJ (1995) The phenomenological movement: Implications for nursing research. *J Adv Nurs* 22: 791–9

# Example number ten: The NPNR National Journal Club, review from the third meeting

> The paper reviewed first appeared in 1997, in the *Journal of Advanced Nursing* (**26**: 125–33), 'Expressed emotion and schizophrenia: the efficacy of a staff training programme' (Willets L and Leff J).

## Abstract/overview

This paper reports on an investigation of the presence of expressed emotion (EE) in five community care facilities. The authors discovered that levels of high EE existed in some staff-client relationships. A training programme was subsequently developed to enable community mental health workers to increase their knowledge about schizophrenia and repertoire of strategies for managing a variety of difficulties. It was hoped that this training would decrease levels of EE present in their relationships with clients. The authors report a small but non-significant increase in knowledge following the training, and an increase in the use of strategies aimed at effecting change. They also report that no significant changes in EE levels were reported.

## Title

Feedback comments indicated that members felt that the title could have been more clear in identifying a nursing interest. Perhaps if the title had indicated specifically which staff the training was for, this would have added to the clarity.

## Abstract

Feedback comments indicated that members felt that the abstract identified the research problem, but did not specify a hypothesis or outline the methodology. Members also acknowledged that the abstract identified the major findings of the report. Concerns were also raised regarding the term 'high expressed emotion' and members felt that this was a rather pejorative expression. What would it mean as a member of a family that is labelled 'high EE'? Similarly, what affects would it have on a single (or several) member of staff to be given this label? In the same way that concerns have been raised regarding assigning labels to clients (Clunn, 1993; Thompson *et al*, 1988), perhaps clinicians and researchers should consider the possible deleterious effects of giving such labels to family carers or members of staff.

## Introduction

Members felt that the introduction and literature review were merged and they struggled to identify easily the point the authors were trying to make. The aims of the study are clear but it was felt that the research question could have been clearer. This was due to the terminology used. For example, the terms 'appropriate intervention strategies' and 'problematic behaviours' were thought to be somewhat ambiguous.

## Literature review

The literature review included appropriate and relevant literature relating to expressed emotion, however, there appeared to be important omissions. A particular oversight was that of Brooker and Butterworth's (1991) study which described the effect on the role and function of the community psychiatric nurse (CPN) after training to deliver psychosocial intervention to families caring for a relative at home. Also, Nolan *et al's* (1997) work on family care which, among other issues, discusses the longitudinal nature of family care.

Members also questioned if one could measure EE within staff in the same way as families. Although staff may be in a position where they are part of the same community as the clients, their relationship is different to that of the family. (For example, they leave that environment and go home to their own families.)

## Method

Members stated that they felt that in places the method and introduction were merged and subsequently lacked clarity. Additionally, the strengths and weaknesses of the chosen approach were not explored. Criticisms were levelled regarding the author's reference to the limited value of naturalistic studies. Many authors, such as Lincoln and Guba (1985), Denzin and

Lincoln (1994), Heideggar (1962), Melia (1982) would construct rigorous arguments for studying people in their natural settings. Obtaining clients' views and the lived experiences of staff caring for these people could have produced useful and valuable data; particularly as, ultimately, it is their care that we are interested in.

## Sample selection

Some reservations were raised concerning the size of the sample, although it should be noted that the authors did acknowledge this limitation. The major concern raised by members regarding the sample was what effect self-selection and the use of a convenience sample may have had on the results (Burns and Grove, 1993). In order to enhance the validity of the findings, the authors could have made some effort to include a control group, perhaps randomly selecting some of the community care staff and not providing them with the training.

## Ethical considerations

There was no indication of the members of staff consenting to participate in this study. It may have been felt that staff did not need to consent, but members expressed an opinion that this was inappropriate. In terms of ethical considerations, members of staff should be treated no differently to clients (Lipson, 1994). The absence of any ethical considerations was felt to be an oversight.

## Results

Members felt that the results could have been presented more clearly. For example, the tables were not properly identified in the text nor properly labelled. There was perhaps an over-zealous use of percentages for small numbers of subjects in the study.

## Data analysis

On the whole, the approach to data analysis appeared to be appropriate yet some members felt that statistical analysis was not clearly indicated. The small sample did not allow sufficient analysis (eg. there were an insignificant number of subjects for a paired t-test) and to determine whether or not significant differences were attributable to variations in other relevant variables.

## Discussion, conclusions and recommendations

Feedback comments indicated that members felt that in this section there were a number of variables which should have been clearly identified from previous studies and that had not been controlled in any way in this study. Perhaps a more useful study would have been for the authors to investigate how the course affected the practitioners' thoughts, feelings and subsequent practice of this particular client group.

Members did state that the paper highlighted some interesting lines of enquiry for possible future enquiries. One such line of enquiry would be to conduct a participation observation study of the practice of the practitioners in order to provide a further source of data. Since in this current study all the data was obtained by interviews and questionnaires and is provided by the practitioners, this third form of data would enable a triangulation of data and have the potential to add to the validity of the findings (Begley, 1996; Nolan and Behi, 1995). The conclusions might be considered to be rather assertive given the size of the sample, and members felt the conclusions drawn did not have the evidence to support them.

## Final comments: what meaning does this have for psychiatric and mental health nurses?

Some criticisms were levelled concerning how this research bridges the 'theory practice gap' and how the results were going to aid nurses in their practice. Perhaps this reiterates the issue of the danger of research being published in journals that are read only by other researchers, and as a consequence practice remains largely unaffected by these studies. A point highlighted by Professor McKenna at the NPNR 1997 Edinburgh conference when he stated :

> *It is better that one nurse implements research findings that produce a positive effect on the quality of care, than a dozen non-commulative research studies which end up gathering dust on a shelf.*

A major issue that arose was that of researchers and practitioners having a dogmatic view of:

❖ Conditions such as schizophrenia and the care associated with people given this diagnosis.

❖ Approaches to researching and understanding care issues for this group of people. For example, Gournay (1996) advocates adopting a more biologically-oriented approach to caring for individuals termed to be 'schizophrenic' and that disorders such as schizophrenia will become clear beyond ambiguity in our lifetime. Other authors highlight that psychosocial intervention for these clients and their families is the way forward (Gamble *et al*, 1994). Whereas other authors have suggested that case management provides answers to some of the problems of providing care for these clients and their families (Ford *et al*, 1995). However, Moorey (1998) draws attention to the number of recent reviews of a large body of evidence which cast considerable doubt on the reliability, construct validity, predictive validity and the aetiological specificity of the diagnosis of schizophrenia. Questions concerned with the cause and treatment of schizophrenia, and the value of interventions for people with this label then become incoherent if the notion of schizophrenia is rejected as a meaningful scientific construct (Moorey, 1998).

Strict adherence to one particular approach to providing care at the expense of all other approaches appears to limit drastically the care options available to client and practitioner. Similarly, to restrict the focus of research to such a narrow subject area when understanding is far from complete appears somewhat premature. This narrow-mindedness appears all the more inappropriate given other author's statements regarding the continued uncertainty surrounding care of such people. Dawson (1997, p. 1) makes this point most clearly when he states:

*The truth of the matter is that we are now as far removed from such a theory as we were twenty or thirty years ago. We have not the faintest notion of what might be occurring in the brain... that is, we do not yet have a model of normal thought processes, let alone 'abnormal' thought processes.*

Opinion was divided regarding the readability of the paper, with some members reporting that they found this to be an interesting and thought-provoking paper. Members also stated that they wondered if the authors had tried to accomplish too much with one study; in that it appeared that the authors were concerned with both evaluating the training course they provided and simultaneously examining change in EE and the change in interaction this may produce.

| Table 7.2: Key points arising from the third review |
|---|
| 1  As laudable as any nursing related research study may be, if it ultimately makes no difference to the care of clients, then how valuable and useful is it? |
| 2  Wholesale adoption of one particular approach to providing care at the expense of all other approaches is at best restrictive and limiting, and at worst damaging and deleterious. |
| 3  Similarly, wholesale adoption of one particular research paradigm at the exclusion of others can only limit the depth of understanding available to the researcher and force him/her to view the world through a particular lens. |

# References

Begley CM (1996) Using triangulation in nursing research. *J Adv Nurs* **24**: 122–8

Brooker C, Butterworth T (1991) Working with families caring for a relative with schizophrenia: the evolving role of the community psychiatric nurse. *Int J Nurs Stud* **28**(2): 189–200

Burns N, Grove SK (1993) *The Practice of Nursing Research: Conduct, critique and utilisation*. 2nd edn. WB Saunders, Philadelphia

Clunn PA (1993) The child. In: Rawlings RP, Williams FR, Beck CK, eds. *Mental Health — Psychiatric Nursing*. CV Mosby, St Louis: 715–48

Dawson PJ (1997) A reply to Kevin Gournay's 'Schizophrenia: a review of the contemporary literature and implications for mental health nursing theory, practice and education'. *J Psychiatr Ment Health Nurs* **4**: 1–7

Denzin NK, Lincoln YS (1994) Entering the field of qualitative research. In: Denzin NK, Lincoln YS (1994) *A Handbook of Qualitative Research*. Sage, California: 1–17

Ford R, A, Ryan P, Repper J, Craig J, Muijen M (1995) Providing a safety net: Case management for people with a serious mental illness. *J Ment Health* **1**: 91–7

Gamble C, Midence K, Leff J (1994) The effects of family work training on mental health nurses' attitude to and knowledge of schizophrenia: a replication. *J Adv Nurs* **19**: 1169–77

Gournay K (1996) Schizophrenia: a review of the contemporary literature and implications for mental health nursing theory, practice and education. *J Psychiatr Ment Health Nurs* **3**: 7–12

Heideggar M (1962) *Being and Time*. Harper Row, New York

Lincoln YS, Guba EG (1985) *Naturalistic Enquiry*. Sage, Newbury Park, California

Lipson JG (1994) Ethical issues in ethnography. In: Morse JM, ed. *Critical Issues in Qualitative Research Methods*. Sage Publications, London: 333–55

Melia KM (1982) 'Tell it as it is' — qualitative methodology and nursing research: Understanding the student nurse's world. *J Adv Nurs* **7**: 327–35

Moorey J (1998) The ethics of professionalised care. In: Barker P, Davidson B, eds. *Psychiatric Nursing: Ethical strife*. Arnold, London

Nolan M, Behi R (1995) Triangulation: the best of all worlds? *Br J Nurs* **4**(14): 829–32

Nolan M, Grant G, Keady J (1997) *Understanding Family Care: The multi-dimensional nature of caring and coping*. Open University Press, Oxford

Thompson IE, Melia KM, Boyd K (1988) *Nursing Ethics*. Churchill Livingstone, Edinburgh

# 8

# The second phase of the NPNR National Journal Club development: Taking shape

Example number eleven: The NPNR National Journal Club, review from the fourth meeting

The paper reviewed first appeared in 1994, in the *Journal of Advanced Nursing* (**19**: 1096–1104), 'How can nurses build trusting relationships with people who have severe and long-term mental health problems? Experiences of case managers and their clients' (Repper J, Ford R and Cooke A ).

## Abstract/overview

This paper reports on a study that investigated how case managers, who worked specifically with people with long-term mental health problems, formed and maintained relationships with their clients. The authors conducted forty-six in depth interviews with these case managers and their clients, and using a qualitative method, analysed the interview data, and produced a framework of themes. They argued that these themes revealed how both clients and case managers focused on the problems and strategies of forming and maintaining relationships. They suggested that case managers adopted a philosophy that enabled both parties to feel positive about the work.

## Title

Feedback comments indicated that members felt that although the paper is five years old, it remains topical and has an appropriate focus that was reflected in the title.

## Abstract

Members felt that the abstract introduced the focus of the study, gave a brief outline of the method and identified the major findings of the report. Concerns were raised regarding the imprecision of the description of the qualitative methodology. Perhaps a summary of the central themes would have enhanced it.

## Introduction

The introduction was felt to include the appropriate background to the study, and a rationale for undertaking the study. Perhaps this section could have been enhanced by including operational definitions of terms such as 'trusting relationship'. Also, it was unclear if the American definition of 'case management' was adopted as the operational definition for this study. Another argument stated that with this paper being published in an international journal, the authors may have benefited from setting the context of the history of case management in the UK.

## The method

Members stated that they felt that the method had several weaknesses. While alternative data collection methods were considered, members argued that the strengths and weaknesses of the chosen approach were not explored in enough detail. A stronger argument could have been constructed drawing on the extensive literature that refers to the value of naturalistic studies (Heideggar, 1962; Melia, 1982; Lincoln and Guba, 1985; Benner and Wrubel, 1989; Denzin and Lincoln, 1994), particularly given the need to uncover the knowledge embedded in the clinical experience of the case managers and the 'lived experiences' of the clients themselves (Benner, 1984; Benner and Wrubel, 1989).

Criticisms were also levelled regarding the incomplete review of the literature. The authors made reference to 'previous studies' without citing these specifically, nor did they include any critique of these studies.

## Sample selection

Members raised concerns regarding the nature of the sampling strategy. The case managers' influence of sample selection is likely to have effected the results, and members wondered if this amounted to a form of internal censorship. While the authors acknowledge this limitation and state they will account for the bias by marking quotations from this group with an asterisk, no asterisk is to be found on any of the quotations. It appears that the authors used purposeful sampling (Patton, 1990; Morse, 1991) yet they do not make this specific, nor do they identify the minimum criteria for inclusion in this sample.

Members feedback indicated that they would have liked to have heard more from the clients. Certain clients were excluded from providing any data at the behest of some case managers and the reasons for this exclusion were highlighted. This desire to see more data from the clients warrants further consideration. Until 1985 relatively little research had been conducted to elicit the views of users of mental health services (McIver, 1991a, b). Researchers appeared to have a concern that the nature of mental illness precluded users of the services from having the ability to express valid and reliable opinion. Arguments suggested that if the user has a distorted state of mind, how can they offer reliable opinions of their service? The case managers may have had similar concerns. However, more recently attempts have been made to obtain the views of mental health service users (MIND, 1986; Elbeck and Fecteau, 1990; Elzinga and Barlow, 1991; Sheppard, 1993; Pickett *et al*, 1993; Babiker and Thorne, 1993; Lovell, 1995; Stephenson *et al*, 1995; Beech and Norman, 1995). The members argument in favour of wishing to see more data from the clients appears to be well founded.

**Ethical considerations**

The absence of any ethical considerations or details regarding ethical approval was felt to be an oversight (Lipson, 1994). The paper contained no mention of ethical considerations, neither those pertaining to the staff nor those to the clients. Members were left wondering did any clients refuse to be interviewed and if so why?

**Data analysis**

Members feedback indicated that they felt the data analysis section lacked detail. The paper is somewhat imprecise with regard to the research design, in that it appears to be using a phenomenological method yet does not make this clear. However, the major criticism of this section was the lack of a comprehensive explanation of how the themes were induced. Members wanted to see how the researchers had moved from labels (initial categorisation) to condensing these into 'main problem areas' to the central themes. Additionally, it would have been useful to see how the themes/ categorisations inter-related with one another.

**Findings**

Members wondered if the findings and the discussion of the findings had been amalgamated into one section. Points of view were raised that argued in favour of a more in depth discussion of the findings. For example, when the authors highlighted the practice of adopting certain perspectives and having understanding and empathy, members wanted to know how the case managers adopted these perspectives? How did they convey this empathy? How did the clients experience it? It should be noted that on the whole the members felt that the findings reflected their understanding of the practice and sentiments of case management. Members also stated that the findings were somewhat obvious, but this does not mean that they were not valuable.

## Discussion, conclusions and recommendations

Members did state that while the conclusions were somewhat generalised, the paper highlighted some interesting lines of enquiry for possible future studies. The addition of some recommendations arising from the findings may have been useful.

## Final comments: what meaning does this have for psychiatric and mental health nurses?

Few psychiatric nurses would argue with the findings of this study regarding the formation of relationships. Establishing a trusting relationship, engaging clients and communicating with clients have been identified as integral aspects of psychiatric nursing in many studies. For example, the review of psychiatric nursing in 1994 (DoH, 1994), reaffirmed the idea of what psychiatric nurses should be doing and summarised these activities under the following headings:

- establishing therapeutic relationships resting in a respect for others
- responding flexibly to changing patient needs
- making risk assessments and judgements.

As long ago as the 1970s, Towell's (1975) study identified several roles for psychiatric nurses in different clinical settings, including having a significant role in treatment within therapeutic communities. Cormack (1983) found that psychiatric staff were effective at, among other activities, staff initiated interactions. More recently, Duffy and Lee (1998) found that the core activities of psychiatric nurses within contemporary trusts included psychosocial interventions and therapies.

Hill and Micheal (1996) used a phenomenological approach and found that a core activity of psychiatric nurses is their ordinary contact which is respectful and empathic. Similarly, Gallop (1997) has suggested, 'the potential power of psychiatric nursing comes from the unique nature of the caring relationship' and the uniqueness is centred on the use of empathy, whereby the nurse comes to know and understand the world of the other and to use that understanding constructively. Consequently, while few psychiatric nurses would disagree with the findings, is the paper under review saying anything new? Is it adding to the understanding or is it simply confirming current understanding? The paper appeared to have the potential to explore these activities and processes in more detail, and this would have added to the extent of the knowledge.

The paper also appears to be saying that it is easy to work with clients with severe and long-term mental health problems, and this may not always be the case. The sometimes complex process of forming ordinary relationships with extra-ordinary people is not always a simple matter (Hill and Micheal, 1996). Again, perhaps this complexity could have been explored more fully if the researchers had included more detail. For example, a dynamic of any psychiatric nurse (including case managers)/client relationship is the extent to which the nurses are prepared to exercise power over clients or to share power with clients (Campbell, 1998). Crucial questions should be asked regarding issues such as, how does the case manager abdicate this potential power to the client? And yet, at the same time, reconcile this practice with the possibility of having to force hospital admission and/or treatment on the client? Such endeavours to maintain the equilibrium and symmetry of power dynamics cannot be easy, particularly when both parties are aware of the potential of the use of power by the case manager as a form of intervention. It is conceivably the situations where major problems occur in forming relationships that reveal most about the complexity of this process. However, there was an absence of such situations within the paper.

It is reasonable to suggest that problems can exist regarding engagement for all clients, not just for the client group featured in this study. Given the qualitative nature of the study, the authors are not attempting to generalise their findings to a wider population, but they do state:

> *There are others for whom the approach and strategies identified in this study offer useful guidelines for their work.*

(Repper *et al*, 1994, p. 1104)

Consequently, the paper can be considered to be brave as it invites others to come on board and debate and discuss. It can be considered to be valuable and relevant to all.

**Table 8.1: Key points arising from the fourth review**

| | |
|---|---|
| 1 | It is a motivational paper and is friendly to read, however, the findings do not appear to be saying anything new, and it had potential to be much richer. |
| 2 | The paper portrays it as easy to work with these clients and this may not be the case. |
| 3 | The paper is brave and ploughs a furrow, inviting others to come on board and debate and discuss and is valuable. |

# References

Babiker IE, Thorne P (1993) Do psychiatric patients know what is good for them? *J Roy Soc Med* **86**: 28–30

Beech P, Norman IJ (1995) Patients' perceptions of the quality of psychiatric nursing care: Findings from a small-scale descriptive study. *J Clinical Nurs* **4**: 117–23

Benner P (1984) *From Novice to Expert: Excellence and power in clinical nursing practice.* Addison-Wesley, Menlo Park, California

Benner P, Wrubel J (1989) *The Primacy of Caring: Stress and coping in health and illness.* Addison-Wesley, Menlo Park, California

Campbell P (1998) Listening to clients. In: Barker P, Davidson B, eds. *Psychiatric Nursing: Ethical strife.* Arnold, London: 237–48

Cormack D (1983) *Psychiatric Nursing Described.* Churchill Livingstone, Edinburgh

Denzin NK, Lincoln YS (1994) Entering the field of qualitative research. In: Denzin NK, Lincoln YS, eds. *A Handbook of Qualitative Research.* Sage, California: 1–17

Department of Health (1994) *Working in partnership: a collaborative approach to care. Report of the mental health nursing review team.* HMSO, London

Duffy D, Lee R (1998) Mental health nursing today: ideal and reality. *Mental Health Practice* **1**(8): 14–16

Elbeck M, Fecteau G (1990) Improving the validity of measures of patient satisfaction with psychiatric care and treatment. *Hospital Community Psychiatry* **41**(9): 998–1001

Elzinga RH, Barlow J (1991) Patient satisfaction among the residential population of a psychiatric hospital. *Int J Social Psychiatry* **37**(1): 24–34

Gallop R (1997) Caring about the client: The role of gender, empathy and power in the therapeutic process. In: Tilley S, ed. *The Mental Health Nurse: Views of practice and education.* Blackwell Science, London: 28–42

Heideggar M (1962) *Being and Time.* Harper Row, New York

Hill B, Micheal S (1996) The human factor. *J Psychiatr Ment Health Nurs* **3**: 245–8

Lincoln YS, Guba EG (1985) *Naturalistic Inquiry.* Sage, London

Lipson J (1994) The Use of self in ethnographic research. In: Morse JM, ed. *Qualitative Nursing Research: A contemporary dialogue.* Sage, London: 73–89

Lovell K (1995) User satisfaction with in-patient mental health services. *J Psychiatr Ment Health Nurs* **2**: 143–50

McIver S (1991a) *An introduction to obtaining the views of users of health services.* King's Fund Centre, London

McIver S (1991b) *Obtaining the views of users of mental health services.* King's Fund Centre, London

Melia KM (1982) 'Tell it as it is' — qualitative methodology and nursing research: Understanding the student nurse's world. *J Adv Nurs* **7**: 327–35

MIND (1986) *Finding our own solutions: Women's experiences of mental health care.* National Association for Mental Health, London

Morse JM (1991) Strategies for Sampling. In: Morse JM, ed. *Qualitative Nursing Research: A Contemporary Dialogue.* Sage, London: 126–45

Patton MQ (1990) *Qualitative Evaluation and Research Methods.* 2nd edn. Sage, London

Pickett SA, Lyons JS, Polonus T, Seymour T, Miller SI (1993) Factors predicting satisfaction with managed mental health care. *Psychiatric Services* **46**(7): 722–3

Repper J, Ford R, Cooke A (1994) How can nurses build trusting relationships with people who have severe and long-term mental health problems? Experiences of case managers and their clients. *J Adv Nurs* **19**: 1096–104

Sheppard M (1993) Client satisfaction, extended intervention and interpersonal skills in community mental health. *J Adv Nurs* **18**: 246–59

Stephenson C, Wilson S, Gladman JRF (1995) Patient and carer satisfaction in geriatric day hospitals. *Disabil Rehabil* **17**(5): 252–5

Towell D (1975) *Understanding Psychiatric Nursing*. RCN, London

# Example number twelve: The NPNR National Journal Club, review of the fifth meeting

The paper reviewed first appeared in 1998, in the *Journal of Advanced Nursing* (**27**:195–203), 'Nurses' responses to people with schizophrenia' (Rogers TS and Kashima Y).

## Abstract/overview

This paper reports on a study that investigated differences between general nurses, psychiatric nurses and lay people. It attempted to identify differences between their personal standards concerning how they should respond, and beliefs about how they actually would respond to people with schizophrenia. Evidence of these differences were examined in each of the three domains; thinking, feeling and behaving. Significant differences were identified between the response types and between the different response domains. Significant interaction effects were also identified based on participants' professional status in nursing. The authors argue that their results support Devine's (1989) theory concerning the automatic activation of stereotypes and their controlled inhibition in favour of different personal beliefs. The authors additionally argue that professional socialisation in psychiatric nursing facilitates this process with relation to people with schizophrenia.

## Title

Feedback comments indicated that members felt the title was somewhat misleading. The study contained an examination of three groups of people, including lay people. However, the title makes no reference to the examination of lay people's responses.

## Abstract

Members expressed that the abstract introduced the focus of the study, gave a brief outline of the method and identified the major findings of the report.

## Introduction

It was felt that the introduction included the appropriate background to the study, and a rationale for undertaking it.

## Background literature

Members stated that they felt that the background literature section was well written, comprehensive, easy to read and thorough. It offered a balanced argument and drew upon a wide range of appropriate literature. Additional comments stated that it might be argued that within the list of terms regarded as positive, in addition to the term 'sensitive', it might be argued that the stereotypical traits 'strong, convincing, active and mysterious' could be construed as positive evaluative statements (Facchia *et al*, 1976).

## The hypothesis

It is reasonable to say that the range of responses regarding the paper's hypotheses were mixed, although there was a range of criticism. Comments ranged from a feeling that the first two hypotheses lead to a confirmation of the obvious, and lead to members wondering, 'what would this confirmation add to the knowledge base?' Additionally, members stated that they felt the third hypothesis could be regarded as somewhat obsolete since the introduction of Project 2000 nurse training programmes and the introduction of common foundation programmes. An alternative view was expressed that asserted that differences in emphasis, philosophical underpinning, attitude, knowledge and skills base still exist between psychiatric and general nurses. Consequently, research into this issue and a hypothesis of this nature might be regarded as entirely appropriate.

## Method

Members stated that they felt that the method was appropriate to the study design and stated research questions, however, it still raised some questions. The first question centred around why the pilot study did not sample the same population as the main study? According to Polit and Hungler (1997), the purpose of a pilot study is to carry out a small scale version or trial run of the major study in order to obtain information for improving the project or assessing its feasibility. Bond (1991) makes similar remarks and indicates that if a pilot study is carried out on a small number of subjects, it may help to answer a number of questions, including whether or not the subjects can understand what is being asked of them. Considering that this questionnaire would need to be completed by lay people, it would appear to have been wise to screen it for nursing jargon and the excessive use of medical terminology. Consequently, members wondered what value would be obtained by conducting the pilot study on a group of fifteen nurse academics?

Another question concerned the methods of data collection, in particular encouraging the respondents to complete the questionnaires in small groups. Members expressed concern that such a method of data collection could have influenced the results due to peer pressure, and wondered why the participants were not encouraged to complete the questionnaires on their own? While the authors may have had a plausible rationale for such a method, this was not highlighted in the paper. A further question related to the collection of the data for the section of the study concerned with 'should *vs* would' responses to people with schizophrenia. It was argued that the design is weakened by the fact that what respondents 'would do', had to be taken on trust. The authors do point out that there was no evidence of the respondents trying to portray themselves in the most favourable light possible, but these criticisms could have been prevented by the inclusion of an observation element, perhaps using simulators (Faulkner, 1994), in that simulated or role played events could be created and the responses to these events observed.

## Sample

Members raised concerns regarding the nature of the sample composition. The authors described the average age of the respondents for each of the three groups sampled and the ratio of male/female. The average age of the psychiatric nurses was five years older than the remainder of the sample. This produced a situation where the psychiatric nurses had significantly more clinical experience than their general colleagues. There was a further difference between the number of males in the different sample groups. Consequently, it could be argued that the authors were not comparing like with like (Parahoo, 1997). Any differences that exist in responses from the different groups could then be attributed to any of the variables and not necessarily the dependent variable. It should be noted that the authors do make some reference to the age difference between the groups and how this could affect the results. However, they do not acknowledge the variation in clinical experience or the proportion of males to females as possible explanations for the differences in response to the questionnaire.

## Ethical considerations

The authors stated that ethical approval had been obtained before the study commenced; however, some of the members stated that they would have liked to have seen some more detail regarding ethical approval. For example, all research involving human subjects is carried out at some cost to the participants. While this cost may be difficult to identify or may appear trivial, humans as subjects need and deserve appropriate respect and protection.

## Data analysis

Members' feedback indicated that they felt the data analysis section lacked detail. The paper is somewhat imprecise with regard to the research design, in that it appears to be using a phenomenological method yet does not make this clear. However, the major criticism of this section was the lack of a comprehensive explanation of how the themes were induced. Members wanted to see how the researchers had moved from labels (initial categorisation) to condensing these into 'main problem areas' to the central themes. Additionally, it would have been useful to see how the themes/ categorisations inter-related with one another.

## Results

The range of responses regarding the results was mixed. Some members reported that they felt it; included the appropriate analysis for the data collected, contained a high number of charts, tables and graphs and used a substantial amount of research terminology. Consequently, members described this section as well written and informative. However, other members felt that the use of terminology and jargon could be regarded as excessive. Comments included concerns regarding how many nurses would be discouraged from reading and assimilating the paper due to the use of terminology. These concerns have been expressed by several authors, eg. Hunt (1981), Miller (1985) and LoBindo-Wood and Haber (1986). The variation of opinion expressed by the members regarding this issue highlights something of a dichotomy facing authors of research reports. It is likely that such authors wish to reach as many people as possible with their research as their findings have an increased chance of effecting thinking and/or practice. They may wish to use a minimum of terminology. At the same time they may feel the need to appear knowledgeable and credible to their academic peers. Consequently, questions and dilemmas exist for authors concerning the issue of how much terminology is excessive.

## Discussion, conclusions and recommendations

Members stated that factors appeared to be omitted from the discussion. They pointed out that they had witnessed the phenomenon of negative stereotypes of mentally ill people present in general nurses being replaced by more positive views as a result of spending time with clients while on clinical placement, supporting the findings of the authors. However, the members described how these positive views were only temporary in that once the general nursing students became re-socialised into their peer group and general nursing clinical placements, the positive views were under- mined and they once more adopted the more negative stereotypes. It appears to be possible that change in people's stereotypes of individuals with mental illness may be related to the length of time of exposure to such people, or the intensity of the exposure. The article highlighted some interesting lines of inquiry for possible future research and recognised some of the study's limitations.

**Final comments: what meaning does this have for psychiatric and mental health nurses?**

The article pointed out differences between general nurses and psychiatric/ mental health (P/MH) nurses in their responses to people with schizophrenia. Some members argued that this was a confirmation of the obvious; namely, that graded exposure to the stereotyped target group decreases negative responses in the thinking and feeling domain (Nolan, 1993). Other members felt that these findings add to the argument that there are differences in emphasis, philosophical underpinning, attitudes, knowledge and skills between general and P/MH nurses. Recent attempts to explicate these differences (Cutcliffe and McKenna, 2000a,b) included the identification of eight alleged elements of the uniqueness of mental health nurses. These included: the ability to work in ordinary ways with extra-ordinary people; the human component of P/MH nursing, best seen as the craft of nursing; forming and maintaining relationships founded on empathy; and the endeavours to form partnerships with clients and work in collaboration with clients.

The findings of the reviewed study perhaps support these elements, in that in order to form empathic relationships, establish partnerships and work in ordinary ways with extra-ordinary people, the P/MH has to first come to terms with his/her own internal prejudices and agendas (Cutcliffe, 1995). As Benner and Wrubel (1989, p. 12) state:

*The nurse has in some sense personally come to terms with the reality of the illness and is able to convey acceptance and understanding to the patient.*

Skilled mental health practitioners can be regarded as people who can acknowledge their personal prejudices, thoughts and feelings; and who can hold such perceptions in abeyance, allowing them to be challenged and re-framed into more positive perceptions, to a degree that they are able to work with people who provoke negative stereotypes.

| Table 8.2: Key points arising from the fifth review | |
|---|---|
| 1 | The paper adds to the debate surrounding the issue of the differences in emphasis between psychiatric/mental health nurses and general nurses, and perhaps indicates a component of the alleged uniqueness of psychiatric/mental health nurses that Nolan (1993) alluded to. |
| 2 | The paper confirms the continuing presence and influence of negative stereotypes of people who suffer from mental illness and provides useful evidence on one method to counteract such stereotypes. |
| 3 | Perhaps the extent of the terminology or jargon included in the text may distance some potential readers, minimising the potential impact of the article. |

# References

Benner P, Wrubel J (1989) *The Primacy of Caring: Stress and coping in health and wellness*. Addison-Wesley, New York

Bond S (1991) Preparing a research proposal. In: Cormack D, ed. *The Research Process in Nursing*. 2nd edn. Blackwell Science, London

Cutcliffe JR (1995) How do nurses inspire and instil hope in terminally ill HIV people? *J Adv Nurs* **22**: 888–95

Cutcliffe JR, McKenna HP (2000a) Generic nurses: the nemesis of psychiatric/mental health nursing? Part one. *Mental Health Practice* **3**(9): 10–14

Cutcliffe JR, McKenna HP (2000b) Generic nurses: the nemesis of psychiatric/mental health nursing? Part two. *Mental Health Practice* **3**(4): 20–23

Devine PG (1989) Stereotypes and prejudices: their automatic and controlled components. *J Pers Soc Psychol* **55**(1): 5–18

Facchia J, Canale D, Cambria E, Ruest E, Sheppard C (1976) Public views of ex-mental patients: a note on perceived dangerousness and unpredictability. *Psychol Reports* **38**(2): 495–8

Faulkner A (1994) Using simulators to aid the teaching of communication skills in cancer and palliative care. *Patient Education Counselling* **23**: 125–9

Hunt J (1981) The process of translating research findings into practice. *J Adv Nurs* **12**: 101–10

Lobindo-Wood G, Haber J (1986) *Nursing research, critical appraisal and utilisation*. CV Mosby, Toronto

Nolan P (1993) *A History of Mental Health Nursing*. Chapman Hall, London

Miller A (1985) The relationship between nursing theory and nursing practice. *J Adv Nurs* **10**: 417–24

Parahoo K (1997) *Nursing research: Principles, process and issues*. Macmillan Press, London

Polit DE, Hungler BP (1997) *Essentials of Nursing Research: Methods, appraisal and utilisation*. 4th edn. Lippincott, Philadelphia

# 9

## The third phase of the NPNR National Journal Club development: Gaining confidence in the approach

### Example number one: The NPNR National Journal Club, review from the sixth meeting

The paper reviewed first appeared in 1997, in the *Journal of Psychiatric and Mental Health Nursing* (4: 285–94), titled 'Case Management: a week in the life of a clinical case management team' (Waite A, Carson J, Cullen D, Oliver N, Holloway F and Missenden K ).

### Abstract/overview

This paper reports on a study that attempted to describe the work of a clinical case management core team. The researchers gathered information through non-participant observation and went on to produce transcripts which were subsequently examined. From these transcripts, the authors produced seven categories of activity which were felt to encompass the range of activities practised by the team: planned client contact; unplanned client contact; family/carer contact; liaison; administration; team information sharing and supervision; training and personal development. The authors also calculated the amount of time engaged in these activities and their results were discussed in reference to Kanter's components and principles of clinical case management.

### Title

Feedback comments indicated that members felt that the title identified the focus of the research study but perhaps could have been improved by including an indication of the methodology used.

### Abstract

Members felt that the abstract introduced the focus of the study, gave a brief outline of the method and identified the major findings of the report.

## Introduction

Some members stated that the introduction included an appropriate background to the study, in that the authors identify problems with case management, particularly in the way researchers have rarely given adequate descriptions of the precise nature of the service they are investigating. Some concerns were expressed over the way the introduction appears to merge with a review of selected literature and consequently they struggled to identify easily the current level of knowledge or understanding of this phenomenon. This has particular implications for the selection of an appropriate method (see below). Other members reported further confusion arising from the introduction. The introduction indicates that the general aims/principles and the core functions of case management have been identified. It goes on to say that few studies provide adequate descriptions. Since the authors have cited these studies, a logical question is, how do these previous studies describe clinical case management and what do they say it is? Would it not have been appropriate to include and then critique such definitions if they exist?

The confusion is perhaps cleared up somewhat in the next section of the paper where the authors highlight the absence of any literature that details the actual process of clinical case management. Some members felt that it may have been more appropriate to use this as the justification for the study, as such arguments appear to be cogent and robust.

## Method

Members stated that they felt that there were several flaws with the method and research design. First, was the issue of precision and clarity. The paper under review appears to have an absence of precision and clarity. All the readers are told is that it used a qualitative method (p. 289). Stern (1994) submitted that although there may be similarities in all interpretative methods, the frameworks underlying the methods differ. Baker *et al* (1992) constructed similar arguments and furthermore, they reasoned that failure to explicate qualitative methodologies is resulting in a body of nursing research that is mis-labelled. Similarly, Morse (1991, p. 15) warned of this mixing of methods and stressed that, 'the product is not good science; the product is a sloppy mishmash'.

By paying attention to the resolution or precision of qualitative research method, the researcher is endeavouring to ensure rigour (Baker *et al*, 1992). Such rigorous studies should 'stand up' better to critique by enabling the reader to examine whether or not the chosen method was appropriate to the nature of the research study. Furthermore, some members questioned whether or not it was accurate to describe this paper as a qualitative study since the handling and presentation of the data provided little insight into the subjective worlds of the participants. This apparent confusion regarding the method may be further evidenced by the authors' use of the terms reliability and validity, and perhaps the presence and influence of Kanter's theory in the minds of the researcher during data collection and analysis.

In considering these arguments, there is a need to examine the philosophical underpinnings of quantitative research approaches. A researcher who adopts a quantitative approach to the collection of data is viewing the world through a particular type of lens. The view suggests that the world can be explained and understood in terms of universal laws and objective truths (McKenna, 1997). Its positivist and empiricist underpinnings suggest that there is only one reality and consequently a measure of the accuracy of this reality is its validity.

However, the qualitative researcher views the world through a very different lens. Key authorities on qualitative research point out that it is inappropriate to attempt to apply positivistic and empiricist views of the world to qualitative research (Benner and Wrubel, 1989; Morse, 1991; Denzin and Lincoln, 1994). Qualitative research are based upon the belief that there is no one singular universal truth, the social world is multi-faceted, it is an outcome of the interaction of human agents, a world that has no unequivocal reality (Ashworth, 1997). It is concerned with describing, interpreting and understanding the meaning people attribute to their existence and to their world.

Qualitative research findings should be tested for credibility or accuracy using terms and criteria that have been developed exclusively for this very approach (Hammersley, 1992). Leininger (1994) makes this point most clearly when she states:

> *We must develop and use criteria that fit the qualitative paradigm, rather than use quantitative criteria for qualitative studies. It is awkward and inappropriate to re-language quantitative terms.*

Some members wondered if the presence and potential influence of Kanter's theory moved the study away from being an inductive study and moved it toward a deductive study. Given the existence of such an existing theory begs questions about the research design. According to Morse and Field (1995):

> *The researcher should selectively and appropriately choose a research approach according to the nature of the problem and what is known about the phenomenon to be studied.*

If a theory already exists that provides definitions, principles and components of clinical case management, was it appropriate to attempt to use a qualitative method? Given Morse and Field's (1995) argument, maybe there would have been more merit in testing Kanter's theory (a deductive study). In some ways that appears to be what the authors have done. Members identified further problems pertaining to the method section.

Some wondered, what constituted an 'activity' for the purposes of this study and suggested the authors could have included a definition. Furthermore, how was the information recorded? What endeavours did the authors make to minimise the impact of the Hawthorne Effect (Polit and Hungler, 1997).

## Data analysis

A criticism raised by the members was the lack of a comprehensive explanation of how the themes were induced. Members wanted to see how the researchers had moved from labels (initial categorisation) to condensing these into 'main problem areas' to the central themes. Also, it would have been useful to see how the themes/categorisations inter-related with one another. Members wondered if this was further evidence of the lack of precision or clarity evident in this paper.

## Ethical considerations

The absence of any ethical considerations or details regarding ethical approval was felt to be an oversight (Lipson, 1994.) The paper contained no mention of ethical considerations. All research involving human subjects is carried out at some cost to the participants. While this cost may be difficult to identify or may appear trivial, the humans as subjects need and deserve appropriate respect and protection (RCN, 1998).

## Results

It is reasonable to say that the range of responses regarding the results section were mixed. Some members reported certain discrepancies in the results. For example, the pie chart indicates a figure of 35% for the total time case managers devoted to client contact. Yet the discussion (p. 292) refers to 38% and the 35% (p. 293). Furthermore, page 292 states that team information sharing and staff support/development accounts for 31% of the case manager's time. However, adding these two figures together from the pie chart figures adds up to 29%.

Other comments indicated the usefulness of the examples (from work outside of the observed week) used to add to the richness of the understanding. It was noted that planned client contact was the only category that has such examples to support the findings and members wondered why this was the case? Was it that no data was available? Arguably, the theory would be richer for such examples (Benner and Wrubel, 1989).

## Discussion, conclusions and recommendations

Opinions were divided regarding this section. The discussion raises some important issues, particularly those pertaining to smaller caseloads and recognising the need to fulfil important additional tasks. Also, comments regarding the need for ongoing clinical supervision were met with over-whelming support from the members. This argument continues to be raised in the literature (Butterworth and Faugier, 1992; Bond and Holland, 1998; Barker and Cutcliffe, 1999). The findings from this paper further add to the qualitative evidence supporting the widespread uptake and use of clinical supervision. Concerns were raised about how the paper appears to move into comparing contact numbers, and towards a quantitative method. Yet such an endeavour falls outside of the stated aim of the paper and added to the overall positivistic 'flavour' of the paper.

Members expressed some concern regarding the use of 'sweeping generalisations' in the discussion, such as 'research shows that working in the community is more stressful than working in hospital settings.' Given that stress is such a personal and individualised reaction (Rawlins *et al*, 1993), it is at best unwise to make such claims. Members did not doubt the accuracy of such findings, but felt that it would have been more appropriate to cite the results in more detail.

## Final comments: what meaning does this have for psychiatric and mental health nurses?

What this paper does do is add to the debate concerning the nature of psychiatric/mental health nurse (P/MH) practice. According to Duffy and Lee (1998), Hopton (1997) and Cutcliffe and McKenna (2000a/b), P/MH nurses in the United Kingdom find themselves in a position of uncertainty and subsequently mental health nursing is deeply immersed in a crisis of legitimacy. Whether or not mental health nurses should lose their specialist status and become generic nurses is based on the argument that there is compelling evidence to support the introduction of multi-skilling and cross training (HMSU, 1996). Yet opponents of such a position maintain that there is something crucial and unique in mental health nursing which is distinct and worth preserving (Nolan, 1993). Nonetheless, the literature is, at best unclear, regarding the precise nature of this uniqueness. Cutcliffe and McKenna (2000a) assert that this lack of precision is one of the problems and if P/MH nurses are unable to articulate what their contribution is and what is the nature of this uniqueness, then arguably it is more difficult to defend this distinctiveness.

Consequently, the paper reviewed can be seen to be attempting to identify elements of this uniqueness, since a key element of this process is describing what these nurses do. Perhaps the problems with the method compromise the credibility or validity of this theory. Further qualitative inquiry is needed to identify the nature of the alleged uniqueness of mental health nurses.

**Table 9.1: Key points arising from review number 6**

| | |
|---|---|
| 1 | The paper appears to have some confusion regarding the method and evidenced by the authors' inappropriate use of the terms reliability and validity, and perhaps the presence and influence of Kanter's theory in the minds of the researcher during data collection and analysis. Members questioned whether or not it was accurate to describe this paper as a qualitative study since the handling and presentation of the data provided little insight into the subjective worlds of the participants. |
| 2 | The paper reviewed can be seen to be furnishing the argument that psychiatric/mental health nurses provide a unique contribution, since a key element of this process is describing what these nurses do. |
| 3 | The paper might have been served by attention to issues of methodological precision. Such mindfulness and the resulting methodological rigour is likely to increase the overall quality of the inquiry and enhance the credibility of the findings. |

# References

Ashworth PD (1997) The Variety of qualitative research: Non-positivist approaches. *Nurse Educ Today* **17**: 219–24

Baker C, Wuest J, Stern PN (1992) Method slurring: the grounded theory/phenomenology example. *J Adv Nurs* **17**: 1355–60

Barker P, Cutcliffe JR (1999) Clinical risk: a need for engagement not observation. *Mental Health Practice* **2**(8): 8–13

Benner P, Wrubel J (1989) *The Primacy of Caring: Stress and coping in health and illness.* Addison Wesley, New York

Bond M, Holland S (1998) *Skills of Clinical Supervision for Nurses.* Open University Press, Oxford

Butterworth T, Faugier J (1992) Supervision for life. In: Butterworth T, Faugier J, eds. *Clinical Supervision and Mentorship in Nursing.* Chapman Hall, London: 230–40

Cutcliffe JR, McKenna HP (2000a) Generic nurses: the nemesis of psychiatric/mental health nursing? *Part One Mental Health Practice* **3**(9): 10–14

Cutcliffe JR, McKenna HP (2000b) Generic nurses: the nemesis of psychiatric/mental health nursing? *Part Two Mental Health Practice* **3**(4): 20–3

Denzin N, Lincoln YS (1994) Introduction: Entering the field of qualitative enquiry. In: Denzin N, Lincoln YS, eds. *Handbook of Qualitative Research.* Sage, London

Duffy D, Lee R (1998) Mental health nursing today: ideal and reality. *Mental Health Practice* **1**(8): 14–16

Hammersley M (1992) *What's Wrong with Ethnography?* Routledge, London

HMSU – University of Manchester (1996) *The future healthcare workforce: the Steering Group report.* Health Services Management Group, Manchester

Hopton J (1997) Towards a critical theory of mental health nursing. *J Adv Nurs* **25**: 492–500

Leininger M (1994) Evaluation criteria and critique of qualitative research studies. In: Morse J, ed. *Critical Issues in Qualitative Research Methods*. Sage, Thousand Oaks

Lipson J (1994) The use of self in ethnographic research. In: Morse JM, ed. *Qualitative Nursing Research: A contemporary dialogue*. Sage, London: 73–89

McKenna H (1997) *Nursing Theories and Models*. Routledge, London

Morse JM (1991) Qualitative nursing research: A free for all. In Morse JM, ed. *Qualitative Nursing Research: A Contemporary Dialogue*. Sage, London: 14–22

Morse JM, Field PA (1995) *Qualitative Research Methods for Health Professionals*. 2nd edn. Sage, London

Nolan P (1993) *A History of Mental Health Nursing*. Chapman Hall, London

Polit DF, Hungler BP (1993) *Essentials of nursing research: Methods, appraisal and utilization*. 3rd edn. JB Lippincott, Philadelphia

Rawlins RP, Williams SR, Beck CK (1993) *Mental Health — Psychiatric nursing, a holistic life-cycle approach*. CV Mosby, St Louis

Royal College of Nursing (1998) *Research Ethics: Guidelines for nurses involved in research or any investigative project involving human subjects*. The Royal College of Nursing, London

Stern PN (1994) Eroding grounded theory. In: Morse JM, ed. *Critical Issues in Qualitative Research Methods*. Sage, London: 210–23

# Example number fourteen: The NPNR National Journal Club, review from the seventh meeting

The paper reviewed first appeared in 1998, in the *Journal of Advanced Nursing* (**27**: 83–90), titled 'The knowledge and attitudes of mental health nurses to electro-convulsive therapy' (Gass JP).

## Abstract/overview

This paper reports on a study that attempted to illicit the knowledge and attitudes of mental health nurses of electro-convulsive therapy (ECT). One hundred and sixty-seven questionnaires containing attitude/knowledge scales were returned from the 345 sent out. The author discovered limitations in the reliability of the instrument and reliable measures of the respondents' knowledge of ECT were not obtained. The authors' findings indicated correlations with higher levels of knowledge, and; a) length of experience, b) area of clinical practice. He also noted significant variations in knowledge of cognitive side-effects. The author concludes that nurses' knowledge of ECT requires improvement in many cases and that this has implications for nurse education.

## Title

Feedback comments from the members regarding the title were mixed, with some saying the title clearly identified the focus of the research, while others felt the title could have indicated something of the research approach, the methodology or the design.

## Abstract

Members expressed that given the limited space the abstract managed to convey the core of what the paper was about. Perhaps the author could have included some detail about the sample, and it said nothing about the context against which the study took place.

## Introduction

Some members stated that the introduction was concise and to the point, whereas others felt that again it provided no context as to why the research was undertaken. It is possible that this section of the text would have been strengthened by including some justification for the study. Members were left wondering: Was the study conducted in response to a national issue or agenda? As a result of some increasing trend in the use of ECT? Or, as a result of the author's particular interest in this subject?

## Literature review

If the bulk of the comments for the preceding sections were positive, it is reasonable to say that the members expressed more criticism of the literature review. In this section the author suggests that ECT can be regarded as a form of punishment. While few would disagree that this can be the case, ECT is clearly not the only 'medical' or even nursing treatment/ intervention that can be regarded in this way, eg. the administration of tranquilising medication (particularly after a violent incident), the use of seclusion rooms, and indeed 'punishment therapy' (Masson, 1992).

Most of the literature focuses on papers that discuss the advantages and disadvantages of ECT. It is only in the last two paragraphs that papers describing similar studies are mentioned. This left members wondering, are these the only studies of this kind? Concerns were expressed regarding the balance of the literature and if this was a comprehensive review, and if important papers had been omitted, for example, Liam Clarke's (1995) paper 'Psychiatric nursing and ECT'. There was, notably, no mention of the complexities associated with attitudinal measurement, little on nurses and nothing much on conscientious objection to healthcare interventions. The literature review made no mention of who receives ECT, and this could be particularly relevant as mental health nurses' attitudes towards ECT may well be dissimilar for different 'conditions' or 'illnesses'.

## Method

The members stated that they felt that there were several flaws with the method. The author selected a convenience sample and while this may have been appropriate, he could have explored the advantages and disadvantages of using such a sample. Additionally, a rationale for choosing this sampling strategy may have been beneficial. The author used a data collection tool which had been used in a previous study. However, the author acknowledges that this tool produced low reliability scores which left the members wondering, if this tool has already been identified as having a low reliability, then why choose this tool and not another one? Perhaps the choice of this tool is linked to an incomplete or limited literature review, in that this may have been the only tool that was uncovered in the literature.

Further methodological difficulties were evident in the adoption of a tool designed to measure attitudes in the United States of America (USA). Attitudes are influenced by the pervading culture and sub-cultures (Hammersley, 1992; Stanfield, 1994) and it is unlikely that nurses in the USA have the same culture to nurses in Britain. Members expressed that insufficient detail was provided on the method used and the rationale for choosing this method. It may have been worthwhile for the author to have explored alternative scoring systems, for example, using questions with visual analogue scales, which have particular value in measuring subjective experiences which would have been more in keeping with measuring attitudes (Polit and Hungler, 1997).

Since the authors sample was comprised entirely from two trusts, it is conceivable that the nurses' attitudes could well have been influenced by another local ECT policy that existed and it may have been useful to see an overview of such policies (if they existed). In terms of the low response rate, the author acknowledges this, and it should be noted, made efforts to increase the response rate with the use of a follow up letter. However, in terms of the research design, members questioned the logic in sending out questionnaires at Christmas time (although this probably coincided with the author's dissertation schedule). Maybe the author's pilot study could have identified certain clinical areas that would be unlikely to provide a comprehensive response to such questionnaires; such as those areas who do not invest heavily in ECT. Yet no breakdown of response rate to the pilot study, according to clinical area is included.

A further problem identified with the method was that respondents were instructed to choose between ECT, pharmacological intervention and psychotherapy. Yet many of the members declared that more often than not, their treatments are concomitant and therefore, deciding between them is not a reflection of practice.

## Ethical considerations

The absence of any ethical considerations or details regarding ethical approval was felt to be an oversight (Lipson, 1994.) The paper contained no mention of ethical considerations. All research involving human subjects is carried out at some cost to the participants. While this cost may be difficult to identify or may appear trivial, the humans as subjects need and deserve appropriate respect and protection (RCN, 1998).

## Findings

It is reasonable to say that the members raised several criticisms regarding the findings section. The demographic details of the sample were described in this section which only served to confuse matters. If the author included these details in order to enable a repeat of his study in the future, members felt that it would have been more appropriate to have included the details of the sample under a separate sub-title. If the author included these details in order to carry out some analysis, for example, to look for correlations between the sex of the respondents and their knowledge/attitudes, it would be entirely appropriate to include the details in this section. Yet no such correlations are examined, leaving some of the members wondering about inattentive construction of questionnaires.

Two surprising, and possibly noteworthy observations are that no Project 2000 (P2K) students were included in the sample and, secondly, that more than half the sample were aged forty years or over. Was it that the study was completed before the advent of P2K or was there some other unstated reason for this omission?

A significant criticism was that, contrary to the author's over zealous attention to the results, no really significant differences between the groups of nurses responding existed. The mean differences in knowledge scores between 'elderly care' nurses and 'acute care' nurses differed very little. Yet the discussion made an awful lot of not very much. Perhaps this does raise an interesting point of, when do differences become significant and who decides? The author's comment on page 86, regarding 'elderly care' nurses having their knowledge based more exclusively on biomedical literature was felt to be inappropriate and inaccurate, especially when one considers Kitwood and Benson's (1995) work, Nolan *et al*'s (1997) research and many 'elderly care' nurses' arguments that they provide holistic, multi-dimensional care rather than bio-medically orientated, physical care (Ross, 1997; Pulsford, 1997).

The relatively small differences in knowledge (less than 1.5) are raised as an issue by the author and he explains these differences in part, as a result of the degree of experience. He also states that the knowledge did not vary according to the nurses' qualifications. It is unlikely that the education/training is responsible for any differences in knowledge. Yet the author suggests that such differences in knowledge could be addressed in nurse education, which is somewhat illogical. The author also argues that exposure to ECT is not associated with differences in knowledge of ECT, yet on page 87 he posits a relationship between choice of ECT and the nurses' clinical area. Members argued that the nurses' level of knowledge is likely to affect whether or not they would select ECT as the treatment of choice. How easy would it be for a nurse to recommend a treatment or intervention of which they had no or limited knowledge? Lastly, members felt that the findings section contained unvalidated opinions which would be better located in the discussion section.

### Discussion, conclusions and recommendations

In his discussion, the author argued in favour of more biological sciences to be taught in nurse education because the 1982 syllabus and P2000 syllabus have a greater psychosocial orientation. Earlier in his paper (p. 86) he argued that the knowledge of ECT as measured does not vary according to the qualification of the respondent. Furthermore, as stated earlier, his sample did not contain any nurses who had undergone the P2K training. It is inappropriate and unwise to base arguments on such small differences and when the sample does not enable potentially important comparisons to be carried out. Members expressed the view that the author appears to have an unwritten, implicit agenda, perhaps that of a return to the 'good old days' of biologically-orientated nurse training, and this appears to have influenced his interpretation of the results.

Additional points included a concern regarding Pippard (1992) as a legitimate reference to support the argument regarding lack of teaching on ECT, as this was only Pippard's impression and personal opinion. Also, that 'length of experience' alone, may not be sufficient explanation of any existing differences. Just because some nurses may have a commonality in their length of experience post qualification does not make them a homogenous group. Different nurses use their post-registration time in different ways. For example, some embrace the notion of 'lifelong learning' and continue to grow and develop after qualifying. Others adopt a less developmental approach and are less enthusiastic about continuous personal and professional development and growth.

### Final comments: what meaning does this have for psychiatric and mental health nurses?

It is important for nurses who are involved with this particular treatment to be aware of the variety of issues involved in ECT. It is reasonable to suggest that the extent of a nurse's knowledge and his/her attitude towards ECT may well have an effect on how the nurse presents ECT to clients. If there are significant deficits in the nurse's knowledge of ECT, then as the author of this research points out, there is a need to address this issue. However, the crucial point is in determining how and where this deficit can be remedied. Unfortunately, this paper does not provide enough valid findings to indicate how this deficit can be rectified.

It does raise some interesting questions for practice. One particular issue is, how can nurses help clients to be fully informed (and give informed consent) if the nurse is unable to provide the client with all the information they need? This paper can be regarded as increasing awareness of this issue and consequently has merit.

**Table 9.2: Key points arising from review number 7**

| | |
|---|---|
| 1 | The mean difference in knowledge scores were not particularly large, no really significant differences between the groups of nurses responding existed. Yet the author's discussion said a great deal as a result of this small difference. Perhaps this raises the issue of, when do differences become significant and who decides? |
| 2 | Members expressed the view that the author appears to have an unwritten, implicit agenda, perhaps that of a return to the 'good old days' of biologically orientated nurse training, and this appears to have influenced his interpretation of the results. |
| 3 | The recommended changes in nurse education are not supported by the findings in the study and arguments to return to a nurse training with greater biological emphasis would need to be much more cogent and robust before such a change should be considered. However, It does raise some interesting questions for practice. In particular, how can nurses help clients to be fully informed (and thus give informed consent) when the nurses themselves are not fully informed? |

# References

Clarke L (1995) Psychiatric nursing and ECT. *Nurs Ethics* 21(4): 321–31

Hammersley M (1992) *What's Wrong with Ethnography?* Routledge, London

Kitwood T, Benson K (1995) *The New Culture of Dementia Care*. Hawker Publications, London

Lipson J (1994) The use of self in ethnographic research. In: Morse JM, ed. *Qualitative Nursing Research: A Contemporary Dialogue*. Sage, London: 73–89

Masson J (1992) *Against Therapy*. Harper Collins, Glasgow

Nolan M, Grant G, Keady J (1997) *Understanding Family Care: A multidimensional model of caring and coping*. Open University Press, Buckingham

Pippard J (1992) Audit of electroconvulsive treatment in two National Health Service regions. *Br J Psychiatry* 60: 634

Polit DF, Hungler BP (1997) *Essentials of Nursing Research: Methods, appraisal and utilisation.* 4th edn. JB Lippincott, Philadelphia

Pulsford D (1997) Therapeutic activities for people with dementia — what, why and …why not? *J Adv Nurs* **26**: 704–9

Royal College of Nursing (1998) *Research Ethics: Guidelines for nurses involved in research or any investigative project involving human subjects.* RCN, London

Ross LA (1997) Elderly patients' perceptions of their spiritual needs and care: a pilot study. *J Adv Nurs* **26**: 710–15

Stanfield J (1994) Ethnic model in qualitative research. In: Denzin N, Lincoln YS, eds. *Handbook of Qualitative Research.* Sage, London: 175–88

# 10

## The fourth phase of the NPNR National Journal Club development: Critiquing with a degree of confidence

Example number fifteen: The NPNR National Journal Club, review from the ninth meeting

> The paper reviewed first appeared in 1990, in *Image: Journal of Nursing Scholarship* (**22**: 32–38), 'The tradition of toughness: A study of non-professional nursing care in psychiatric nursing settings' (Morrison EF ).

### Abstract/overview

This paper reports on an exploratory study that attempted to identify aspects of the care organisation that may affect the violent behaviour of clients. Having noted that violence in psychiatric settings is a significant problem, the authors pointed out that there was a dearth of literature that examined the influence of the organisation in relation to violent client behaviour. Using a grounded theory method, a theory of non-professional nursing care was induced which had a core variable entitled 'the tradition of toughness'. Further social norms and roles were identified that operationalised the theory. The norms were: a) the need for physical restraint; and b), 'it's not you we don't trust'. The nursing role of 'enforcing', included the strategies; 'policing', 'supermanning' and 'putting on a show'.

### Title

Feedback comments from the members was mostly favourable. The title was regarded to be explicit and concise. Perhaps the inclusion of the word violence may have added to the clarity and it may have been worthwhile for the title to say what type of study it was. For example, the title could have stated that it was a grounded theory study. However, the title was felt to capture the imagination of the reader.

## Abstract

Even though it was untitled, the paper did contain a succinct abstract. (Perhaps the absence of a title to the abstract was an idiosyncrasy of the particular journal and not an oversight on the part of the author.) Members felt that the abstract contained the essential components of the paper and gave the reader the necessary synopsis. Criticisms included the view that the abstract may have been a little brief and said little about the methodology. Additionally, a summary of the main discussion points arising could have strengthened the abstract.

## Introduction

Feedback about the introduction was predominantly favourable. The introduction was felt to set the relevant background to the study and identified the then current 'gaps' in the theory. The introduction contained a definition of violence (which appeared to be the definition of violence provided by the American Psychiatric Association in 1974), and the members response to this definition was mixed. Some members expressed that since violence is such a subjective phenomenon, ie. what one individual regards as violent, another would regard as assertive (Cutcliffe, 1999), the definition provided can be regarded as imprecise. Other members felt that having a definition was necessary for the study, as in order to explore the social processes involved in violence within certain psychiatric healthcare settings, it may be necessary to have an understanding of what is meant by the term 'violence'.

An alternative view was posited that suggested it was not necessary for a precise definition in that the researcher can work with whatever conceptualisations of violence the interviewees used. Indeed, in one of his many texts on grounded theory methodology, Glaser (1992) declared that the grounded theorist approaches the area of study with only an abstract wonderment of what is going on. Yet, it is also worth noting that in this day and age, where economics and the drive towards evidence-based practice have a significant influence on the research agenda within health care, justifiable concerns and/or questions could be raised of a researcher who attempted to begin a study by stating that they have an interest in a particular area but no concept of what they should be researching. The process of writing a research proposal currently inhibits potential researchers from making such a decision. Consequently, it is no surprise that the member feedback to the inclusion of such a definition in a grounded theory study was diverse.

Members did express some concerns that the introduction appeared to be blended with the literature review section. Given that the author used a grounded theory method, and Glaser and Strauss' (1967) position on the use of literature prior to commencing data collection, it would have been appropriate for the author to justify the use of a review of the literature at this stage in the study. Furthermore, as a result of this literature review it may have been prudent for the author to state that they used a modified version of grounded theory and not grounded theory (Glaser, 1992).

## Methods

Members stated that as the author was investigating an area of practice where little theory existed, the use of a grounded theory method was appropriate. The choice of obtaining data from three different settings raises the issue of the choice between a wide diverse sample or a more 'focused', narrow, concentrated sample in grounded theory. Arguments in favour of the use of a wide, diverse sample suggest this method ensures extensive data that cover the wide ranges of behaviour in varied situations (Lincoln and Guba, 1985; Munhall and Boyd, 1993).

Another point of view could be constructed that reasons in favour of a more narrow or focused sample, rather than maximum variation. Since in grounded theory, the researcher is concerned with uncovering the situated, contextual, core and subsidiary social processes, the processes need to be shared and experienced by the individuals who make up the social group. Otherwise, if an individual has no experience of the social or psychosocial process, how can they comment on it? Indeed, Lincoln and Guba (1985) pointed out that grounded theory has been termed 'local theory' as it brings together and systematises isolated, individual theory. Selection of a sample of participants who have only a limited experience of the process, or put another way, a sample that is not local, will only provide data and a subsequent theory that has a partial or limited understanding of the process being studied. Consequently, in the paper reviewed it is possible that the emerging theory amalgamates the commonalities of three local theories, each one belonging to each individual ward. Additional member comments point out that it may have been interesting too, if the observation of the ward staff had been carried out covertly. Additionally, further related insights may have been gained by interviewing senior figures in the organisation (eg. nurse managers, policy makers) and medics. Although it was noted that such individuals may well be regarded as falling outside of the particular social process under investigation.

The section titled 'Setting', contained a thorough description of the people and places of the hospitals. Members indicated that this section contained some judgements on the part of the author, which could have been supported or substantiated by including references/evidence.

## Ethical considerations

Members stated that the paper reported that formal access had been granted by the academic institution's human subjects committee and the hospital institutional review board. As the members were not familiar with the nuances of gaining ethical approval for a research study in an American hospital, the members were unable to ascertain whether or not the correct and proper ethical considerations had been deliberated upon. The author indicates that individual consent was gained from each participating client.

## Subjects

More detail on how the sample was selected may have been useful. In particular, members wondered if the author had used theoretical sampling as this would have been in keeping with the methodology (Glaser and Strauss, 1967; Glaser, 1992). It is possible that the author felt, having made it clear that she was using grounded theory, that readers would automatically assume that this included theoretical sampling. Nevertheless, some additional information regarding the sampling choices indicated by the emerging theory may have been useful. The paper contains some information regarding the evolution/development of the interview content, which is also appropriate for grounded theory.

## Analysis

Members reported how the author makes it clear how the different sources of data provided information on different issues. This triangulation of data sources can be perceived to add to the confirmation and completeness of the research findings (Nolan and Behi, 1995; Begley, 1996). An argument supported by Redfern and Norman (1994) who posit that a specific advantage of using a triangulated study in nursing relates to the increased confidence in the results and a more complete understanding of the domain or process. The means to establish the credibility of the findings were rigorous and that is to the betterment of the paper. One of the methods used was to verify the truthfulness of a patient's account of an incident. In the cases where the stories were corroborated, one could argue that the truthfulness is enhanced. Where the stories were not corroborated, data was not used. A possible outcome of using this method of corroboration is that even though the client's story was true and may have added to the in-depth understanding, where the story was not corroborated, the data was not used.

The author states that she enlisted the help of two 'external experts or consultants' in order to carry out external audits and an ongoing critique of the theoretical process. According to Cutcliffe and McKenna (1999), this approach as a method of establishing credibility of qualitative research findings has several philosophical and epistemological difficulties. Firstly, since qualitative studies are normally indicated when there is an absence of theory pertaining to the specific phenomenon or area of study being examined, how likely is it that such 'experts or consultants' will exist? Indeed, the author justifies the need for this study, in part, due to the dearth of studies in the specific area. Furthermore, the author fails to describe what defined these individuals as experts or if they have been subjected to any criteria in order to determine the extent of their alleged expertise. If such individuals do exist, this leads to the second difficulty (Cutcliffe and McKenna, 1999). The process of data analysis and theory induction in grounded theory depend upon the creative processes between the researcher and the data (Glaser, 1978; Glaser, 1992; Munhall and Boyd, 1993). It is unlikely that two or more people will interpret the data in the same way or induce precisely the same categories/core variable.

**Findings**

Feedback from the members indicated that the findings were presented in a clear and well structured style which included illuminating and interesting insights into the social processes which were present on the unit. These findings contained rich description and analysis supported by statements from the interviewees. The findings highlighted how the culture of the units and the nurses populating the units had a clear influence on the resulting (violent) behaviour of the clients. The abuse of the power inherent in the institution, by certain individuals, perpetuates the incidence of violence. Since this study was carried out in the United States, and used a qualitative method, it would be inappropriate to generalise these findings. It is possible that the behaviours and social processes witnessed on the psychiatric unit are indicative of a wider cultural phenomenon. Perhaps a national cultural phenomenon that encourages the 'tradition of toughness'. (As might be evidenced by such cultural norms as the constitutional right to bear arms, or the 'Hollywood' perpetuated image of masculinity.)

Glaser and Strauss (1967) asserted that substantive theories are usually induced from the data and formulated first and then these substantive theories are followed by formal theories. Consequently, as the conceptual generality of the grounded theory moves from substantive to formal theory, the scope of the theory is widened. There may well be elements of the theory induced from an American psychiatric unit that resonate with nurses from other countries and other psychiatric units.

The findings in this paper are echoed in the experiences of many psychiatric/mental health nurses from around the world, where some nurses are allowed to behave in an inappropriate manner. Some of the members reported having witnessed similar processes within Australian psychiatric units, British psychiatric units and British Secure Hospitals (Smith and Hart, 1994; Crichton, 1995; Harbourne, 1996; Rees and Lehane, 1996; Whittington and Wykes, 1996).

## Discussion, conclusions and recommendations

Members noted that the discussion highlighted the relevant, supporting empirical literature and discussed the implications of the findings. It should be noted that the conclusions and recommendations were presented under the discussion heading and members felt that there may have been merit in presenting each of these in separate sections.

## Final comments: what meaning does this have for psychiatric and mental health nurses?

Feedback from the group members suggested that they felt this was a clear, comprehensive, interesting and illuminating paper, which highlighted an important aspect of clinical practice. Furthermore, it added to the empirical evidence in this area (and stimulated a great deal of debate in the journal clubs).

Even though the paper is ten years old, it draws attention to fundamental behaviours and dynamics within mental healthcare systems that need consideration and addressing. The findings (and similar experiences echoed by some of the members) suggest that the practice of some mental health nurses appears to remain embedded and strongly influenced by the medical model. The paper reiterates that many clients with mental health problems continue to be medicalised and it reminds us of the inherent capability of a 'care system' to be more concerned with exerting power and control over the people it is supposed to be caring for. It reminds psychiatric/ mental health (P/MH) nurses of the issue of empowerment. If P/MH nurses are genuinely concerned with empowering clients, then these findings serve as a crucial and valuable insight into a mode of practice that needs to be abandoned as a matter of urgency. In addition to a culture that appears to perpetuate and glorify a 'tradition of toughness', it perhaps highlights the discomfort that some P/MH nurses may have with the expression of certain emotions, eg. anger and frustration. In addition to these clinical issues, despite being ten years old, it serves as a good example of one way of writing a qualitative research study report. Additionally, the paper contains rigorous attempts to establish the credibility or authenticity of the qualitative findings, and such endeavours are to the betterment of the paper. It should be noted that the technique of enlisting external experts, used by the author, has several philosophical and epistemological difficulties.

**Table 10.1: Key points arising from review number nine**

| | |
|---|---|
| 1 | The paper reiterates that many clients with mental health problems continue to be medicalised and it reminds us of the inherent capability of a 'care system' to be more concerned with exerting power and control over the people it is supposed to be caring for. |
| 2 | It serves as a crucial and valuable insight into a mode of practice that needs to be abandoned as a matter of urgency and at the same time, despite being ten years old, serves as a good example of one way of writing a qualitative research study report. |
| 3 | The paper contains rigorous attempts to establish the credibility or authenticity of the qualitative findings, and such endeavours are to the betterment of the paper. However, the technique of enlisting external experts, used by the author, has several philosophical and epistemological difficulties. |

# References

Begley CM (1996) Using triangulation in nursing research. *J Adv Nurs* **24**: 122–8

Crichton J (1995) The response to psychiatric inpatient violence. In: Crichton J, ed. *Psychiatric Inpatient Violence: Risk and response*. Duckworth, London

Cutcliffe JR (1999) Qualified nurses lived experiences of violence perpetrated by individuals suffering from enduring mental health problems: a hermeneutic study. *Int J Nurs Stud* **36**: 105–15

Cutcliffe JR, McKenna HP (1999) Establishing the credibility of qualitative research findings: The plot thickens. *J Adv Nurs* **30**(2): 374–80

Glaser BG (1978) *Theoretical Sensitivity: Advances in the methodology of grounded theory*. Sociology Press, Mill Valley, California

Glaser BG, Strauss AL (1967) *The Discovery of Grounded Theory: Strategies for qualitative research*. Aldine, New York

Glaser BG (1992) *Basics of Grounded Theory Analysis: Emerging vs Forcing*. Sociology Press, Mill Valley, California

Harbourne A (1996) Challenging behaviour in older people: nurses' attitudes. *Nurs Standard* **12**(11): 39–43

Lincoln YS, Guba EG (1985) *Naturalistic Inquiry*. Sage, London

Munhall PL, Boyd CO (1993) *Nursing Research: A qualitative perspective*. 2nd edn. National League for Nursing Press, New York

Nolan M, Behi R (1995) Triangulation: The best of all worlds? *Br J Nurs* **14**(10): 587–90

Redfern SJ, Norman IJ (1994) Validity through triangulation. *Nurse Researcher* **2**(2): 41–56

Rees C, Lehane M (1996) Witnessing violence to staff: a study of nurses' experiences. *Nurs Standard* **11**(13–15): 45–7

Smith ME, Hart G (1994) Nurses' responses to patient anger: From disconnecting to connecting. *J Adv Nurs* **20**: 643–51

Whittington R, Wykes T (1996) An evaluation of staff training in psychological techniques for the management of patient aggression. *J Clinical Nurs* **5**: 257–61

## Example number sixteen: The NPNR National Journal Club, review from the tenth meeting

NB: The following review comments were originally compiled by Ian Beech, Ann Fothergill and Ben Hannigan, University of Wales.

---

The paper reviewed first appeared in 1999, in the *International Journal of Nursing Studies* (**36**: 105–16), 'Qualified nurses' lived experiences of violence perpetrated by individuals suffering from enduring mental health problems: a hermeneutic study' (Cutcliffe JR).

---

### Abstract/overview

This paper reports on a study that attempted to discover the lived experiences of nurses who experience violence perpetrated by individuals suffering from enduring mental health problems. Consequently, it adopted a hermeneutic, phenomenological method which produced an emerging theory comprised of the three key themes; personal construct of violence, feeling equipped, and feeling supported. As a result of his findings, the author suggested relationships between exposure to violent incidents, the ability to deal with incidents therapeutically and how formal support systems influence this relationship.

### Title

There was a mixed view from the reviewers on whether or not the title adequately explained the content and focus of the paper. The majority agreed that the title gave a clear indication of what the paper was about, however, some groups felt it was too long, and jargonistic. Suggested alternatives included, replacing 'hermeneutic' with 'phenomenological' or 'qualitative'. Counter arguments noted that if these terms were used, some criticism could be levelled at the title for not offering a precise description.

### Abstract

There were some mixed views of the abstract. Many members thought that the abstract was good, in that it was concise, clearly written and gave an adequate overview of the study. Others, however, wanted more of the detail of the study, while some described the abstract as jargonistic. Those who felt this added that it could have been strengthened by the addition of further information. For example, some members wanted more background information on the sample and explanations on the meaning of some of the concepts used in the paper. It is likely that given this level of detail it would have been difficult given word limits within abstracts.

## Introduction

Generally, members felt that the introduction to the paper was a good one. A sound justification for the study was given, and previous literature was presented and discussed. There was agreement that finding out about the experiences of nurses in relation to violence was an important topic, which merited research investigation. Violence within the National Health Service remains a significant cause for concern. This concern has been reiterated recently by the Department of Health, who require all NHS Trusts to monitor and act to reduce violence against staff (Turnbull and Paterson, 1999) and it is reasonable to suggest that 'quick fix' solutions do not appear to be the answer. Clearly, what is needed is a deeper and more thorough understanding of the variables and inter-relationships involved, in order to construct effective, workable and affordable strategies and interventions.

## Methodology

The study was identified as being based on a hermeneutic, pheno-menological approach. The majority of members experienced difficulty understanding the philosophy used and felt that a clearer description of what phenomenology and hermeneutics is, was needed. Most members were unclear about the relationship between the section of the paper which discussed phenomenological philosophy and the research study. Other groups, however, felt that the phenomenological approach added to the overall precision and clarity of the method. Several key authors (Glaser, 1978; Lincoln and Guba, 1985; Morse, 1991; Hammersley, 1992) have argued that methodological precision is a hallmark of high quality research. Failure to include such precise descriptions may result (quite correctly) in criticism of the paper. However, it is incumbent upon the researcher to include clear descriptions and explanations of the method and consequently, not only address issues of methodological rigour, but additionally, increase the 'readability' and/or 'accessibility' of the paper.

## Data collection

Data were collected in this study using 'semi-structured conversations'. Some members commented favourably on the attention given in the paper to the description of this method, and were particularly pleased to see the inclusion of questions used in the study. The method was felt to be congruent with the aims of the research. However, some members wanted the author more clearly to demonstrate how the use of a hermeneutic approach was reflected in his research questions, design and analysis. While acknowledging that there is no one singular 'correct' way to write a qualitative research report (Dreher, 1994), members felt that the strength of the author's 'methodology and research design' section was the detailed account given of what he did and how he did it. For example, the author was praised for giving details of questions used to start each of the semi-structured conversations. Some members felt that the strengths and limitations of the method needed to be included here.

**Sample**

Many groups commented on the sample used in the study. The sample was chosen from a ward in which staff had experienced an unusually high level of violence. Some members felt, in this respect, that the study participants would not have been typical of most P/MH nurses. However, since generalisation of the findings from representative populations to wider populations is not the purpose in qualitative research (Morse and Field, 1995; Morse, 1998), perhaps the selection of a sample who can provide the richest and deepest understanding of the phenomenon/process is a reasonable choice. Some members reflected this viewpoint when they commented that the paper included a good account of why this unit had been chosen.

Perhaps an alternative strategy for sampling may have been to access a P/MH population who experience a more 'usual' level of violence and gain an understanding of their 'lived experiences' of violence first. Following this, the lived experiences of P/MH nurses who experience the unusually high level of violence could be obtained, and a comparison of the two emerging theories may indicate some useful insights. For example, further understanding of the proposed relationship between exposure to violence, the number/severity of incidents encountered, the level of support and the subsequent level of stress and/or experiential learning. All those who participated in the interviewing were described as having been full-time qualified mental health nurses. For some, the study would have been strengthened by the inclusion of unqualified nurses, and part-time staff.

**Ethics**

There were differences of opinion with respect to the ethical dimensions of the study. Some members were critical over what they saw as a general lack of attention to this area, while others praised the study for the attention given to the process through which informed consent was obtained. Since ethical committee approval is required when the study occurs within NHS property (Beauchamp and Childress, 1994; RCN, 1998) it would have been necessary to gain ethical approval prior to conducting this study. The absence of such approval can be regarded as a deficiency of this study.

## Findings

There was general praise for the systematic way in which data were analysed. Members commented on the detail given to the description of the process of thematic analysis. One group added that this level of detail was relatively rare in reports of qualitative studies. The main findings were presented around three key themes: 'personal construct of violence', 'feeling equipped' and 'feeling supported'. Some members commented favourably on the use of data extracts to illustrate the themes. A number of the groups expressed the view that the figures used to illustrate the possible relationship between clinical supervision and stress caused by experiencing violence were unhelpful, and did not clarify the points that were being made.

For some members, the findings added little in the way of new knowledge. As one group put it, 'we already knew this'. Others, however, took the view that the fact that the findings were in keeping with what was already known about the experience of violence added to their 'face validity', and that a 'lived experience' of violence had been arrived at. Some members felt that this type of study is valuable for psychiatric/mental health (P/MH) nursing; in that they make explicit elements of theory which are implicit in the practice of many P/MH nurses. Several authors have identified the need for nursing research to shift its attention away from quantitative studies into uncovering the unique knowledge embedded in nursing practice. According to Pearson (1992, p. 222):

> *Much of our scholarly theorising is only distantly related to the real world of practising nurses, especially when it utilises the most rigorous methods of positivism, the mechanistic application of problem solving or attempts to reduce or categorise the phenomena encountered in nursing.*

Benner (1984) made similar remarks, asserting the need for a new paradigm of nursing research that is concerned with understanding the knowledge embedded in clinical expertise and inducing theory from this knowledge. Such theory is central to the advancement of nursing practice and the development of nursing science. Consequently, studies of this type appear to be making some attempt towards uncovering the unique knowledge embedded in P/MH nursing practice.

Many of the groups discussed the contribution of the paper to clinical practice. While some felt that not much new had come from the study, others felt that this research strengthened the case for education and training. In particular, the need for greater attention to training and clinical supervision with regards to the management of violence was identified.

Other members felt that the paper highlighted the need for formal policies to be implemented in the workplace in order to have comprehensive strategies for dealing with violence, debriefing and staff support.

## Final comments: what meaning does this have for psychiatric and mental health nurses?

Members felt that the paper addressed an important and interesting topic, which had relevance for P/MH nurses. For some, however, the paper was marred by what they saw as too much jargon, and a lack of succinctness. The issue of the overuse of jargon within the NHS has been raised recently (Buggins, 1995; Casey, 1995; McGlade *et al*, 1996), culminating in the establishment of a nationwide group that has the remit of examining the language used by health professionals, and considering the implications of this language for clients and their carers (see Client Representative group for the NHS Centre for Coding and Classification, Buggins, 1995). More recently, Scott (1998) drew attention to the overuse of jargon within nursing, and suggested that jargon can be regarded as the language of the insecure. While the issues surrounding the use of jargon in nursing are not immediately and totally transferable to nursing research, there are parallels and consequently, lessons to be learned. If a research report contains so much jargon that the potential audience it intends to reach are repelled, then the impact of the research paper on practitioners (and practice) is likely to be diminished. However, as stated previously, precise description of the research method is a hallmark of quality, and writers of research reports may need to include some terminology in an attempt to provide this precision. It appears that a balance of these positions should be aimed for and that the result of this may be methodologically precise research reports that reach the widest possible audience.

**Table 10.2: Key points arising from the tenth review**

| | |
|---|---|
| 1 | Given that violence within the National Health Service remains a significant cause for concern, and that there is a need for a deeper and more thorough understanding of the variables and inter-relationships involved, the study may be regarded as timely. |
| 2 | The overuse of research 'jargon' in places, perhaps reduces the accessibility of the paper to a wider readership and could be regarded as 'off putting'. While the author appeared to make some efforts to explain certain research terms, perhaps this issue highlights the dilemma facing writers of research reports; finding the correct balance between the use of clear, accurate terminology which adds to the methodological clarity of the research and the overuse of such terms, to the extent that some readers find this 'off putting'. |
| 3 | While some members felt the paper was not saying anything new, others felt that this type of study is valuable for psychiatric/mental health (P/MH) nursing; in that they make explicit elements of theory which are implicit in the practice of many P/MH nurses. |

# References

Beauchamp TL, Childress JF (1994) *Principles of Biomedical Ethics*. 4th edn. Oxford University Press, Oxford

Benner P (1984) *From Novice to Expert: Excellence and power in clinical nursing practice*. Addison Wesley, Menlo Park, California,

Buggins E (1995) Communications: Mind your language. *Nurs Standard* **10**(1): 21–22

Casey A (1995) Standard terminology for nursing: Results of the Nursing Times Project. *Health Informatics* **1**: 41–3

Dreher M (1994) Qualitative Research Methods from the reviewer's perspective. In: Morse JM, ed. *Critical Issues in Qualitative Research Methods*. Sage, London: 281–97

Glaser BG (1978) *Theoretical Sensitivity*. Sociology Press, Mill Valley, California

Hammersley M (1992) *What's Wrong with Ethnography?* Routledge, London

Lincoln YS, Guba EG (1985) *Naturalistic Enquiry*. Sage, London

McGlade LM, Milot BA, Scales J (1996) Eliminating jargon, or medicalese, from scientific writing. *Am J Clin Nurs* **64**(2): 256–7

Morse JM (1991) Qualitative nursing research: A free for all? In: Morse JM, ed. *Qualitative Nursing Research: A Contemporary Dialogue*. Sage, London: 14–22

Morse JM (1998) What's wrong with random selection? *Qualitative Health Res* **8**: 733–5

Morse JM, Field PA (1995) *Qualitative Research Methods for Health Professionals*. 2nd . Sage, London

Pearson A (1992) Knowing nursing: Emerging paradigms in nursing. In: Robinson K, Vaughan B, eds. *Knowledge for Nursing Practice*. Butterworth Heinemann, London

Polit DF, Hungler BP (1997) *Essentials of Nursing Research: Methods, Appraisal and Utilisation*. 4th edn. Lippincott, Philadelphia

Royal College of Nursing (1998) *Research Ethics: Guidance for nurses involved in research or any investigative project involving human subjects*. RCN Publishing, London

Scott H (1998) Nurses must start writing so as to be understood. *Br J Nurs* **7**(14): 812

Turnbull J, Paterson B (1999) *Aggression and Violence: Approaches to effective management*. Macmillan Press, London

# Section four: Future considerations

# 11

# The future of psychiatric and mental health nursing research?

All too often researchers, and not just those working in nursing, are accused of being out of touch with the reality of what goes on in the real world. Whether this is correct or not is probably unimportant, but what is clear is that research often does not benefit from the same level of credibility as a person's own experience of the work place. This is entirely understandable when you consider the cognitive mechanisms in place to help us frame our thought processes and decision-making activities. If we were to try to survive solely on our instincts within a professional arena, it would not be long before we were overwhelmed with questions for which we simply did not have any answers. Trial and error may be all right for the developing child, but nurses are adults, dealing, in the main, with adult problems and as nurses we have to have access to adult solutions. It would be professionally arrogant to assume that our practical experience alone could place all the answers at our finger tips and besides, mental health care has become so sophisticated over the last thirty years that, working exclusively from past or observed experience would gradually reduce, not increase, our body of collective knowledge. If mental health nursing is to meet the challenge of providing appropriate and complex care it has to have more at its disposal than myth and legend. The reality is that our future success lies in combining all the evidence resources at our disposal, including research, with the spontaneity of our intuitive actions and subjecting both to the same level of critical evaluation. In short, raising the level of our professional thinking to a more mature status.

To enable this to happen certain key issues have to be addressed and it is more than simply individual practitioners reading more research, or researchers doing more practice-based projects. No, the route to success involves understanding what part the science and art of nursing have to play in this development process and attributing to them suitable responsibilities and expectations (Bekker et al, 1999). In the space available to us within this chapter we cannot possibly deal with the whole of this agenda and will therefore, address the part that should be played by research and evidence. We also recognise that research alone cannot function in a vacuum and that for it to be effective, reciprocal influences must come from the areas in which it is to be considered and used. We have divided the chapter into two sections:

- the responsibilities of research in relation to nursing
- the responsibilities of nursing in relation to research.

# The responsibilities of research in relation to nursing

On the face of it, any research endeavour has one major objective: to provide information that answers questions. Research linked to a professional discipline is no different. The major difference between professional researchers and those undertaking research within a profession is that in most cases researching itself will be a secondary function to some other professional role. This is not just the case within nursing. If one looks at the evidence base generated within psychiatry, it is almost exclusively the work of practising psychiatrists and the same applies within the fields of social work and other disciplines allied to medicine. There are implications for this form of practice and we will address them later in this chapter, however, the point is that in most cases, those undertaking discipline-related research should have a good understanding of the work of that discipline and be well grounded in the questions for which it needs answers. The main question need not necessarily be whether the researcher has the ability to link research with practice but whether or not the research they choose to undertake is of a good enough quality to have relevancy for other practitioners. If it can be established that the design, method and robustness of the research activity reach the necessary standard, there is the question of how, and in what form, the research reaches others for use as an intelligence source. Finally, there is the question of how that work finds its way into practice and its impact evaluated. From these questions we can identify five themes that collectively sum up the responsibilities of research in relation to any chosen subject that it purports to represent:

1    The appropriateness of the research topic and its relevance to other members of the profession or users of their services.
2    The quality of the research activity, including the identification of appropriate methods and designs.
3    The coherence of the writing and dissemination strategy associated with a specific piece of research.
4    The attention given to the practical application of the research and how this is expressed within the researcher's reports.
5    The effectiveness of the evaluative feedback loop between researcher and practitioner/user.

These five themes will now be considered in more detail.

## The appropriateness of the research topic

If you were asked to explain why it was that you had arrived late for work, you would be regarded with a certain amount of suspicion if you began your excuse by venturing the belief that there was life on the planet Mars. Similarly, if you were asked by an anxious relative to explain why it was that a patient who almost perpetually self-harmed by using razor blades to cut tracks into her arms, was being allowed the freedom to repeat such activities even though she came under the seemingly protective umbrella of in-patient care, your response would be of little use if it did not specifically address, not just the question, but the concern behind its asking.

We have already stated that all too often practitioners see research as answering the wrong questions, but there is also the other issue of whether it provides the right answers. If you undertake a review of mental health nursing research papers printed over the last thirty years you will discover that they follow a particular trend. The intensity of that trend is more marked as we reach the current day. In the early 1970s most nurses undertaking and reporting research (though certainly by no means all) were either working as research assistants for medical staff or were researching topics which were of a medical or psychiatric nature. Diagnostic activities, illness presentations and drug actions research were both the domain of medical as well as nursing staff. In the main, the research methods used by both disciplines were often similar though there was at times stark contrast between the totally quantitative approaches of psychiatry and the predominantly qualitative ones adopted by nurses. Arguably, the main difference between the research activities of the two disciplines was that psychiatry was building a knowledge base that was to constitute the foundations for its present work and research activities, while nursing was replicating psychiatry and doing little to establish an evidence foundation upon which to build knowledge for nursing. As one comes closer to the present day, we find that nursing has increasingly concentrated its efforts on researching issues that are central to the work of its own discipline. However, the legacy of those earlier years can still be seen and the future challenge will be to re-focus nurse researchers' endeavours on to nursing related research issues (Ward, Cutcliffe and Gournay, 1999).

The **nurse-oriented research focus** should be what drives the uni-disciplinary research agenda, but it is important that nurses do not simply select nursing topics on which to concentrate (Crowe, 1998; McCabe, 2000). True, if nurses are to be recognised as equal partners within the multi-disciplinary team they have to be able to articulate their own evidence in support of their decision-making activities, but to be genuine team members they need to take part in team activities. Much of contemporary psychiatry is based around group decision-making and this has to be driven by group research. Service delivery cannot exist without nurses and it follows that nurses must be involved in the research that establishes the nature, organisation, resourcing and evaluation of that care. Equally, the care itself cannot function isolated from the work of other disciplines, so nursing research has to both dovetail and collaborate with the research activities of those disciplines. Compared to thirty years ago, perhaps the major change is that nurses must take the lead in their own research rather than allowing others to do it for them. In the case of multi-disciplinary research, there is also no reason why a nurse should not take the lead as long as they are suitably qualified to do so (for examples of this approach see: Onyett, Pillinger and Muijen, 1995; Ward, Armstrong, Lelliott, and Davies, 1999; Wooff, Goldberg and Fryers, 1988).

It would be inappropriate for us to state what we consider to be the **research priorities** for psychiatric and mental health nursing. Such things are determined by individuals, groups and organisations in relation to the local context (Barker, Jackson and Stevenson, 1999). There does, of course, have to be a balance between what the individual wants to do and what needs to be done; what the individual thinks is important and what contributes to the general good; what develops the individual and what develops their professional group. Such decisions should be made in collaboration with others and we would strongly recommend that no research project be undertaken solely on the strength of one individual working alone. However, within psychiatric and mental health nursing there are areas of general concern that appear to influence service thinking no matter where the individual works, and nursing research has to continue to address these issues in the future if it is to contribute to the process of defining nursing responsibilities. These include:

❦ Nurses' use of traditional management techniques such as control and restraint, seclusion and PRN medications (Bowers *et al*, 2000; Chien, 1999; Mason, 1997).

❦ The use of special observations for those who are deemed to be at risk of harming themselves or others (Cleary *et al*, 1999; Barker and Cutcliffe, 1999; Jones, Lowe and Ward, 2000; Jones *et al*, 2000; Neilson and Brennan, 2001).

❦ Risk assessment and management (Gournay and Bowers, 2000; Hazelton, 1999; Raven and Rix, 1999).

❦ The evaluation of psychotherapeutic interventions (Marks, 1977; Gournay *et al*, 2000; Reilly, 2001).

❦ Nurse prescribing (Allen, 1998; Cutcliffe and Campbell, 2002; Gray and Gournay, 2000; Kaas *et al*, 2000).

❦ The roles and responsibilities of those working as independent practitioners specifically within community settings (Atkinson, 1996; Bennett, Done and Hunt, 1995; Wilkinson, 1992; Ward *et al*, 1999; Ward and Jones, 1997; White and Brooker, 2001).

❦ Working in different care settings, and increasingly the problems facing in-patient care (Gournay, Gray, Wright, and Thornicroft, 1997; Ward, Cutcliffe, and Gournay, 2000).

❦ Working with different diagnostic and age groups (Gournay and Beadsmoore, 1995; Akhtar and Samuel, 1996; Cole, Scoville and Flynn, 1996; Conrad, 1998; Barker, 1999; Stordeur, Vandenberghe and D'hoore, 2000).

❦ Working with different ethnic and cultural groups (Rodriguez, Lessinger and Guarnaccia, 1992; Lutzen and Nordin, 1995; Takeuchi and Cheung, 1998).

❀ Philosophical issues in relation to care (Lutzen and Nordin, 1994; Nolan, Brown and Crawford, 1998; Carlsson, Dahlberg and Drew, 2000; Cutcliffe and Goward, 2000).

❀ Clinical decision making (Carpenter, 1991; Alty, 1997; Narayan and Corcoran, 1997).

❀ User involvement (Valimaki, Leino-Kilpi and Helenius, 1996; Forchuk *et al*, 1998; Rogers *et al*, 1997).

❀ Nursing leadership (McGleish, 1996; Murrells and Robinson, 1997).

❀ Clinical supervision (Cutcliffe and Poctor 1998a/b; Cutcliffe *et al*, 1998, Cutcliffe, 2000; Ashmore and Carver, 2000; Coffey and Coleman, 2001; Edwards *et al*, 2000).

❀ Educational issues, particularly the preparation of psychiatric and mental health nurses (Hardcastle, 1999; Sainsbury Centre for Mental Health, 1997; Lakeman, 1999).

❀ National and international collaboration (Chiu, 1999; International Society of Psychiatric-Mental Health Nurses, 1999; White, 1998).

❀ The future of psychiatric and mental health nursing, including the debate concerning generic and specialist workers (Allen, 1998; Butterworth, 1991; Barker *et al*, 1999; Cutcliffe and McKenna, 2000a/b; Ward *et al*, 1999).

It is also important for nurse researchers to ensure that their work is appropriate to the needs of both the other nurses and service users. This should always entail discussion and decision making with others and specifically those from within the practice domain. Similarly, it is the responsibility of researchers to ensure that they are not carrying out work that has already been completed by others. There are, of course, occasions when this is important, either to establish if the original findings were accurate or if they can be replicated in other areas or time frames. There is also the need to maintain interest in research once it has been completed. The completion of a project and the resultant scientific paper should not constitute the end of the research. Invariably, research recommendations suggest that further work is needed to make more sense of the total picture, yet rarely do nurse researchers follow this through themselves. There is a need for research to be part of a programme of work, or at least to fit into an overall strategy of inquiry. Longitudinal studies are rare in nursing generally and even more so in mental health. Follow up studies have been undertaken (Gournay *et al*, 2000; Newell and Gournay, 1994) but again these are not often tackled. For mental health nursing to develop its research and evidence base the research itself has to be more than just individuals 'shooting in the dark'. Establishing research priorities that give a sense of purpose to all this effort has to come from nurses and be driven by the skills of researchers. More importantly, it has to become part of the strategic thinking of nursing and its leaders, embedded in the desire to improve and be accountable to a collective vision of the future. Only by co-ordinating our research efforts will nursing ever be able to 'join up' all its resources into an accessible body of knowledge (Butterworth, 1991).

Mental health nurses must also contribute to **multi-disciplinary research activities,** otherwise the whole nature of nursing will become insular and detached from mainstream psychiatry and care service thinking (Gournay, Plummer and Grey, 2001; Ricard, 1999). There are benefits to being a strong and relatively large minority group, but specialisation has its price. If nurses only pursue nursing research they may eventually run out of ideas, creativity and imagination (Walters, 1990). Exposure to others only enhances diversity and so it should if nursing research is to flourish. Areas where nurses can contribute to this agenda are only limited by the degree of commitment nurses have to it. Whether nurses take the lead on these ventures will be determined by several factors, not least the relationship between individuals and their research experience. The reality is that at present very little published material exists around the developing face of twenty-first century psychiatry and its organisation. The following represents a small percentage of the areas where nurses need to consider being involved, not just as practitioners but also in researching both the effectiveness and development of change:

- the development of evidence-based care
- clinical governance and quality control mechanisms generally
- care pathways
- service configuration
- formal and rigorous practice development
- mental health and human rights legislation and their implication for practice and service delivery
- therapeutic interventions
- multi-agency working
- evaluations of existing service provision and establishing benchmarks for future change
- introduction of government policy initiatives
- clinical leadership.

## The quality of nursing research

Quality is more than establishing the right fit at the right price. In relation to research it covers a much broader set of items. It is not acceptable to say that research produced results are viable or up to standard if we are only seeking to support our own arguments or contentions. Research has to play a far more independent role. For it to be genuinely credible it has to be impartial, not simply proving a point. Good research is designed to find out, not prove. This can only be achieved by ensuring that the **research methods** to be used are suitable to the subject being researched: that the choice between qualitative or quantitative (or a combination of both) approaches is appropriate to the question; that the tools selected (if any) are both reliable and valid; that the sample is sufficient to produce the data necessary and that its analysis follows accepted scientific principles; that conclusions from the analysis are not driven by personal agendas and that the shortcomings, as well as the successes of the research, are recorded for others to make their own judgement about its quality.

Another trend that appears in the mental health nursing research literature over the last thirty years is that of the use of qualitative research. Unlike the topics themselves, which have tended to move away from psychiatry, the more contemporary literature shows a marked increase in the use of different methodologies with a definite move towards far more qualitative work being undertaken, in line with psychiatry itself. Many nurse researchers argue that nursing has become far more adult in its use of research methods and it now has enough knowledge of these to be able to use those appropriate to the study, rather than choosing studies appropriate to their knowledge (Burnard and Hannigan, 2000; Croom, Procter and Couteur, 2000). The literature itself is testimony to this with research from mental health nurses using any number of different approaches (Bowers, Gournay and Duffy, 2000; Carlsson *et al*, 2000; Gournay and Bowers, 2000; Gournay, Veale and Walburn, 1997; Tang *et al*, 2001).

Quality can only be achieved by researchers learning from and reporting their mistakes. One way of achieving this is through **research supervision**. All too often inexperienced researchers undertake potentially significant pieces of work without approaching other, more experienced, researchers for guidance and support. So much effort can be wasted simply for the sake of spending a little more time in preparing the study properly. Nurses who have as their main job some other form of professional activity other than research, carry out most of the research undertaken within psychiatric and mental health nursing. This is not the case with many other disciplines. For many of those carrying out projects the work may well be part of their own professional development, as is the case with those completing higher degrees. Certainly, these individuals are very much on the increase (Ward *et al*, 2000), which bodes well for the future. However, the fact remains that their skills base cannot be considered to be as broad or as in-depth as those who undertake research for a living and have consequently received appropriate supervision, on-going training and feedback about their performance. In effect, amateurs, no matter how talented, undertake most nursing research, as is the case for psychiatry sometimes with dire consequences (Prior *et al*, 2001). Without the proper guidance from an experienced supervisor, 'amateurish' will be the tag attributed to their work. Nursing cannot afford to be so entrepreneurial.

All too often, of course, the results of poorly developed research are reported in professional journals as fact, leading practitioners to consider inaccurate findings as possible drivers for their own practice. Rarely do such papers ever get past the rigorous review processes of research and scientific journals, but it is fair to say that these are not the popular day-to-day reading material of working nurses so the likelihood of such bad science influencing change is increased. As we have discussed at length, the necessity for nurses to be able to critique both poor as well as good research is crucial if this situation is to be avoided.

## Reporting and disseminating research

Many people find that having completed a piece of research, especially those for academic courses, they are reluctant to write up the work for publication. There are several reasons for this: the fact that there is no longer any pressure to complete the task and it is easy to keep on saying, 'I will do it next week'; the individual may not have experience of writing for publication and the activity is a daunting one that they are not prepared to tackle; the absence of a supervisor to help with the production of a manuscript or simply that the individual feels that their work would not be of value to others. Waddell reports that too little research finds its way into press and even then it is not read or used properly (Waddell, 2001); while Kempster contends that evidence-based journals are either not prepared to publish work in mental health or do not receive papers which are of a good enough standard to be published (Kempster, 1998).

It should go without saying that all research has to be published or at least made available for public consumption. If researchers keep information to themselves, even if they are unsure as to its value, it means that others cannot benefit from it. There are several questions that have to be asked when considering writing for publication and future researchers must ensure that they answer them and follow them through.

❖ Has the research project specifically allocated time at the end of the work for write-up?

❖ Has the research material been prepared with a view to being easy to convert into a published paper, ie. is it accessible?

❖ How many different papers can the research support?

❖ Should the paper be sent to a professional or a scientific journal, or both using different styles?

❖ Have the specific styles of the targeted journal been considered so that the paper can be written to their contributors' criteria?

❖ Has the researcher contacted the editor of the targeted journal beforehand to establish that the intended paper is appropriate and that the journal would be interested in receiving it?

❖ What format does the journal want the manuscript to be sent in, ie. hard copy, floppy disk, etc. and how many copies need to be sent?

❖ Does the researcher need to get help from a supervisor to write the paper?

❖ Have time frames been set to complete the work?

❖ Is there someone who can read and critique the paper before it is sent to a journal for consideration?

❖ Is the researcher aware that some journals are stricter than others in terms of peer review and that in many cases papers will be returned for editing, correction and, in some cases, major re-write? If so, has time been allocated to this work?

❖ What happens if the paper is rejected completely?

Of course, writing for publication is only part of the dissemination process. Once work is complete it has to be championed by the researcher, those involved in the work and those who supported it. This means conference presentations and teaching sessions and the researcher has to be prepared to defend their work within those environments and, if need be, obtain the skills to do so. This is not an easy task for many people and should be considered when planning research. Too few inexperienced researchers appreciate that the dissemination strategy must be integral to any research proposal or outline and carry as much importance as the quality of the research itself.

## The practical application of research

While it may be assumed that once research has been completed, the papers written and the dissemination strategy undertaken, that the job of the researcher is complete, this is not necessarily the case. Even when potential research is being considered, thought has to be given to its applicability to the practical environment and though not all research is designed for implementation, especially that of a philosophical nature, work stimulated by observations from practice certainly should be. The **implementation strategy** is often no more than the purpose of carrying out the project in the first place, though in more sophisticated programmes it will be the driving force for completing the work. In many cases, the application of research into practice has to be the responsibility of the researcher, but obviously it has to involve others because culture change or practice developments cannot be successful if they do not engage all those who will be affected by it (Cutcliffe *et al*, 1998c; Jackson *et al*, 1999a; Jackson *et al*, 1999b).

Research should not be undertaken for its own sake; we cannot afford the time to be that self-indulgent. It has to serve a purpose and in a professional environment dominated by clinical practice this must provide the rationale for such activities. Practitioners need to take much of the responsibility for ensuring the quality of any research adoption, but the researcher should take an active part in the process by ensuring initially that the work undertaken provides the sort of material that those practitioners need. **Practice development** should be as rigorous as the work that under-pins it, but if research outcomes are inconsistent with the demands of practice developers it is a failure of research planning (Ward *et al*, 1998). Discussion and outcome clarification needs to be undertaken at the start of an intended project, revisited throughout and evaluated as part of its terminal activities.

**Research feedback**

If a piece of research is completed, published and disseminated properly the opportunities are there for the researcher to gain invaluable feedback from others about the nature of the work. These lessons have to be learnt for, as we have already described, the majority of mental health nursing research is not undertaken by professional researchers. Researchers are sometimes accused of being arrogant and much of this stems from either their unwillingness or inability to listen to what others say about the quality or appropriateness of their work. The work of the NPNR National Journal Club involves just that process and by publishing the aggregated critiques of over 500 nurses about specific published papers it would be unwise of their authors not to take note, and learn from, those reviews. In theory, nurse research should improve as we progress through this century. We have a growing body of knowledge, we have an increasing number of individuals equipped to carry out good quality and suitable research, and a culture that values research and evidence far more than ever before. No one expects every piece of research to be perfect, indeed, very little of it ever is. What is expected is that mistakes form the basis of development and that researchers acknowledge those mistakes when presenting their findings. There is always room for improvement and professional egos should not stand in the way of progress. It has to be the responsibility of a researcher, once a project is complete, to seek actively the informed feedback of others about the nature of their work. By doing so we can expect better quality work, more individuals equipped to provide research supervision, a more focused research agenda as well as a better informed nursing workforce. The feedback loop is an essential component of an upwardly spiralling quality improvement programme.

## The responsibilities of nursing in relation to research

Though it is true that researchers have to take responsibility for their own research, the terminal feedback loop discussed above is not the only point at which nurses have a responsibility to support research and researchers. There are various times within both the planning and the life of projects where the involvement of those outside of the direct research process can make a genuine contribution to its success and quality. The whole purpose of this book is to bring to nursing's attention a mechanism for one form of feedback, but it is by no means the only one. Research critiquing certainly encapsulates the essence of professional awareness but invariably it is a process carried out after the work has been completed. It could even be argued that research papers do not tell everything about the research itself and as such much of what goes on within the research world could still be hidden from the critical eye of nurses. It is crucial that all nurses are involved in some way or another with the development of the mental health nursing knowledge base because, in truth, it has to belong to them if it is to have any meaning. If individual nurses do not take advantage of those possibilities, nurse researchers could quite rightly take the opposing view to that described at the beginning of this chapter and accuse nursing itself of being out of touch with the reality of what goes on in the real world. We have to be quite clear about this: however or wherever the evidence is gathered, developed and disseminated, the future of psychiatric and mental health nursing, along with all other disciplines delivering mental health care, will centre upon proof that its actions are the best and most appropriate for service user needs. If nurses feel removed from the source of that evidence it will be very difficult for them to take an active part in its adoption and, as such, will offer care which is either unsubstantiated or not of the best quality. If, by contributing to the research or evidence generating process, nurses can get a sense that they own that knowledge for themselves, it will cease to be vested with the mystical qualities historically attributed to research activities. In doing so, evidence generation and implementation becomes a dynamic process and twenty-first century psychiatric and mental health nursing practice the main beneficiary. Let us consider those areas where nurses can make a difference within this agenda.

**The appropriateness of the research topic**

In an ideal world each practitioner would undertake their own research work, rendering the necessity to communicate his or her needs to others completely superfluous. Of course, such a situation is totally impractical and would in itself be very counterproductive. If we examine this highly improbable situation in more detail, it provides us with ideas as to what needs to be considered for non-researchers to be able to maintain research quality.

Some people have to research, others have to inform research decisions and in a reciprocal process use the research findings to inform their practice. Not everyone wants to be a researcher. Not everyone has the skills to undertake research. Not everyone has the work opportunities or allocated time to be able to commit themselves to researching. This does not mean that research is the domain of researchers or a minority of the 50,000 plus psychiatric and mental health nurses registered in the UK alone. Being committed to research does not mean you have to undertake it, but it does mean you have to support it. It also means de-mystifying its language, its activities and methods so that those who do not use these things regularly can at least understand what their researching colleagues are doing. The first task in maintaining quality is the ability to recognise it when you see it and that can only be achieved if you have a reasonable knowledge of the specialist vocabulary. As you will have seen from the review chapters and, in particular, while exploring the different critiquing approaches, this does not mean having an intimate working knowledge of research. It means that you can picture what it is that the researcher is talking about and shape an impression of their work and intentions. It also gives some clues as to how they intend to achieve their outcomes and makes reading and understanding their findings more of a possibility. To do this it is necessary to organise your thoughts into patterns so that you concentrate on the specific aspects of the paper, looking for things that should be there and those that should not.

Secondly, having de-mystified the language you have to desensitise yourself to the fact that research is something which can only be understood by other researchers. There is a commonly held belief that research is only published for the benefit of other researchers and this is, or at least should be, totally untrue. Research, when published, enters the public domain and is free to all who read it. Contained within those papers is the 'stuff of kings', if only their secrets could be unlocked. But, this is not as difficult as it seems, as we have already shown in the previous chapters. What is important is for non-researchers to lose their suspicion of research as a 'not for them' entity. Half the battle is overcoming the psychological barrier of so-called academic snobbery. Once that has been achieved then research, no matter in how much depth it is read, becomes far more accessible.

Thirdly, the process of communicating information is all important. We have already considered the role of the researcher writing about their research, but what we are suggesting here is something that happens long before decisions about potential projects take place. Non-researchers, in effect, practitioners, are also guilty of not writing about their clinical practice. There are any number of professional journals representing mental health nursing to which papers about practice could be sent. Yet a brief analysis of these shows that much of what they contain centres around policy, legislation, personal views and research. Very few articles describe service structures or discuss clinical issues. This is a turnaround from the situation thirty years ago when the vast majority of these articles addressed just such issues. Nurses need to write about their clinical practice for researchers to have an anchor or benchmark to begin the inquiry. For many researchers this is where their ideas about research activities come from. For others it is discussions, collaboration, practice links and supervision. But these too are the responsibility of other nurses. If, as we have suggested, most researchers in nursing have some link with the clinical base, then it is the conversations that occur within them that shape people's thoughts and ideas about the subject matter for their intended research. Equally, when research has been published, all too often having read a paper a nurse will think to themselves that this was inappropriate or could have been done in a different way that would have been more beneficial to them. Writing to the journal is one way of registering this fact and all journals have a letters section. The fact is that nurses need to be more proactive in their support of research and lodge their dissatisfaction at what they see as being invalid. If no one tells a journal that what they published is not what they want, then the journal has no way of knowing this except through its circulation figures. If in those letters nurses tell the journal what they actually want, then over time this will begin to shape the publishing agenda and ultimately, the research one as well. Our experience of letters to journals is that this very seldom happens.

Fifthly, the selection of research topics must be linked to actual research need. Who is best at describing this if it is not those who do the actual work? Nurses have to take part in local discussions about strategic planning, clinical decision-making and service configuration. They need to know what others are thinking and be politically aware as well as clinically so. They need to make a contribution to these discussions so that their professional opinions are heard, then talk about them to each other on a clinical level to ensure that there is debate about change and development. They need to be supported by their clinical leaders and managers and to do this they have to communicate what it is that they want to achieve. This does not mean that they simply table a shopping list but learn to construct reasoned arguments, backed up by evidence that clearly identifies the necessity to undertake certain courses of action. Part of that action will be the research topics necessary to make appropriate changes. They also need to work with multi-disciplinary colleagues to ensure that the aspirations of nurses are not in conflict with others, and, if they are, to find a way of combining the efforts so that different levels of outcomes can be achieved. Researchers who work outside of the clinical situation should be invited to development meetings so that they can get a flavour of the discussion. Follow-up meetings with individuals or groups then bring about clarification of the topics and the researcher and practitioners can work together as a team to develop the research project or programme.

Lastly, nurses must take part in the research work of others. While this is not necessarily part of the selection process it is still a method of ensuring that nurses own the research in some way, get used to making decisions about research activities and are better equipped at a later stage to inform others about their requirements of the research process.

## The quality of nursing research

Much of what we have discussed above relates also to the quality agenda. However, ensuring that the research of others is carried out to an acceptable standard, when you are not researching yourself can be fraught with difficulties, not least that the researcher might accuse you of not understanding what it is that he or she is trying to achieve. The first thing that readers of research must do is equip themselves with a suitable critiquing tool, like those used within this book. The use of that tool has to be practised. You cannot expect to be an expert at finding the hidden meanings within papers at the first attempt, though it has to be said that surprising results can be achieved very quickly. It is also important that you try to undertake critiques with others, either a friend or a colleague in the clinical area. Discuss each section and compare notes. Gradually your separate reliability measures with that tool will improve and you can begin to use it more often on your own.

Quality in research can mean different things to different people. We understand it to be that the correct research method was used, that an appropriate sample was selected, the data was collected in line with the excepted practice of the method, that data was analysed appropriately and the results made sense. Hidden within these few statements however, are any number of different possibilities and these can often only be teased out by a careful unpicking of the work. For example, a project was undertaken which explored the application of Parse's theory of human becoming to an in-patient psychiatric setting in the USA (Northrup and Cody, 1998). The method used, descriptive evaluation, was appropriate, while the data gathering methods too were sound. Data was analysed and recommendations made in relation to the successful implementation of the theory within the clinical setting. On the face of it, an interesting and robust piece of research with relevance to mental health nursing practice. Careful scrutiny of the paper reveals that the implementation of the theory and the subsequent pre-mid and post data gathering sections were carried out over such a small period of time that genuine implementation simply could not have taken place (Jackson *et al*, 1999a,b). Therefore, the recommendations which initially had seemed perfectly acceptable, were in fact misleading. While the research was robust, the researched phenomenon was not. Consequently, the recommendations were invalid. Had nurses attempted to implement this work themselves based upon those recommendations they may well have become very disillusioned with their own performance had it not matched their expectations, and valuable time and effort could have been wasted. Establishing the truth behind research reporting is at the heart of quality controlling research itself.

It is often far easier to find fault with the work with others than to find the good in it. Just because one aspect of a project is suspect does not mean that lessons cannot be learnt from it or that other aspects that are perfectly reliable and valid cannot be considered as useful. Critiquing does not mean being hypercritical. It is a balanced process of establishing what is good and what is not, learning from the mistakes and using the successes. All this can occur in a single paper.

## Reporting and disseminating research

If nurse researchers in the future are to continue to improve upon the effectiveness of their report writing and dissemination activities, those who are the audience for these must read and listen carefully to what is being said and feed back their responses. All scientific journals, and many professional ones, provide a contact address for the lead author of a paper. It is there to enable people to contact them, yet all too often this never happens. If researchers have taken the time to write, it is the responsibility of the reader to report back what they thought of the work, be it critical or complimentary.

Similarly, it would be unfair to expect potential readerships to read everything that is written. The following represent the basics of a reading strategy that combines quality with coverage:

❖ Choose journals that publish papers that fit your areas of interest or practice, only read those ones and do not read any others unless a particular paper is recommended.

❖ Speak with your local librarian about finding papers for you on specific topics and requesting searches to be carried out at regular intervals.

❖ Identify the journals you and your colleagues or a team have access to, either in the library or through personal subscriptions, and allocate responsibility to each person for reading different journals. Report back to each other on a regular basis those of interest and those requiring specific attention, for whatever reason.

❖ Keep a reference record of those papers that were relevant to your needs, gradually building up a catalogue you can refer back to at a later date. Try to avoid reading and discarding. There is nothing worse than being unable to find a paper that you know has the answer you seek. It is almost worse than never having read it in the first place!

❖ Use a notice board in the clinical area to display copies of new and relevant material.

❖ Talk to your colleagues about what you find.

❖ Organise a journal club in your ward, unit or team and try to ensure that it has a multi-disciplinary attendance.

❖ Don't restrict yourself to nursing journals alone.

❖ Learn how to decide quickly what should be read now, what can wait till later and what needs to be discarded straight away. It will save you valuable time.

❖ Allocate yourself regular periods of quiet time when you can read.

❖ Always make notes while reading and attach these to the paper, or place them in the journal, when you have finished.

❖ Check the references used by the author in relevant papers, find them at the library or request them from the librarian. They will enhance your understanding of the paper and the subject matter.

## The practical application of research and research feedback

We have chosen to combine these two sections because in reality, for the non-researcher, they constitute similar processes. We have already addressed many ways that readers can report back to writers about their thoughts on a paper, but feedback is not just about a person's reaction to a paper. Consider one last important strategy. The main objective of writing up research for publication has to be that someone will read the work and be inspired enough to want to use what they found within their own practice (Hanily, 1995). **Practice development** is no easy activity and requires careful planning and supervision (Cavanagh and Tross, 1996). If research has been carried out in a robust way, so too must the practice development that implements it into practice. Seeking the advice and opinion from the researcher may be one way of ensuring continuity between the two activities. Even if this is not plausible, nurses using the work of others to enlighten their practice ought to write to the original authors before they begin their development work informing them of their intentions, at intervals during the implementation phases and again once the work is finished and evaluated. Positive feedback of this type does wonders for the researcher's confidence and gives far more meaning to their own work. It might just be the incentive they need to carry on with their endeavours. Of course, once the development work has been carried out, and this may take several years, it too will need to be written up for public consumption; so the cycle of publishing feedback continues, as it should if we are to progress our knowledge.

## Concluding remarks

Research, its reporting and adoption into clinical services and practice has to be seen as a joint effort between those who undertake it and those who use it. Increasingly, within psychiatric and mental health nursing these two groups are not mutually exclusive with more and more practitioners carrying out their own investigation. The apparent rift between the two groups is slowly closing and to a certain degree the aspirations of both groups are common ground. The activities of critical thinking and enquiry are not simply the domain of researchers, just as the processes of clinical decision making and service delivery are not exclusive to practitioners. For mental health nurses to build on their obvious successes to date, these facts have to be recognised by all and research has to become an active component in the professional lives of all those who aim to deliver quality mental health care. As we have shown, being active in research does not necessarily mean that you are undertaking the work itself, but likewise being a researcher should never mean that your research is not driven by the demands of the practice environment.

Nurse researchers have to embrace all aspects of the nursing agenda; from the so-called soft activities of philosophical and phenomenological enquiry to those of the, equally incorrectly titled, hard research of randomised controlled trials and meta analysis. In reality, they are all part of the same family, simply different methods chosen to suit the form of investigation required and the subject content to which they will be applied. Whether we are predominantly qualitative or quantitative is immaterial to the main aim of producing a theoretical basis for psychiatric and mental health nursing that is sound, scientific and applicable. Future discipline specific research will have to show that it meets all these requirements if it is to converge with the demands of an ever more critical professional audience.

Embarking upon research programmes that are exclusively nursing is one goal of nurse-researchers but there has to be a commitment to the multi-disciplinary research agenda as well. Increasingly, nurse-researchers are becoming more sophisticated in their methodological knowledge and their contribution to the wider activity of 'whole community' enquiry is imperative to the successful outcomes of such work. Psychiatric research needs nurses just as much as psychiatric services. The two are interwoven and research that attempts to exclude one or more of the other parties is bad science, and even worse politics.

Non-researchers also have a responsibility to make their contribution to the research process, although in different ways to the researcher. We have shown throughout this book that critically reviewing research is an essential ingredient of the research process itself. The selection of appropriate research topics, the evaluation of the outcomes of that endeavour and the competent application of them into clinical practice and/or professional thinking are all the domain of the non-researcher. Ultimately, being research/evidence-aware must be a guiding factor in the work of all those who aspire to delivering effective care and treatment to those who suffer the debilitating, soul destroying effects of mental ill health.

# References

Akhtar S, Samuel S (1996) The concept of identity: developmental origins, phenomenology, clinical relevance, and measurement. *Harv Rev Psychiatry* 3: 254–67

Allen J (1998) A survey of psychiatric nurses' opinions of advanced practice roles in psychiatric nursing. *J Psychiatr Ment Health Nurs* 5: 451–62

Alty A (1997) Nurses' learning experience and expressed opinions regarding seclusion practice within one NHS trust. *J Adv Nurs* 25: 786–93

Ashmore R, Carver N (2000) Clinical supervision in mental health nursing courses. *Br J Nurs* 9: 171–6

Atkinson MM (1996) Psychiatric clinical nurse specialists as intensive case managers for the seriously mentally ill. *Semin Nurse Manag* 4: 130–6

Barker P, Cutcliffe JR (1999) Clinical risk: a need for engagement not observation. *Ment Health Practice* 2(8): 8–12

Barker P (1999) Therapeutic nursing for the person in depression. In: Clinton M, Nelson S, eds. *Advanced Practice in Mental Health Nursing*. Blackwell Science, Oxford:137–57.

Barker P, Jackson S, Stevenson C (1999) What are psychiatric nurses needed for? Developing a theory of essential nursing practice. *J Psychiatr Ment Health Nurs* 6: 273–82

Bekker H, Thornton J, Airey C, Connelly J, Hewison J, Robinson M et al (1999) Informed decision making: an annotated bibliography and systematic review. *Health Technol Assess* 3: 1–156

Bennett J, Done J, Hunt B (1995) Assessing the side-effects of antipsychotic drugs: A survey of CPN practice. *J Psychiatr Ment Health Nurs* **2**: 177–82

Bowers L, Gournay K, Duffy D (2000) Suicide and self-harm in inpatient psychiatric units: a national survey of observation policies. *J Adv Nurs* **32**: 437–44

Bowers L, Jarrett M, Clark N, Kiyimba F, McFarlane L (2000) Determinants of absconding by patients on acute psychiatric wards. *J Adv Nurs* **32**: 644–9

Burnard P, Hannigan B (2000) Qualitative and quantitative approaches in mental health nursing: moving the debate forward. *J Psychiatr Ment Health Nurs* **7**: 1–6

Butterworth T (1991) Generating research in mental health nursing. *Int J Nurs Stud* **28**: 237–46

Carlsson G, Dahlberg K, Drew N (2000) Encountering violence and aggression in mental health nursing: a phenomenological study of tacit caring knowledge. *Issues Ment Health Nurs* **21**: 533–45

Carpenter MA (1991) The process of ethical decision making in psychiatric nursing practice. *Issues Ment Health Nurs* **12**: 179–91

Cavanagh SJ, Tross G (1996) Utilising research findings in nursing policy and practice: considerations. *J Adv Nurs* **24**: 1083–88

Chien WT (1999) The use of physical restraints to psychogeriatric patients in Hong Kong. *Issues Ment Health Nurs* **20**: 571–86

Chiu L (1999) Psychiatric liaison nursing in Taiwan. *Clin Nurse Spec* **13**: 311–4

Cleary M, Jordan R, Horsfall J, Mazoudier P, Delaney J (1999) Suicidal patients and special observation. *J Psychiatr Ment Health Nurs* **6**: 461–7

Coffey M, Coleman M (2001) The relationship between support and stress in forensic community mental health nursing. *J Adv Nurs* **34**: 397–407

Cole BV, Scoville M, Flynn LT (1996) Psychiatric advance practice nurses collaborate with certified nurse midwives in providing health care for pregnant women with histories of abuse. *Arch Psychiatr Nurs* **X**: 229–34

Conrad BS (1998) Maternal depression symptoms and homeless children's mental health risk: Risk and resiliency. *Arch Psychiatr Nurs* **XII**: 50–8

Croom S, Procter S, Couteur AL (2000) Developing a concept analysis of control for use in child and adolescent mental health nursing. *J Adv Nurs* **31**: 1324–32

Crowe M (1998) Developing advanced mental health nursing practice: a process of change. *Aust N Z J Ment Health Nurs* **7**: 86–94

Cutcliffe JR (2000) To record or not to record: Documentation in clinical supervision. *Br J Nurs* **9**(6): 350–55

Cutcliffe JR, Proctor B (1998a) An alternative training approach in clinical supervision. Part one. *Br J Nurs* **7**(5): 280–5

Cutcliffe JR, Proctor B (1998b) An alternative training approach in Clinical Supervision. Part two. *Br J Nurs* **7**(6): 344–50

Cutcliffe JR, Epling M, Cassedy P, McGregor J, Plant N and Butterworth T (1998a) Ethical dilemmas in clinical supervision: The need for guidelines. *Br J Nurs* **7**(15): 920–3

Cutcliffe JR, Epling M, Cassedy P, McGregor J, Plant N and Butterworth T (1998b) Ethical dilemmas in clinical supervision: The need for guidelines. *Br J Nurs* **7**(16): 978–82

Cutcliffe JR, Jackson A, Ward MF, Cannon B, Titchen A (1998c) Practice development in mental health nursing: Part One. *Ment Health Practice* **2**: 27–31

Cutcliffe JR, McKenna H (2000a) Generic Health Care Workers: The Nemesis of Psychiatric/Mental Health Nursing? Part one. *Ment Health Practice* **3**(9): 10–14

Cutcliffe JR, McKenna H (2000b) Generic Health Care Workers: The Nemesis of Psychiatric/Mental Health Nursing? Part two. *Ment Health Practice* **3**(10): 20–23

Cutcliffe JR, Goward P (2000) Mental health nurses and qualitative research methods: a mutual attraction? *J Adv Nurs* **31**: 590–8

Edwards D, Burnard P, Coyle D, Fothergill A, Hannigan B (2000) Stress and burnout in community mental health nursing: a review of the literature. *J Psychiatr Ment Health Nurs* **7**: 7–14

Forchuk C, Jewell J, Schofield R, Sircelj M, Valledor T (1998) From hospital to community: bridging therapeutic relationships. *J Psychiatr Ment Health Nurs* **5**: 197–202

Gournay K, Beadsmoore A (1995) The report of the clinical standard advisory group: standards of care for people with schizophrenia in the UK and implications for mental health nursing. *J Psychiatr Ment Health Nurs* **2**: 359–64

Gournay K, Bowers L (2000) Suicide and self-harm in in-patient psychiatric units: a study of nursing issues in 31 cases. *J Adv Nurs* **32**: 124–31

Gournay K, Denford L, Parr AM, Newell R (2000) British nurses in behavioural psychotherapy: a 25-year follow-up. *J Adv Nurs* **32**: 343–51

Gournay K, Gray R, Wright S, Thornicroft G (1997) *Mental health nursing in inpatient care: A review of literature and an overview of current service provision.* Institute of Psychiatry, London

Gournay K, Plummer S, Grey R (2001) The dream team at the Institute. *Ment Health Practice* **4**: 15–17

Gournay K, Veale D, Walburn J (1997) Body dysmorphic disorder: pilot randomised controlled trial of treatment implications for nurse therapy research and practice. *Clin Effectiveness Nurs* **1**: 38–46

Gray R, Gournay K (2000) What can we do about acute extrapyramidal symptoms? *J Psychiatr Ment Health Nurs* **7**: 205–11

Hanily F (1995) A new approach to practice development in mental health. *Nurs Times* **91**: 34–5

Hardcastle M (1999) Assessment of mental health nursing competence using level III academic marking criteria: the Eastbourne assessment of practice scale [in process citation]. *Nurse Educ Today* **19**: 89–92

Hazelton M (1999) Psychiatric personnel, risk management and the new institutionalism. *Nurs Inq* **6**: 224–30

International Society of Psychiatric-Mental Health Nurses (1999) *A Position on the Rights of Children in Treatment Settings.* International Society of Psychiatric-Mental Health Nurses, Philadelphia

Jackson A, Cutcliffe J, Ward M, Titchen A, Canon B (1999a) Practice development in mental health nursing: Part Three. *Ment Health Practice* **2**: 24–27, 30

Jackson A, Ward MF, Cutcliffe J, Titchen A, Canon B(1999b) Practice development in mental health nursing: Part Two. *Ment Health Practice* **2**: 20–25

Jones J, Lowe T, Ward M (2000) Inpatient's experiences of nursing observation on an acute psychiatric unit: a pilot study. *Ment Health Care* **4**: 125–29

Jones J, Ward M, Wellman N, Hall J, Lowe T (2000) Psychiatric inpatients' experience of nursing observation: a United Kingdom perspective. *J Psychosoc Nurs Ment Health Services* **38**: 10–20

Kaas MJ, Dehn D, Dahl D, Frank K, Markley J, Hebert P (2000) A view of prescriptive practice collaboration: perspectives of psychiatric-mental health clinical nurse specialists and psychiatrists. *Arch Psychiatr Nurs* **14**: 222–34

Kempster M (1998) Evidenced-based medicine in mental health. *Evidence Based Nursing* **1**: 40

Lakeman R (1999) Advanced nursing practice: experience, education and something else. *Nurs Prax NZ* **14**: 4–12

Lutzen K, Nordin C (1994). Modifying autonomy — a concept grounded in nurses' experiences of moral decision-making in psychiatric practice. *J Med Ethics* **20**: 101–7

Lutzen K, Nordin C (1995) The influence of gender, education and experience on moral sensitivity in psychiatric nursing: a pilot study. *Nurs Ethics* **2**: 41–9

Marks I (1977) Costs and benefits of behavioural psychotherapy: a pilot study of neurotics treated by nurse-therapists. *Psychological Med* **7**: 685–700

Mason T (1997) An ethnomethodological analysis of the use of seclusion. *J Adv Nurs* **26**: 780–9

McCabe S (2000) Bringing psychiatric nursing into the twenty-first century. *Arch Psychiatr Nurs* **14**: 109–16

McGleish A (1996) Leadership in practice: developing leadership in forensic mental health nursing. *Nurs Standard* **10**: 14–5

Murrells T, Robinson S (1997) Developing the nursing contribution to the management of the mental health services. *J Nurs Manag* **5**: 325–32

Narayan SM, Corcoran S (1997) Line of reasoning as a representative of nurses' clinical decision making. *Res Nurs Health* **20**: 353–64

Neilson P, Brennan W (2001) The use of special observations: an audit within a psychiatric unit. *J Psychiatr Ment Health Nurs* **8**: 147–55

Newell R, Gournay K (1994) British nurses in behavioural psychotherapy: a 20-year follow-up study. *J Adv Nurs* **20**: 53–60

Nolan PW, Brown B, Crawford P (1998) Fruits without labour: the implications of Friedrich Nietzsche's ideas for the caring professions. *J Adv Nurs* **28**: 251–9

Northrup DT, Cody WK (1998) Evaluation of the human becoming theory in practice in an acute care psychiatric setting. *Nurs Sci Q* **11**: 23–30

Onyett S, Pillinger T, Muijen M (1995) *Making Community Mental Health Teams Work*. The Sainsbury Centre for Mental Health, London

Prior C, Clements J, Rowett M, Taylor D, Rowsell R et al (2001) Atypical antipsychotics in the treatment of schizophrenia. *Br Med J* **322**: 924

Raven J, Rix P (1999) Managing the unmanageable: risk assessment and risk management in contemporary professional practice. *J Nurs Manag* **7**: 201–6

Reilly D (2001) Obsessive compulsive disorder: cognitive behavioural interventions and the role of the nurse. *Ment Health Practice* **4**: 16–19

Ricard N (1999) The new challenges of mental health nursing research and practice. *Can J Nurs Res* **31**: 3–15

Rodriguez O, Lessinger J, Guarnaccia P (1992) The societal and organizational contexts of culturally sensitive mental health services: findings from an evaluation of bilingual/bicultural psychiatric programs. *J Ment Health Adm* **19**: 213–23

Rogers ES, Chamberlin J, Ellison ML, Crean T (1997) A consumer-constructed scale to measure empowerment among users of mental health services. *Psychiatr Serv* **48**: 1042–7

Sainsbury Centre for Mental Health (1997) *Pulling together: The future roles and training for mental health staff*. The Sainsbury Centre for Mental Health, London

Stordeur S, Vandenberghe C, D'Hoore W (2000) Leadership styles across hierarchical levels in nursing departments. *Nurs Res* **49**: 37–43

Takeuchi DT, Cheung MK (1998) Coercive and voluntary referrals: how ethnic minority adults get into mental health treatment. *Ethn Health* **3**: 149–58

Tang WK, Chiu H, Woo J, Hjelm M, Hui E (2001) Telepsychiatry in psychogeriatric service: a pilot study. *Int J Geriatr Psychiatry* **16**: 88–93

Valimaki M, Leino-Kilpi H, Helenius H (1996) Self-determination in clinical practice: the psychiatric patient's point of view. *Nurs Ethics* **3**: 329–44

Waddell C (2001) So much research evidence, so little dissemination and uptake. *Evidence Based Mental Health* **4**: 3–5

Walters K (1990) Critical thinking, rationality and the vulcanization of students. *J Higher Educ* **61**: 448–67

Ward MF, Armstrong C, Lelliott P, Davies M (1999) Training, skills and caseloads of community mental health support workers involved in case management: evaluation from the initial UK demonstration sites. *J Psychiatr Ment Health Nurs* **6**: 187–97

Ward MF, Cutcliffe J, Gournay K (1999) *A review of research and practice development undertaken by nurses, midwives and health visitors to support people with mental health problems*. United Kingdom Central Council for Nurses, Midwives and Health Visitors, London

Ward MF, Cutcliffe J, Gournay K (2000) *The Nursing, Midwifery and Health Visiting Contribution to the Continuing Care of People with Mental Health Problems: A review and UKCC action plan*. United Kingdom Central Council for Nursing, Midwifery and Health Visiting, London

Ward MF, Jones J, Gorton S, Reed J (1999) The future of mental health nursing. *Nurs Times* **95**: 51–4

Ward MF, Jones M (1997) Evaluating the impact of in-patient bed reduction and community nurse increases in one English Mental Healthcare Trust. *J Adv Nurs* **26**: 937–45

Ward MF, Titchen A, Morrell C, McCormack B, Kitson A (1998) Using a supervisory framework to support and evaluate a multiproject practice development programme. *J Clin Nurs* **7**: 29–36

White E (April 1998) Methodological issues in national census research: The case of community mental health nursing in the UK, *Leading Edge. International Nursing Research Conference*. Edinburgh

White E, Brooker C (2001) The Fourth Quinquennial National Community Mental Health Nursing Census of England and Wales. *Int J Nurs Stud* **38**: 61–70

Wilkinson G (1992) The role of the practice nurse in the management of depression. *Int Rev Psychiatry* **4**: 311–15

Wooff K, Goldberg DP, Fryers T (1988) The practice of community psychiatric nursing and mental health social work in Salford. Some implications for community care. *Br J Psychiatry* **152**: 783–92

# Appendix: Key points

## Example one: Parahoo (1999)

❖ The study identified the limited familiarity with and use of research by many psychiatric/mental health nurses; yet it also highlighted the same nurses' enthusiasm to make use of research. Consequently, the need for support/facilities (of various types) to help these nurses become 'research-based' practitioners is reiterated.

❖ Members felt that the differences between 'evidence-based' and 'researched-based' practice were not made clear in the paper, and this important difference needed to be highlighted.

❖ Members were uncomfortable with the implicit assumption concerning the hegemony of RCTs and it was felt that it would have been more appropriate to point out that different research methods produce different types of knowledge and are suitable for different research questions. With no one method being 'better' than another.

## Example two: Pullen *et al* (1999)

❖ Given the wide range of confounding variables and interactions of variables that could impact on patterns of drug/alcohol use, and its alleged relationship with religiosity, it may not be wise to posit such relationships as a straightforward 'cause and effect' hypothesis.

❖ Given the well established relationship between drug/alcohol abuse and 'religiosity', the value or purpose of another study to confirm further what already appears to be known to be in question. Particularly, when many unanswered, yet relevant questions within this substantive area remain.

❖ While there is an abundance of literature that lends support to the argument of attending to one's 'spiritual' needs and there is evidence that such needs can be met by engaging in 'religious' activities, it would be inaccurate to consider religious activities as the only way of meeting such needs.

# Example three: Hannigan (1999)

❖ Members stated that the sampling strategy could be regarded as one of the strengths of the paper since it sampled the total population (ie. each education centre that provided the CPN course). Furthermore, it achieved a response rate of 82%, which is high for a postal return survey: the members felt that such results could be taken to be indicative or representative of the total population.

❖ While the paper included some discussion of the findings, there was a distinct view that perhaps the author had not asked certain 'big' questions within the discussion, and perhaps the study missed an opportunity.

❖ Members felt that the apparent honesty of the author, both with regard to the limitations and reporting of the study could be regarded as one of the strengths of the paper, as this honesty was evident throughout the paper.

# Example four: Fletcher (1999)

❖ The paper draws further attention to the potential problems associated with 'custodial' methods of 'constant observations', re-emphasises the difficulties some nurses have with such methods of 'care' and illustrates the potential value of care approaches that focus on engaging such clients. Furthermore, it reiterates that care of the suicidal client is a particularly skilful, yet demanding activity.

❖ Consideration must be given to ethical issues in all research, and research with vulnerable groups (eg. mental health clients) may present particular ethical concerns which must be addressed. Failure to do so can be seen to be undermining the credibility of the research.

❖ The paper adds support to the argument that service user feedback/data should be included in studies that are concerned with service evaluation or research.

# Example five: Allen (1998)

❖ While the author claimed to have undertaken a qualitative analysis of the comments written in response to the questions, members felt that the author did not appear to have undertaken, what could accurately be described as qualitative research. Of particular concern was the authors claim that counting the same word or phrase constituted qualitative data analysis.

❖ While the research did not uncover any new insights with this research, the findings did reiterate theoretical (and valuable) positions, in particular the importance in ensuring that advanced nursing roles do not become a 'dumping ground' for practices no longer desired by medics.

❖ Members acknowledged that the conclusions were partially justified by the results. However, in the light of the methodological limitations, the possible unrepresentative nature of the sample; the absence of any reliability or validity measures; and the cross-sectional nature of the study, it may have been more appropriate for the author to phrase his conclusion in a tentative manner, rather than the 'assertive' manner used in the paper.

## Example six: Pejlert *et al* (1998)

❖ The structure and arrangement of the information contained in the paper was thought to be somewhat equivocal and confusing.

❖ The study highlighted an important issue that is repeatedly highlighted. In that a study that discusses the opinions or elicited the experiences of recipients of care, illustrates that nurses who were kind and understanding, were equated with providing good care.

❖ The paper contains too much tautological and unnecessary text and consequently this text may diminish the impact of the overall message of the paper.

## Example seven: Veeramah (1995)

❖ There is evidence of only limited discussion of the implications for nursing practice/theory/research. Members highlighted that there are so many relevant issues relating to this matter and the findings of the research, and felt that the researcher rather 'sold himself/herself short.'

❖ The paper does make specific recommendations and these were felt to have sense and value. However, while they appear to have some resonance with the results, they do not appear to have been uncovered through the research process. That is, many of the recommendations do not appear to have evolved directly from the results and consequently, the members felt that some of these had an element of impracticability.

❖ The paper was reasonably well written and it appears to have been written purposefully to enable the reader's understanding. (Indeed, the author makes such claims within the paper.) Consequently, one of the strengths of the paper can be considered to be the absence of unnecessary jargon or tautology.

# Example eight: Whittington and Wykes (1994)

❖ While the paper raises some interesting points and perhaps indicates several possible directions for future research, the model presented and subsequently tested (in part) in the paper was felt to be somewhat simplistic and provided little understanding of the complex interplay of processes, dynamics and variables which appear to be involved in client violence, nurses' behaviours and nurses' feelings.

❖ The paper addresses an important substantive issue and was considered to be 'brave' for its willingness to broach these potentially awkward and often emotive subjects, such as client violence and the nurse's role in perpetuating this violence.

❖ The paper contains important implications for psychiatric/mental health nursing practice, yet these were largely implicit in the paper, and perhaps would have benefited from being made explicit and from undergoing a more rigorous discussion.

# Index

**Sarah Mallory** grew up in the West Country, England, telling stories. She moved to Yorkshire with her young family, but after nearly thirty years of living in a farmhouse on the Pennines she has now moved to live by the sea in Scotland. Sarah is an award-winning novelist, with more than twenty books published by Mills & Boon Historical. She loves to hear from readers, and you can reach her via her website at: sarahmallory.com.

# THE NIGHT SHE MET THE DUKE

Sarah Mallory

MILLS & BOON

First published in Great Britain 2023
by Mills & Boon, an imprint of HarperCollins*Publishers* Ltd,
1 London Bridge Street, London, SE1 9GF

www.harpercollins.co.uk

HarperCollins*Publishers*, Macken House, 39/40 Mayor Street Upper, Dublin 1, D01 C9W8, Ireland

The Night She Met the Duke © 2023 Sarah Mallory

ISBN: 978-0-263-30510-4

04/23

## Chapter One

Midnight, and Prudence Clifford was still wide
awake. It was exceptionally warm for April and the
drawing room curtains had not been drawn, allowing a welcome draught of cool air to come in through
the open window, stirring the muslin under-curtains.

It had been a busy day. Pru had spent the morning assisting the doctors at the Bath Infirmary before joining her aunt to go shopping in Milsom Street.
Mrs Clifford had retired soon after dinner, but Pru
remained in the drawing room, reading the book she
had recently chosen from the circulating library. The
plot might be silly but she always enjoyed the adven-
tures that befell the heroines of Gothic novels. Her
own world seemed very dull in comparison. She was
dull, too. She knew that because she had been described as such.

The incident had happened at the last assembly
she attended before coming to Bath. It was almost
four years ago, but she had never forgotten it. She

had danced with a young gentleman who was visiting Melksham and later heard him talking about her to his fashionable friends: 'Ah, you mean Miss Prudence Clifford, a lady as dull as her name!'

Pru had just come out of mourning for her beloved brother, Walter, which somehow made the gentleman's words even more painful.

Walter had died following a riding accident shortly after his twenty-first birthday and it had been a blow to them all, but especially to Pru. Barely twelve months separated them and it was Pru who nursed Walter through the final weeks of his life. The pain and grief of his death had never left her. Also, with the loss of the heir, Papa's estate would now pass to a distant cousin and Pru's parents expected her, as the eldest of four daughters, to make a good match.

Prudence never shone in a crowd. Her height made her shy. She was too reserved, and the young man's words rang only too true with her. When, some weeks later, Aunt Minerva, relict of Papa's only brother and with no family of her own, declared she was going to hire a companion to live with her in Bath, Pru offered her services, thus giving her younger and far more lively sisters their chance to enter society.

Pru had never regretted her decision. Two of her sisters were very soon betrothed and she was genuinely happy for them. Now, at five-and-twenty, she had given up all hopes of marriage and life in Bath suited her very well. Aunt Minerva was kindness itself and a most undemanding companion. She made no objection to her niece's efforts for the Parish Widows and Orphans Fund or her other charitable causes. She even allowed her to spend two mornings each week helping at the infirmary. Now Pru was not only dull but *worthy*. A very lowering thought.

Deep in her book, an exciting point where the heroine is alone in a haunted house, Pru was disturbed by a sudden noise. The dull thud sounded very much as if it had come from Mrs Triscombe's house, a few doors away. The dashing widow was notorious for holding regular card parties that went on well into the morning. Pru would have dismissed the noise, except that the thin muslin at her windows moved with a soft sigh, as if an outer door had been opened.

She glanced at the clock. It was nearly one, but despite the hour she did not immediately conclude that the disturbance was intruders or a ghostly spectre. She thought, quite sensibly, that one of the servants had slipped in or out of the house. However, she could not be easy until she had been downstairs to make sure they had not left the door unlocked.

Lighting her bedroom candle, she made her way downstairs to the hall. The main door was securely bolted and she went on down to the basement. There was just one bedroom below stairs and that was allocated to their only manservant, Nicholas. Light spilled out from his open door and when Pru glanced in she saw the man lying fully dressed on the bed, one arm hanging down towards the empty brandy bottle on the floor.

She stepped into the room and shook Nicholas by the shoulder, but he merely shrugged her off and went on snoring gently. Pru felt a spurt of irritation. He must have come down the area steps and in through the kitchen. A quick glance showed her the ribbon of light along the bottom of the kitchen door and her irritation turned to anger. If the man had left the kitchen lamps burning, it was very likely that he had also left the door unbolted. Pursing her lips, Pru gripped the candleholder a little tighter and went into the kitchen.

The outer door was firmly closed, which would have been a relief, if there had not been a stranger sitting at the table.

## Chapter Two

'What is the meaning of this?'

At Pru's outraged exclamation the stranger looked up. Her first thought had been that he was a friend of Nicholas, but she quickly changed her mind. A fashionable curly brimmed beaver hat lay beside him on the table and his dark coat was perfectly tailored to fit over his broad shoulders. His white silk waistcoat was exquisitely embroidered and as he raised his head, the candlelight glinted on the diamond nestling in the folds of his dishevelled neckcloth. Despite his craggy features and the dark stubble covering his face, this was no servant.

He did not get up, merely glowered at her from beneath his black brows.

'The gate to your area steps was open.'

'That may well be so, but it does not excuse your coming in here.'

'I fell down the damned steps! Since the door was

open, I thought I might as well come in this way, rather than go back up to the front door.'

'But it is *one o'clock in the morning*!' she retorted.

'Aye. The night is still young.'

From the faint slurring of his words, she suspected he was not quite sober. She blew out her candle and placed it on the table.

She said coldly, 'I would be obliged if you would leave the way you came. Immediately.'

'Oh, I don't think so. You see, I am in dire need of diversion.'

He pushed himself to his feet and Pru quickly stepped aside, keeping the full width of the kitchen table between them.

'Go,' she commanded. 'Get out!'

'Ah, you are thinking I have no money.' He glanced down at his clothes. 'I grant you I am a little dusty from the fall, but be assured, I can afford to pay for my pleasures.' He threw a heavy purse upon the table. 'There, does that make my presence more acceptable?'

'Not in the least,' Pru retorted. 'If you were a gentleman, you would go away this minute.'

'Well, I'm not. I am a duke—'

She gave a scornful laugh. 'Even worse!'

'For heaven's sake, ma'am, I have only come here to play.'

He took a step towards Pru and she snatched up the poker from the hearth behind her.

'Stay away from me!' she warned him. 'Get out now, or, or I will call my manservant.'

The stranger scowled. His black hair had fallen across his brow and he pushed it back with an impatient hand.

'Hell and damnation, woman, I have no designs upon your virtue! I want to play *cards*.'

'Cards!' Enlightenment dawned, but Pru did not lower the poker. 'Then you have the wrong house.'

His dark eyes stared at her. 'This is not Sally Triscombe's house?'

'It most certainly is not.'

'I'll be damned.'

She winced at his language but replied in chilling accents. 'Very likely, but not here. Now please, go away.'

He ignored her.

'This *is* Kilve Street, is it not?' He rubbed a hand across his eyes. 'And Sal Triscombe has a house here. A widow lady,' he added. 'Very attractive and... accommodating, I am told.'

'How dare you suggest I would know any such creature.'

'Are you telling me you don't?'

Pru bit her lip. She had heard rumours, of course, but no lady would discuss such matters with a strange man. He was looking at her, expecting an answer.

She said carefully, 'I believe such a person might live in the house two doors along.'

He nodded, but the effort seemed to weaken him. He staggered.

'I beg your pardon,' he said, leaning on the table to support himself. 'I am damnably drunk you know.'

'I gathered that much.' Good heavens, what was she doing, talking with this man?

'I have been drinking with my friends since dawn.'

'I have no wish to know about your celebrations.'

'Oh, I wasn't celebrating,' he told her, his lip curling. 'Drowning my sorrows. Although I didn't tell my friends that.'

But Pru was no longer listening. His head was bowed and he was clearly struggling to stay on his feet.

'When did you last eat?' she demanded.

'I cannot remember. Not today. We broke our fast with wine this morning...'

'Good heavens.' She waved him back towards the chair. 'Sit down.'

'What?'

'You need sustenance before you go anywhere.'

'Nonsense!'

'Believe me you *do*,' she told him. 'I would not wager on you getting more than a few yards in your present state. You are far more likely to collapse and be set upon by footpads. Sit down and I will find something for you to eat.'

With an effort he raised his head and looked at her. 'Why should you do that?'

'Because I would not want your death on my con-science!'

With a shrug he lowered himself gingerly onto the chair and Pru bustled about, fetching various foods from the larder. She set before him a knife, fork and a plate upon which she had placed the remains of a game pie. She found bread, cheese and a few jars of pickles and put them on the table before going off to retrieve a ham from the larder.

'Are you going to join me?' he asked, as she began to carve the ham.

'No.'

'But you are going to watch me.'

'I certainly do not intend to leave you alone here. Who knows what mischief you might make?' She placed two thick slices of ham on his plate. 'There. Make a start on that and I will fetch you a tankard of ale.'

'What, no wine?'

'I wish to make you sober, not more drunk.'

'Then at least pour a drink for yourself.'

Pru was about to make some cutting reply, but she stopped, realising that she would indeed like some-thing to fortify herself.

Five minutes later she was sitting opposite the stranger at the table, sipping at a glass of small beer while her companion feasted on the cold meats and pickles she had provided. How prosaic she was. How ordinary. The heroine of her novel would have fainted off to find an intruder in her house. She would not have *fed* him.

'What do you find so amusing?' Her companion's voice cut through these wry thoughts. She looked up to find him watching her.

He waved a knife in her direction. 'You were smiling.'

'Not intentionally.'

'Perhaps not.' He studied her. 'Ah, I see now. Your mouth curves up naturally at the corners.'

'Yes.' She looked away, saying with a faint sigh, 'It is a fault.'

'It is as if you are always on the edge of laughter. How can that be a bad thing?'

'My mouth is too wide.'

'I do not think so.'

Pru realised this was not a proper conversation to be having with a strange man and did not reply.

'May I know to whom I am indebted for this supper?' he asked her presently.

'To my aunt, Mrs Clifford. This is her house.'

His eyes narrowed. 'It is your name I wish to know.'

'I am Miss Clifford.'

He raised his brows and Pru firmly closed her lips, determined not to tell him her first name. However, after a few moments curiosity got the better of her and she broke the silence.

'And who are you, sir?'

'Garrick Chauntry. Duke of Hartland.'

'So, you really are a nobleman.'

'You did not believe me?'

'You are an intruder. And very drunk.'

'Yet you do not appear to be afraid of me.'

With a start Pru realised he was right. Even when she had snatched up the poker it had been in anger not fear. How foolish, when she had been warned since birth about the dangers of being alone with any man other than a relative. She should have been terrified and screamed for help. Although, what good would that have done? The only manservant was lying in a drunken stupor in the next room. She was clearly lacking in imagination.

*...as dull as her name!*

The echo taunted her and she replied with some asperity. 'Do you prefer females who fall into hysterics at the first hint of danger?'

'Not at all. I find them a damned nuisance.'

That sounded as if he had a great deal of experience in the matter. Pru wanted to ask the question, but quickly squashed the idea. It would be safer to change the subject.

'What happened to your friends? You said earlier you were drinking with them.'

'I had another engagement. Said I would meet them at Mrs Triscombe's.'

'And you are only now on your way there?'

'I decided to fortify myself in a tavern before my appointment, then realised I was too drunk to keep it.'

He paused, his mouth thinning to a grim line. Pru had the impression he was looking inside himself and did not like what he saw there. After a moment he shrugged.

'I dashed off a note, excusing myself and saying I would call in the morning. Then I broached another bottle. Or perhaps two, I can't remember. I thought the walk to Kilve Street would sober me. Clearly it did not work.'

'I am astonished you are not lying unconscious in a gutter!'

'I deserve to be.'

She was aware of a sudden stab of pity.

She said, 'Would it help to tell me about it?' He looked up at that, surprised, and Pru flushed. 'I work with a number of charitable bodies who deal with… distressed persons. Some people find it easier to talk to a stranger, someone they will never meet again. I assure you I am very good at keeping confidences.'

'Is that part of your good works, listening to other people's tales of woe?'

'Yes. Sometimes it helps them.'

'What a saint you are.'

He smiled unexpectedly, softening his harsh features and looking suddenly much younger. Much more attractive. Pru felt something contract, deep inside and she quickly pushed back her chair.

'Your tankard is empty,' she said, rising. 'Let me refill it.'

When she returned, he took the tankard with a word of thanks and glanced up at her.

'Do you really wish to know how I come to be in this state?'

*No. Go back to your friends. You are no concern of mine!*

Pru stifled her uncharitable thoughts, and the alarm bells clamouring in her head. She sat down, folding her hands in her lap.

'If you wish to tell me.'

Silence followed. The duke stared into his tankard for a long, long moment.

'I was celebrating my forthcoming betrothal,' he said at last. 'Yesterday—no, the day before—I spoke to the lady's father and received his permission to pay my addresses. I was to go back yesterday and make my offer to the lady.'

'That was the appointment you spoke of.'

'Yes.' A muscle worked in his cheek. 'I was too much the coward. I got damnably drunk instead.'

Pru hesitated.

'Forgive me,' she said slowly, 'but if you are so reluctant...'

'Why offer for her?' He huffed out a breath. 'We had an agreement. The poor girl has been waiting for me to propose these past ten years.'

'I see.'

The look he threw at her said he doubted it.

He went on. 'The match was arranged when Annabelle was in her cradle. It is a common enough tale, two families joined in a marriage of convenience. When she reached sixteen, I raised the matter with Miss Speke herself, to confirm she was happy with the arrangement.' He stopped to take a long draught from his tankard. 'We agreed I should propose on her next birthday.'

'What happened?'

'I was...*obliged* to go abroad.'

'And that was ten years ago?' Pru frowned. 'You have been out of the country for ten years?'

'Yes.' His shrug was eloquent of dejection, despair. 'I had nothing to come home for. I had been a damned fool and I assumed Annabelle's parents had dismissed any thought of an engagement between us. Viscount Tirrill was always a stickler for propriety. Then, two months ago, I received a letter from Lady Tirrill. She informed me that her daughter was still waiting for me to propose. That is why I came to Bath. The family are staying here at present. Do you know them?'

Pru shook her head. 'I know *of* them. The viscount is a subscriber to the infirmary.'

'The what?'

'The Bath Dispensary and Infirmary. It provides medicine and treatment for the poor and destitute of Bath. I am one of the volunteers there. However, I have never met Lord Tirrill or his family. My aunt and I do not move in such exalted circles.'

'No matter. The point is that Miss Speke thinks herself as good as engaged to me and, after talking with her father, we agreed the betrothal must go ahead.'

Pru could not help giving a little whisper of dismay. The duke flicked a derisive glance in her direction.

'You disagree, ma'am?'

'I think,' she said, choosing her words carefully, 'your behaviour this day shows you do not want this union.'

'It is not a case of what I *want*. The woman has remained single upon my account for the past ten years. At six-and-twenty it is highly unlikely she will receive another offer. I cannot in honour do anything *but* marry her!'

He dropped his head in his hands. Pru waited in silence. After a few moments he recovered. He sat up and straightened his shoulders.

'I have ignored my obligations for too long. It is time I faced up to them. Tomorrow I shall call in Royal Crescent. I will beg Miss Speke's forgiveness and do my duty.'

Pru thought that he was far more at ease now he had made his decision. He began to refill his plate and appeared to have forgotten she was sitting opposite. The food was also having an effect, for he looked much better than when he had first arrived. The harsh lines around his mouth had softened and that lock of black hair had fallen back across his brow, softening his rugged face.

It was easy to imagine him as a youth, wild and impetuous. Pru guessed that even now he was no more than thirty. Society would consider him to be in his prime, while a woman was unmarriageable by five-and-twenty.

'You look very serious.' He interrupted her reverie. 'What are you thinking?'

She smiled. 'That you have probably lived a very interesting life.'

'Not the term I would use for it!'

'But I have never left England,' she told him. 'You spend ten years on a Grand Tour—'

'It was hardly that! I was in France when the Treaty of Amiens ended in '03. Fortunately, I had good friends and sufficient funds to escape to Austria.' He grimaced. 'It was far from a pleasure jaunt.'

'Then why did you go abroad?' she asked, puzzled. 'And why stay away for so long?'

He pushed his empty plate away and raised his eyes to hers.

'Do you not know? I killed a man.'

# Chapter Three

Garrick saw the lady recoil in surprise and horror. Confound it, he need not have told her that. He must be a great deal more intoxicated than he had thought.

He should finish his beer and quit this house. An apology for the intrusion, a word of thanks for the food and he could go. He could leave this peaceful room and the woman sitting so quietly across the table from him. Strange, he felt more at home here than he had anywhere else for the past ten years.

She said, quietly, 'Was it a duel?

'Yes. No. Not exactly. It was my father.' His hand clenched hard around the tankard. 'I killed my father.'

He looked up to find she was regarding him with painful intensity. She looked very pale in the candle-light but it was not revulsion he read in her clear grey eyes, it was bewilderment.

*Get out, man, now. No need to torture yourself with all that again.*

'Go on, Your Grace.'

Her soft voice prompted him like a priest in the confessional and he found the words spilling out.

'I grew up like so many of my kind, too much money and no occupation. At nineteen I was in town and living solely for pleasure. I took a lover. Or rather, she took *me*. I was too naive to see the trick.' He broke off and glanced at the woman sitting opposite. 'You are not married. I should not be telling you this!'

Her shoulders lifted a little. 'I have lived in Bath for almost four years and the gossipmongers here have no such scruples. I doubt your tale will be any worse than the salacious stories I have heard from them. Continue, sir.'

He hesitated but she nodded to him to go on and he wanted to do so. Odd, that he should now trust a stranger with secrets he had kept for a decade.

'Her husband found us *in flagrante* and challenged me to a duel. He hinted that we could settle the matter, for a large sum. Naturally, I refused.' His lip curled in self-disdain. 'I was too besotted to pay him off. I thought...' He took another draught of ale. '*All for love and the world well lost.* Ain't that the saying? I thought it was love. I knew the fellow was a crack shot but was determined not to back down. His wife begged me to pay. She said if I did not have the funds I should go to my father, but I could not do that. He was not in good health and I could not burden him. Even when she said she would rather give me up for ever than see me dead, I was not to be swayed from what I saw as a matter of honour. We met on the Heath and... I shot him. A freak chance, I suppose. I was certainly no expert in those days.'

Garrick stopped, reliving the chill of that misty morning, the bone-melting fear that had almost crippled him as he faced his opponent. His stupefaction when his bullet found its mark while he was unscathed.

He went on. 'Word was all over town within days. The fellow was not expected to live and my father insisted I fly the country. I delayed only long enough to beg my mistress to come with me.' He stopped. 'Damme, but this is a sordid business!'

'Having heard thus much I should like to know the rest,' she replied placidly. 'Did she agree to go with you?'

Her calm, melodious voice was like balm upon his spirits.

'No. I found out *la belle* Helene was nothing but a—' He drew in a breath. 'I discovered the whole affair had been a sham. I was a credulous fool, besotted by a scheming woman. She was not unhappy in her marriage, but she was damned furious with me for wounding her husband! It turns out they had been filling their coffers for years by duping young men and then allowing the young fools or their families to buy them off.'

'That is dreadful. But why were they allowed to do it—did no one stand up to them?'

'No. Most preferred to pay up, or they asked their

families to do so. Those who did agree to a duel paid a heavy price. At best they were wounded, at worst… either way no one wanted their humiliation made public.' His lip curled in disdain. 'And the devil looks after his own, it seems. The husband recovered. He inherited a baronetcy a few years ago, and a fortune to go with it. He and his lady live in London now, the height of respectability.' He scowled. 'On the surface, at least.'

'Never mind them. What did *you* do after the duel?'

'What could I do? I fled to Paris. I had intended to return if the fellow survived, but by the time my mother wrote, telling me the fellow was expected to make a full recovery we were at war with France again and I was stranded in Austria. Also.' He swallowed, forcing the words out. 'She told me my father was too ill to suffer any more worry. She said I should remain abroad. I was never more to darken their doors.'

'But surely that was written in the heat of the moment,' she exclaimed. 'She could not mean it.'

'Oh, she meant it.' He ground the words out between clenched jaws. 'After that, all my letters were returned unopened, and when the old duke died two years ago, I learned of it via the lawyers, who also informed me of my mother's wish that I should not return to Hartland Hall before she had removed to the Dower House. It is clear she blamed me for the old duke's death.'

'Forgive me, but you said he was already in poor

health when you left the country,' she pointed out, adding gently, 'It was not your fault, sir.'

'I should have been there.' It was the first time Garrick had spoken of his regrets to anyone. He went on, 'Rather than raising hell in town I should have been a more responsible son.'

'You were very young—'

He interrupted her sharply. 'Pray do not try to excuse my actions, madam. You know nothing about it!' He saw her eyes widen and it sobered him a little. 'I beg your pardon, I should not have ripped up at you like that.'

'No, but it is understandable.' She replied calmly. 'Pray go on. What did you do, after you received the letter from your mother?'

'What could I do? I took her at her word and remained in Vienna. Although I confess it suited me to stay.'

He fell into a brooding silence and Pru observed the play of emotions flickering across his countenance. She guessed his memories were painful and her heart went out to him.

'And now you are in Bath,' she prompted him.

He started, as if he had quite forgotten her presence.

'Yes. I came to England after receiving the letter from Lady Tirrill and now I am in Bath to do my duty.' He picked up his ale. 'There, now you have the whole, unedifying tale.'

'I am so very sorry.'

His lifted a hand, as if to brush away her words.

'It is your turn to talk, Miss Clifford. Tell me about yourself.'

She shook her head. 'There is nothing to say that would not bore you.'

'Humour me.'

'I have done nothing of interest.'

He looked at her over the rim of his tankard.

'Come now, having given you my life history, it is only right that you should do the same! Let us begin with your name.'

Realising he was trying to lighten the mood, she capitulated.

'It is Prudence.'

'And why are you unwed, Prudence?'

'I am too old for marriage.'

He sat forward in his chair, frowning at her. 'That I will not allow.'

'I think you must, Your Grace. I am five-and-twenty.'

'Positively ancient.' His eyes gleamed with gentle amusement.

'Yes. I am but a year younger than Lord Tirrill's daughter.'

He acknowledged that with a nod. 'You have no family, save your aunt?

'On the contrary. My aunt needed a companion and I was happy to fill that role, leaving my parents to concentrate upon finding husbands for my three younger sisters. There are no living sons, you see, and it is imperative that the girls should marry. Or at least, that one of them marries well.'

'And has it worked?'

She smiled. 'Yes. The older two are married and the youngest, Jemima, is now betrothed to a very respectable gentleman of good fortune.'

'Well done, Jemima. And well done you, Miss Prudence Clifford, for your noble self-sacrifice.'

'It is nothing of the kind,' she retorted. 'You are not to think I am unhappy. Aunt Minerva is very good to me and we go on extremely well. There is plenty to entertain one in Bath, you know. We visit the theatre regularly and go to the Pump Room, where my aunt drinks the waters.'

'And do you attend the balls at the Assembly Rooms?'

'Yes, occasionally.'

'Then I do not understand why you are still single.'

Her chin went up. 'Not every young lady is looking for a husband.'

'That has not been my experience, whenever I have been obliged to attend a ball.'

'But you are a duke,' she replied sweetly. 'And therefore *extremely* eligible.'

'That's put me in my place!' he retorted, grinning. 'But tell me truthfully, do you not want to marry?'

'Why should I? My aunt and I live here very comfortably. I have my friends, plenty to entertain me. I have no wish to be paraded like a brood mare before every man on the lookout for a wife. Besides that, I have a little money saved and my aunt has made me her heir. I need not fear the future.'

The duke was frowning at her. Pru met his eyes steadily, refusing to admit that she did sometimes hope that life had more in store for her than dwindling into a lonely old maid. When at length she did look away, she noticed that the darkness outside the window had lightened to grey.

'Goodness, it is almost dawn! You should go, before the maids come downstairs.' She jumped to her feet, gesturing towards the table. 'And take your purse with you.'

'Keep it. For your trouble.'

'I have no need of your money.'

'Then give it to one of your charities,' he retorted, rising. 'It would have cost me a great deal more than that tonight, had I reached Mrs Triscombe's house.'

'You do not intend to go there now?'

'No, I am going back to the Pelican.' He straightened his shoulders. 'I need to make myself presentable for my interview with Miss Speke. I cannot change the past, but I can put right the ill I have done her. Once the knot is tied, I can go to Hartland and set my estates to rights.'

'Then I wish you good fortune, Your Grace.'

'Thank you. And I beg your pardon.'

'For what?'

'Burdening you with my story.'

Pru said lightly, 'It is forgotten already.' She walked over to the outer door and opened it. 'You may trust me, no one shall ever hear of it from my lips.'

He took her hand and held it, causing an unfamiliar fluttering in her breast.

'You are a remarkable woman, Miss Prudence Clifford.' He grinned suddenly. 'If I were not about to propose to another woman…'

The teasing glint in his eyes turned the fluttering to a drumbeat, robbing her of breath. In the early morning light, she could see that his eyes were not black, but a deep green, like the light in a forest at the height of summer. She wanted to stand there for ever, with him holding her hand, smiling down at her.

The fanciful thoughts unsettled Pru and she shook her head to dispel them.

'Goodbye, Your Grace,' she said, exerting every nerve to keep calm.

'Farewell, ma'am.' He brushed her knuckles with his lips. 'And yet, Bath is a small place. It is possible we may meet again.'

The kiss on her fingers made her heart leap most alarmingly and she hastily pulled her hand free.

'It is better we do not,' she told him. 'How would we explain our acquaintance?'

'Yes, that could ruin everything, could it not? However, you do not have much to fear. I shall not be in Bath long. Lord Tirrill has already drawn up plans for the marriage. He wants a quiet ceremony, as soon as possible, at his country seat in Hampshire. Understandable, when my reputation is so badly tarnished.'

'And you have no say in the proceedings?' asked Pru, unable to stop herself.

His mouth twisted. 'It matters little to me when or where we marry. In fact, the less pomp the better! But I should not be troubling you any further with my concerns. Goodbye, Miss Clifford.'

With that he jammed his hat on his dark head, ran lightly up the area stairs and disappeared.

Prudence stood in the doorway, looking up at the now empty pavement. A single star was visible in the morning sky, a tiny spot of silvery light. She pressed the back of her hand to her cheek, remembering the soft touch of his lips on her skin. Then, with a sigh, she stepped inside and closed the door.

## Chapter Four

Garrick strode back to the Pelican feeling much better than he had any right to be. He had spent a whole day drinking as a way of avoiding an unpleasant duty. He had felt like a scoundrel, the heartless rogue his mother accused him of being. By the time he reached Kilve Street and fell down those steps he had concluded it would be better for everyone if he jumped off Pulteney Bridge and put paid to his existence.

Then he had been visited by an angel, a tall, graceful woman with kind grey eyes and a warm smile. He should have known immediately this was not the house he sought. The lady's demure gown covered her from neck to ankle, although the thin green muslin could not disguise her excellent figure. Did she know that? he wondered. No, Prudence Clifford used no arts to attract a man. She wore her light brown hair wound neatly about her head. It was a plain, no-nonsense style, but he had noticed how the candles sparked the occasional glint of gold from those soft tresses.

He thought back to the way she had defended herself. By heaven, she had wielded that heavy poker in fine style! Her outrage at finding a strange man in her house was understandable, what was not so clear was why she had then sat him down and fed him. Did she not know what a dangerous situation she was in, alone with a drunkard in the middle of the night?

'Damned foolish,' he muttered, casting his eyes up to the single star twinkling in the lightening sky. 'That was not very sensible at all, despite your name, Miss Prudence Clifford!'

Prudence. A smile tugged at his lips. Was there some morally uplifting tale about Prudence and Despair? If not, there should be. She had listened to him patiently, not judging, and by the time he had finished telling her his woes he realised just how pathetic he sounded, and what he must do about it. He had not only wasted ten years of his life but Annabelle Speke's life, too. It was time to face up to his responsibilities.

As he reached the end of the street he slowed, wondering if he should go back and check that Prudence had bolted the door against any further intruders. No, he decided. The best thing he could do for Miss Prudence Clifford was to keep away from her.

The maids were already at work in the Pelican when Garrick returned to this room. He locked his door and went to bed, expecting to sleep at least until noon.

However, by ten o'clock he was awake again, refreshed and eager to get on with what must be done.

An hour later he was on his way to Royal Crescent, dressed in a new coat of Bath superfine over fresh white linen with tight-fitting pantaloons and glossy Hessians. His curly brimmed beaver had been brushed clean and now sat on his head, which was still a trifle heavy from yesterday's excesses. How much worse it would have been, had he not been rescued by the angelic Miss Clifford. He wanted to thank her in some way, but reluctantly dismissed the idea, knowing that any communication risked being misinterpreted.

He was admitted to Viscount Tirrill's house by a harassed-looking footman who escorted him up to the drawing room. As he crossed the hall, Garrick was aware of voices coming from His Lordship's study. He could hear the shrill tones of a female and felt a trickle of apprehension run down his spine. Was his non-appearance yesterday the cause of such discord?

The footman left him alone in the empty drawing room. Garrick walked across to the mirror, running a nervous finger around his collar. Having assured himself that his cravat was unsullied and that his countenance bore no sign of his drunken revelries, he moved restlessly across to the window, unable to shake off the feeling that something was amiss.

At that moment the door opened and Viscount Tirrill came in.

'My lord Duke. Good day to you, sir!'

Garrick bowed, trying to ignore the obsequious formality of the greeting.

'Thank you, although I do not deserve such a warm welcome after my failure to present myself yesterday. I am sure you must be wondering—'

'Oh, no, Your Grace, not at all. Your note explained everything. Urgent business…unavoidably detained.' The viscount gave a nervous laugh. 'Happens to us all. Think nothing of it.'

'But I do think of it, sir. It was very wrong of me to disappoint you. And your daughter.' He forced his stiff lips into a smile. 'I trust I can persuade Miss Speke to forgive me, if I might have the honour of a few words with her.'

'Yes, yes, all in good time,' replied his host, clearly ill at ease. 'Will you not sit down, Your Grace. A glass of wine, perhaps?'

'Thank you, but no.' Garrick hesitated, then he said bluntly, 'My lord, has Miss Speke changed her mind?'

'Changed her mind? No, no, Your Grace. Nothing like that, I assure you.' The viscount gave a nervous laugh and there was no doubting his relief when the door opened and Lady Tirrill entered the room. 'Ah, there you are, dear lady. Do come and greet His Grace!'

The viscountess was a sharp-faced woman of decided opinions and Garrick had always considered her the stronger of the two. Now, however, she came towards him twittering nervously. He refused her offer of refreshment but allowed himself to be persuaded to sit down. She was clearly labouring under some strong emotion and began to chatter on about the weather. In this she was diligently assisted by her husband and Garrick felt a traitorous flicker of hope in his chest as he interrupted the flow of inanities.

'Forgive me, but is something amiss? Could it be that Miss Speke no longer wishes to receive my addresses?' The look that passed between them confirmed his suspicions and he nodded. 'If that is the case, then it may be easily remedied…'

'No, no, we are all eager for the match, Your Grace, believe me,' cried Lord Tirrill, jumping to his feet. 'I am sure it can all be resolved in a twinkling, just as soon as Annabelle returns.'

'Returns?' Garrick pounced on the word. 'She is not here?'

The viscount glanced nervously at his wife, who was glaring at him. Garrick frowned. He had been very drunk when he wrote that message crying off from the first appointment, but he was sure he had said he would be calling again today.

'She—she was obliged to go out,' stammered Lady Tirrill, twisting her hands together. 'Quite, quite unexpected, but if you could call again tomorrow—'

Garrick said gently, 'Ma'am, are you quite sure Miss Speke is not avoiding me?' She made no reply and Garrick rose. 'I see. Then I shall not detain you any longer.'

The viscountess gave an angry cry.

'It is all your fault,' she shrieked at him, hunting for her handkerchief. 'If only you had called yesterday, this would not have happened. Everything would have been well!'

'My dear, hush.' Lord Tirrill cast an uneasy glance at the duke.

'I will *not* hush! Annabelle understood what was expected of her. She was perfectly resigned—I mean—'

Garrick interrupted her. 'I beg your pardon, ma'am, but I understood Miss Speke was expecting my offer. That she was very happy to accept it. I think it will be better for me to return again and speak to your daughter myself.' He added firmly, 'Alone.'

'That may not be possible!' snapped my lady, two spots of angry colour appearing on her thin cheeks.

An ominous silence followed and Garrick looked from her to the hapless viscount.

'Do you mean,' he said slowly, 'has she run off with another man?'

'No, no, Your Grace, nothing like that,' Lord Tirrill made haste to assure him, although he had to raise his voice to make himself heard over his wife's angry mutterings. 'She, um, she has gone into the country. With a friend.'

'Emily Undershaw!' Lady Speke fairly spat out the name. 'I knew that woman would be trouble, leading poor Annabelle astray with her independent ways!' She turned her angry countenance towards Garrick.

'She followed us here from Hampshire, Your Grace, filling Annabelle's head with silly notions!'

'A rich spinster,' explained her husband. 'Quite eccentric, of course.'

'And now they have gone off to W-Wales!' cried his lady.

'Wales!' Garrick's brows snapped together. 'Is she so anxious to avoid me?

'Yes!' Lady Speke buried her face in her handkerchief. 'And now they have some silly notion of setting up home together.'

'Hush, hush, my dear, it is all nonsense,' put in Lord Tirrill, hovering anxiously around his wife. 'It is all a tarradiddle designed to vex us.'

'Yes, yes, of course.' Lady Speke dried her eyes and turned to the duke. 'You have no need to worry, Your Grace, all this can be hushed up. We will fetch her back and beat some sense into her.'

'You will do nothing of the sort on my account, ma'am,' Garrick retorted. 'If Miss Speke is not minded to wed me then so be it. We shall say no more about the matter.'

He took his leave with the viscount following him down the stairs, repeating his ever more desperate assurances that it was all a misunderstanding.

'Please! My lord Duke, will you not reconsider?' he begged when they reached the entrance.

A wooden-faced footman handed Garrick his hat and gloves before jumping to open the door. The fellow must have heard every word his master had uttered. If Lord Tirrill had no qualms about speaking plainly in front of his servant, then neither did Garrick.

He said, 'I am very sorry, my lord. It is evident that Miss Speke has no wish to receive my proposal and there's an end to it.'

'But I have already drafted the announcement, Your Grace. What will people *say* if you cry off now?'

'How many have you told?'

The viscount wrung his hands. 'No one!'

'Then you may rely upon my discretion, sir. If word gets out it will not be from me. I shall not mention what has occurred here today to anyone. Good day to you, my lord.'

Garrick set off down the hill to the Pelican, feeling as if a heavy weight had been lifted from his shoulders. He did not doubt there would be some gossip, but it mattered little to him if everyone in Bath knew his prospective bride had run away rather than accept an offer. The main thing was that he was not obliged to marry a woman he did not care for.

He would go to Hartland, as soon as he had concluded his affairs in London. Once he had ascertained that his mother had removed to the Dower House, he could take up residence at Hartland Hall and begin to put the place in order. Heaven knows it needed some attention, if the reports he had received from his steward were correct. His other properties, too, must be inspected. There must be enough work to keep him occupied for years to come and, suddenly, he relished the challenge.

When he passed the end of Kilve Street he thought of Miss Clifford. He would dearly like to see her. To tell her what had happened, but it was impossible. He had given Lord Tirrill his word that he would not speak of it. Besides, Miss Clifford would not want to see him again. Much better that he leave Bath immediately and forget all about this sorry interlude.

# *Chapter Five*

Green eyes, smiling at her. Green eyes in a rugged face and an unruly lock of dark hair that insisted on flopping over his brow...

Prudence sighed as the dream faded and she opened her eyes to face another day. Not quite a dream. She had actually met such a man just a few short hours ago. A duke, no less. She smiled at the memory. A very brief encounter, no more than a few hours. They had done nothing but talk, and yet she felt that something had shifted inside her. She felt lighter, somehow. As if the cloud that had engulfed her since her brother's death had lifted a little.

Pru told no one about the duke's visit to the house, although her conscience was sorely tried when she sat down to breakfast and Aunt Minerva launched into a diatribe against the errant footman.

'Nicholas left the kitchen in *such* disorder last night, Pru, Cook was most put out! The best part of the ham was gone, as well as the last of the game pie and some of the cheese. To say nothing of the small beer, which is seriously depleted! Nicholas denies it, but since he does not remember anything, we cannot set any store by that.'

'Oh, dear,' murmured Pru.

She had done her best to tidy the kitchen, but clearly not well enough for her aunt's eagle-eyed cook, and there was nothing to be done about the missing food. She listened as her aunt continued.

'Cook also told me she found Nicholas unconscious on his bed this morning, having drunk the best part of the bottle of brandy we keep for medicinal purposes! He has begged her to give him a second chance but, really, Cook is adamant that he should go and I agree with her!'

'If he is truly repentant, then perhaps we might give him the benefit of the doubt this once,' suggested Pru, stifling a stab of guilt at not confessing the whole. 'We could impress upon him that he must mend his ways or be turned off.'

'No, no, Cook has the right of it. Why, what is the good of having a manservant if he is too drunk at night to protect us?'

'There is that,' agreed Pru, with feeling. After all, Nicholas had left the outer door open, which had resulted in the whole sorry business.

'Yes,' Aunt Minerva went on. 'We might have all

been murdered in our beds and Nicholas none the wiser.'

Prudence could not refute that argument, but her conscience insisted she defend the man. She suggested they should keep him on as long as he promised not to drink anything stronger than small beer in future. It took her some time to persuade Aunt Minerva, but eventually she succeeded. After that she tried to put the events of the night out of her mind, but it was difficult, because it was the most exciting thing that had ever happened to her.

For the next several days Prudence was constantly looking out for the Duke of Hartland. She went about her business as usual but when she accompanied Aunt Minerva to the Pump Room or strolled with her along Milsom Street, Garrick Chauntry was constantly on her mind.

She was torn between wanting to see him and hoping they would not meet. If anyone should guess they were acquainted and discover the truth it would be disastrous for her and it might also jeopardise the duke's betrothal to the Honourable Miss Speke. Not that there had been any news of that, but she recalled the duke had said the family did not look favourably upon their future son-in-law's reputation.

At the end of the week Pru bought the latest edition of the *Bath Chronicle* and took it off to the morning room, where she scanned it carefully.

'At last!'

She found a small paragraph announcing that Viscount Tirrill and his family had quit Bath and returned to their home in Hampshire. There was no mention of the Duke of Hartland, but she thought that was by design. From everything he had told her, she guessed that Miss Speke was determined to have him but, given his scandalous reputation, her loving parents were far less eager for the match, despite his rank. It was not an ideal situation, but she truly wished him well.

'Oh, my dear Prudence, such news!' Aunt Minerva came in, waving a letter. 'You will never guess!'

Smiling, Prudence laid aside the newspaper. 'No, so you must tell me.'

'I have this minute received a letter from my dearest friend, Jane Borcaster.'

Pru raised her brows. She knew of Lady Borcaster, a friend her aunt had known since girlhood, but she had never heard her mentioned in such glowing terms before. Aunt Minerva glanced at the letter again, as if reminding herself of its contents.

'She has invited us to London! You will recall that her daughter is married to a diplomat, Sir Timothy Flowers, and they are gone out of the country until at least the spring of next year. Jane is therefore alone in town and thought we might like to join her, to see all the celebrations that are planned to take place in the capital this summer.' She hurried across the room to sit down on the sofa beside Pru. 'As you know, a host of foreign dignitaries is coming to London in June to celebrate the defeat of that monster, Bonaparte. And then there is the Grand Jubilee in August, for the centenary of the House of Hanover! Dear Jane has invited us to remain with her for the duration!'

Pru smiled politely. Privately she thought London in summer would be even more uncomfortable than Bath, where the streets could be white-hot. Aunt Minerva went on.

'I quite understand when she says that she does not want to be rattling around in her London house all alone. She lives in Brook Street, you know. The western end, of course, almost Grosvenor Square!'

She stopped, clearly waiting for a reaction from Prudence, who murmured a few words which she hoped would indicate that she was impressed.

'Well, Prudence, what do you say, shall I accept?'

She fixed her niece with a look in which excitement and hope were clearly mingled and Pru shook her head, laughing.

'My dear aunt, this must be your decision, you have no need to consult with me!'

'But I do so want you to come, and dear Jane has kindly mentioned you in her letter, begging me to bring my little niece with me.'

That made Pru laugh. 'Hardly *little*, Aunt, I am taller than most females in Bath. However, if you want me to come with you, then of course I should be delighted.'

'Thank you, my love.' Aunt Minerva sighed and patted Pru's arm. 'You have been such a godsend these past few years. I do not know how I would go on without you.'

Pru disclaimed, blushing, 'My dear, ma'am, I do very little.'

'Nonsense, you virtually run my household, organise any journeys I wish to make, to say nothing of bearing me company with patience and good humour. In fact,' she went on, dabbing at her eyes with a wisp of lacy handkerchief, 'you are like the daughter I never had!'

Pru was touched by her aunt's words, and a trifle guilty. She knew she was very lucky to have such a comfortable home with very few duties and a generous allowance. Yet sometimes she felt stifled by her life in Bath. She had been more aware of it recently. Even with all her charity work she was conscious of a creeping boredom that was making her restless. Perhaps a visit to London was just the tonic she needed.

She said now, 'My dear aunt, pray do not cry. You have been exceedingly good to me and if you want me to come with you then there is no question. I shall accompany you, and enjoy myself prodigiously!'

Mrs Clifford's tears were banished. After hugging Pru and announcing that she was the kindest, most obliging girl, she went off happily to pen her acceptance of Lady Borcaster's invitation.

Prudence was anything but bored for the next few weeks; there was far too much to do. The house in

Kilve Street would be shut up for the summer months, which gave her the opportunity to give notice to most of the staff, including the hapless Nicholas, who was failing miserably in his attempts at sobriety. Then there was the arranging of their journey to London. A post chaise must be hired, and accommodation found along the route. On these points Mrs Clifford's many friends in the Pump Room were invaluable, recommending the best posting establishments and inns to ensure their comfort and security throughout the journey.

There was also the very pleasurable task of buying new clothes and for that the ladies needed no advice. They spent many hours browsing in Milsom Street and it was only Prudence's gentle reminders that they would have the pick of the most fashionable modistes once they reached London that prevented Aunt Minerva from buying far more than could be transported, even allowing for the fact that she had been persuaded to hire a second vehicle to carry Norris, her very superior lady's maid, as well as extra baggage.

Pru's final task was to withdraw from her charitable work. She gave notice at the infirmary that she would not be available to help them for the rest of the summer. After that she turned her attention to the task of packing everything needed for a prolonged stay in London.

At last, all was in readiness and one late May morning the little cavalcade left Kilve Street, waved off by Cook, the two maids and the scullery maid, who had been retained to look after the house until their mistress's return.

Prudence sat back with a sigh as the carriage bowled out of Bath. Her view from the front window was somewhat obscured by the bobbing figure of the postillion but that did not matter. She had done everything required of her and now she was going to enjoy a holiday.

Mrs Clifford was not a good traveller. They spent three nights on the road, arriving in London on the first day of June and pulling up in Brook Street in the late afternoon. Prudence, who had thoroughly enjoyed the journey, looked out eagerly at their home for the next three months. Lady Borcaster's residence was a handsome, three-storey house with a stone pediment around the freshly painted door.

It was clear they were expected. A servant ran out to open the carriage door and by the time they had alighted, Lady Borcaster herself had appeared on the front step.

'There you are at last! Come in, my dears, come in! Cotton will see to everything.'

They were shown into a spacious hall where Mrs Clifford presented her niece to her hostess.

'Delighted to meet you at last, Prudence—I may call you that, I hope? It is how Minerva always refers to you and I feel I already know you so well from her letters! Now, as soon as you have shed your coats, we will go upstairs to the drawing room. Come along.'

As they followed their hostess up the sweeping staircase, Pru glanced back. An army of footmen was carrying in their luggage, overseen by Lady Borcaster's butler, Cotton, while Norris, Aunt Minerva's dresser, darted around giving instructions as to where each trunk should be taken. With so many servants in the house, Pru thought there would be little to do here, save enjoy herself. She followed the other ladies into the elegant drawing room, where two long windows looked out over the street.

'Well,' declared Lady Borcaster, once they were all seated. 'I cannot tell you how delighted I am to have you here! I hope you are not too tired to take a little wine and some cake with me?'

'No, no, not at all,' murmured Minerva, her eyes widening at the sight of the laden table.

Pru had to admit it held more cakes, biscuits and sweetmeats than her aunt would order for a week of dinners. While they were served with wine or cordials from a selection of decanters standing on a side table, she took the opportunity to observe her hostess. Lady Borcaster had been a widow for many years and a generous pension allowed her to indulge her love of comfort and fashion. She was a large, handsome woman and, like Aunt Minerva, she was nearing her fiftieth year. Unlike Mrs Clifford, who was neatly dressed in a plain gown of sober colours, Lady Borcaster clearly favoured ornamentation.

Gold tassels shimmered from the short sleeves and bodice of her red-and-cream-striped gown while an elaborate gold necklace filled the space between her throat and the low-cut bodice. Rings sparkled on every finger and her improbably dark curls peeped out beneath a large turban fashioned from the same cloth as her gown.

A greater contrast to her aunt Pru thought it would have been hard to find. She could understand why Minerva preferred to live in quiet, genteel Bath rather than the bustling metropolis, but as she listened to the two ladies chattering she realised that there was indeed a strong bond between the two. Lady Borcaster had a ready laugh and was clearly very fond of Aunt Minerva. She seemed determined to make their stay an enjoyable one.

'And what about you, my dear?' Pru's wandering thoughts were recalled by the question from her hostess. 'What would you most like to see while you are in town?'

'Really, ma'am I am happy to join in with whatever you and my aunt wish to do,' she replied. 'I have never been to London before, so everything will be a novelty.'

'What, never?' the lady sat forward, her pencilled brows raised in astonishment. 'But this will not do!

Minerva, we must produce vouchers for her for Al-mack's!'

'Oh, no, no,' cried Pru in alarm. 'Truly, Lady Borcaster, I have no wish to make a spectacle of myself!'

'Nonsense! Every gel likes to dance.'

'Not at the Marriage Mart!'

'Ah, so you do know of it, then.' Lady Borcaster gave a fat chuckle. 'Very well, if you are set against it, let us forget the matter. There are enough young debutantes vying for attention and another country miss could find it difficult to make an impression.'

'Unless she is head and shoulders taller than all the rest, as I am,' said Pru bluntly.

'That would make it difficult to ignore you, of course,' conceded her hostess. 'Although under my *aegis* I think we might achieve something for you. A pretty gel like yourself shouldn't be hiding away in Bath.'

'I have tried to tell her as much, very often,' put in Minerva with a heavy sigh.

Realising the two friends were uniting against her, Prudence knew she would need to assert herself.

'I am not hiding away, ma'am. I enjoy my life in Bath, very much.' She raised her chin and added firmly, 'I assure you, Lady Borcaster, I have no wish for a husband so I pray you will not try to find one for me!'

For a moment she thought she might have offended

her hostess, but instead the lady put back her head and laughed.

'Well, well, I think we would both agree that life is much better without a husband, ain't that so, Minerva?'

'Oh, no, no, how can you say so, Jane?' protested Aunt Minerva in her mild way. 'I was devoted to Pru's uncle. Such an excellent man, so kind. I will not hear a word against him!'

'Aye, well, that's all very good, but I believe neither of us would want to marry again,' said Lady Borcaster, not a whit abashed. 'Of course, it helps that we both have sufficient pin money to do as we please. And to buy whatever we fancy!' She turned her twinkling eyes towards Prudence. 'And even if you don't want me to find you a husband, I hope you will let me to buy you a few trinkets, Miss Prudence. It will not take much to give you a little town bronze, and you will look all the better for it when you return to Bath, take my word!' Her smile faded and she gave a gusty sigh. 'I do miss my Susan. She is gone off to the Continent now with Sir Timothy and I have no one to spend my money on, save myself.'

Pru caught a glimpse of the lonely woman behind the glitter and felt sorry for her. It was impossible to dislike her hostess.

'My dear ma'am, I am very willing to be spoiled a little, if it makes you happy,' she said, reaching for a biscuit. 'Although you must grant me permission to say nay, if I think you are being too generous.'

'Excellent! That is capital! 'The smile returned and the dark eyes regained their twinkle. 'Oh, we shall have such a pleasant time of it together, although it will be such a sad crush in the streets, I fear, with so many people driving in to see the spectacles that have been arranged in the parks for the Jubilee. There is to be a Temple of Concord, and a re-enactment of the Battle of the Nile…oh, all sorts of excitement, including fireworks!'

'I do so love fireworks!' exclaimed Minerva, her eyes shining.

'And, before that, we have the Allied Sovereigns,' declared their hostess. 'They have finally arrived in London!'

It was Minerva's turn to sigh. 'I confess I have a great fancy to see the Russian emperor. I hear he is very handsome!'

'Ah yes, Tsar Alexander.' Lady Borcaster nodded. 'He is here, and what a fuss there has been! He declined to stay at Cumberland House, which had been refurbished for his stay, and instead chose to put up with his sister at the Pulteney! Quite a snub to poor Prinny.' Lady Borcaster's chins wobbled as she gave another fat chuckle. 'I am told he is very gentlemanly, quite unlike our Prince Regent. But you shall see for yourself, Minerva, for we are all invited to the levée he is holding on tomorrow.'

'Heavens, what an honour,' gasped Mrs Clifford. 'Pru, do you hear that? A levée!'

'I do, Aunt,' said Pru. 'I am sure we shall find it vastly interesting. But, Lady Borcaster, I am amazed that you were able to obtain the invitation for us at such short notice.'

Their hostess smiled and preened, just a little.

'Well,' she said, straightening one of the gold tassels on her sleeve, 'There is no point in having a diplomat in the family if he cannot be of some use! Sir Timothy arranged the whole before he and Susan went off. Of course, *then* I did not know who I would be taking with me, but that was a minor detail. It is quite a coup, my dear Minerva. We shall be the envy of all my acquaintance! Now, let me tell you what else I have in mind for your visit!'

Prudence let her thoughts wander while the two older ladies gossiped. It occurred to her that the Duke of Hartland might be in town with his bride. If that was the case then she would see him again, as it was very likely that the newlyweds would attend some of the grand parties Lady Borcaster was presently describing.

Garrick Chauntry had often been in her thoughts since their brief meeting and she was curious to know how he would look, without the dark stubble and his deplorably dishevelled clothes. Not that he would acknowledge her, thought Pru, reaching for another macaroon. It would not be right, and she did not wish for it, but that did not prevent her wanting to see him. After all, a cat might look at a king.

# Chapter Six

'Good heavens, this is impossible!' Mrs Clifford stepped off the path to avoid the bustling throng coming towards her. The tracks and paths of Hyde Park were overflowing with sightseers and Prudence was already walking on the grass. After attending the levée at Cumberland House the previous day she was not surprised by the crowds. The Russian emperor was immensely popular and it seemed everyone in London was eager to catch a glimpse of him.

'The world and his wife are out today,' she remarked.

'They are indeed, my dear. I am sorry I suggested leaving the carriage!' declared Lady Borcaster.

'We had no choice, my dear Jane, with the roads so crowded and everything at a standstill. Besides, it is a lovely day, and everyone is in such good spirits, I am very happy to be out of doors!'

'You are always so cheerful, Minerva,' observed Lady Borcaster, moving her parasol to avoid hitting a rough-looking man who surged past with a small child on his shoulders. 'I never thought there were so many people in London!'

'Word is out that Tsar Alexander will be riding in the park today with the grand duchess,' said Pru. 'They have come to see him. As have we, ma'am.'

'Yes, but the emperor does not want to be troubled by all the scaff and raff of the town,' declared my lady, eyeing the crowds with disfavour. 'If we did not have Thomas with us, I should be afraid to be walking here.'

Pru glanced behind at the tall footman who was following at a respectful distance. She had to admit it was comforting to have such an impressive manservant in attendance.

'It is the price the Tsar must pay for being so popular, ma'am,' remarked Aunt Minerva. 'But it is not only the scaff and raff,' she added, seeing a colourful group of fashionably dressed ladies approaching. 'Jane, did we not meet that lady at the tsar's levée?'

'Where?' Lady Borcaster looked up. 'Ah yes, it is Lady Applecross. And her sisters, the Countess of Fauls and Mrs Johnby! They were all there last night, but I had no opportunity to introduce you. Well, well, the morning has not been wasted after all. These ladies are most influential in town, my dears. It will do you a great deal of good to be acquainted,' she added before looking up and hailing the approaching ladies with a cheerful, 'Good morning.'

The two parties stopped, greetings were exchanged and Pru and her aunt were introduced. The countess graciously extended her hand to Mrs Clifford while Mrs Johnby asked Prudence how she was enjoying her visit to town.

'It is not always like this, Miss Clifford, and thank goodness,' she went on. 'We were planning to go to the Ring, to see the emperor, but it is impossible in this crush. We have abandoned the attempt and are going to stroll by the river instead. Perhaps you would like to join us?'

Pru, who had no burning desire to see the emperor again, or to fight her way through the crowds, decided to speak up.

'I for one would like to do that. I believe the Serpentine is a fine body of water, and it might be a trifle cooler there.'

It was agreed and the two groups walked away together to the riverbank. It was by no means deserted but only a few people were strolling there and the ladies could talk uninterrupted. They had reached the eastern end of the Serpentine and were making their way back towards the park gates and their waiting carriages when the conversation turned to last night's levée.

'It was a most glittering occasion,' declared Lady Applecross. 'Such a prestigious beginning to your visit, Mrs Clifford. You will be received everywhere now.'

'Which reminds me, Elizabeth,' remarked Mrs

Johnby, turning to the countess. 'Have you invited them to your musical soirée tomorrow evening?'

'I was about to do so, my dear.' Lady Fauls beamed. 'My dear Lady Borcaster, you must bring your delightful guests with you to Fauls House tomorrow night.'

Lady Borcaster speedily agreed, and Pru listened as her aunt expressed her gratitude for the honour bestowed upon them.

'Just a small, select gathering, of course, Mrs Clifford,' said the countess. 'I assure you there will be no one there you would not wish to introduce to your niece.'

'Indeed not,' declared Mrs Johnby. Something caught her eye at that moment and she added, in quite a different voice, 'There is *one* person who will not be crossing the threshold!'

'Oh, who?' asked Minerva, as all eyes turned to follow Mrs Johnby's stare.

'That creature over there.'

A sudden chill ran down Pru's spine. She did not know if it was caused by Mrs Johnby's words, uttered with such revulsion, or the sight of the large, athletic man striding across the grass in their direction. He was too far away to be sure, but he looked frighteningly familiar.

'Well!' Lady Fauls actually huffed. 'The nerve of the man!'

Minerva turned to Lady Borcaster, who shook her head. 'I do not know him.'

'Nor should you. It is Hartland,' declared Mrs Johnby, confirming Pru's suspicions. 'He may be a duke but no respectable persons will recognise him now.'

Mrs Clifford stared at her, eyes wide. 'Oh, goodness, what has he done?'

'What hasn't he done!' declared Lady Fauls. 'He was banished for his scandalous behaviour as a youth, but even now he has returned he is no better!'

'Why?' Pru could not help herself. 'What is his crime?'

The duke was still a considerable distance away, but she recognised him now. The rugged features and broad shoulders, the powerful body and long strides exuding energy.

'Oh, I do not know where to start.' Lady Fauls waved a hand. 'He narrowly avoided being hanged years ago and was disowned by his family in consequence, I recall. It quite broke his poor father's heart. Then, when he became duke, he did not take up his responsibilities, but left his estates to go to rack and ruin while he enjoyed himself on the Continent.'

'Yes, a true rakehell.' Lady Applecross lowered her voice and Pru strained to hear. 'I have heard he spent his time abroad *conspiring* with Bonaparte!'

'Then why is he at large?' asked Prudence. 'Why has he not been arrested?'

'There is not sufficient evidence, but it is all over town. Heavens, what else is one to think when the man has been living in France for the past ten years? And here he is now, walking around in public, as arrogant as you like!'

'And that is not the least of it,' added Mrs Johnby, with obvious relish. 'He is the very worst of jilts! As good as offered for a poor gel before he went off to the Continent and kept her dangling for ten years. *Ten years*, can you imagine? She was faithful as a nun all that time although he quite ignored her!'

Minerva gasped. 'That is outrageous.'

'Aye, ma'am, never a word, I'm told! But that is not the end of it. Earlier this year he called upon the poor lady and jilted her most cruelly. Cried off. Just like that!'

'But...can it be true?' asked Prudence slowly. 'Could this not be merely conjecture?'

Lady Applecross shook her head. 'No, no. You may ask Mrs Burchell. She knows the family and had it from the mother herself. Naturally she would not divulge the gel's name, poor innocent, but she was happy to denounce the duke for his wicked behaviour!'

Pru thought back to that night, sitting at the kitchen table with Garrick Chauntry. He had been resolved to act honourably. She could not believe he had changed his mind, he had been so determined to do his duty. Surely there must be some mistake.

Lady Applecross exhaled, a long sigh. 'It is so very distressing for the lady. The family know there is little chance of finding her a husband after all this time.

They are bereft and have withdrawn from all society. The young lady herself has gone off to the country to live in seclusion, her life and her prospects quite, quite ruined. I wouldn't be surprised if she went into a decline and perished before too long.'

'But that is scandalous!' exclaimed kind-hearted Minerva. 'Such villainous behaviour should be punished.'

Pru was more cautious. 'Certainly, if it is true.'

'My dear Miss Clifford, how can it be otherwise?' cried Mrs Johnby. 'Mrs Burchell had it from the poor gel's mother.'

'And the information about his activities,' said Pru, 'the accusations of his conspiring with the French?'

'You know the saying,' put in the countess. 'There is no smoke without fire. And if there is no truth to any of this, why does the duke himself not refute it? No, I believe Hartland is a rogue. And you may be sure, Mrs Clifford, that although his rank ensures he continues to be invited everywhere, all *respectable* society has shunned His Grace. He may be a duke but none of *my* friends will receive him!'

'No, nor mine,' declared Lady Applecross. 'Pray, Mrs Clifford, do not look at the man. We must pretend we have not seen him and give him the cut indirect.'

The conversation moved on to other matters but Prudence did not join in. The picture they painted of Garrick Chauntry was nothing like the opinion she had formed of his character and she felt a growing sense of injustice on his behalf. Be he a prince or a pauper she would not judge a man on mere hearsay.

The duke was almost within hailing distance now and he had seen them. She noticed a change in his countenance. It was very slight, but enough to convince Pru he had recognised her. His gaze flickered over her companions, who all studiously avoided him. His brows dragged together and Pru noticed how his lip curled in scorn. He gave her the briefest nod before looking away again.

Something in Pru snapped. She stepped across and blocked his way.

'Good day to you, Your Grace.'

He stopped, his frown deepening, but he touched his hat and gave her a polite bow.

'Perhaps you do not remember me,' she persisted. 'I am Miss Prudence Clifford.'

'How could I forget?'

'I should like to introduce you to my aunt, Mrs Clifford.' She ignored his cold tone and beckoned to Aunt Minerva who hesitated, glancing at the outraged faces of the ladies around her, before stepping over to join her niece.

'The duke and I met in Bath,' said Pru, once the introduction had been made. Mrs Clifford stared at her in amazement and Pru was forced to improvise. 'You will recall that occasionally I went to the Pump Room with Mrs Haddington.'

'Did you, my love?'

Aunt Minerva looked startled, the duke sardonic.

'Such a good-natured soul,' Pru trilled. 'She knows everyone!'

'I do not…oh, yes…' murmured her aunt, edging away to rejoin the other ladies.

Pru smiled at the duke. 'Mrs Haddington will be so delighted when she learns we have met again, Your Grace. I must tell her too, that I have formed the habit of walking in Green Park with my maid every morning, as she suggested.' She fixed him with a stare and added, pointedly, 'Before breakfast.'

There. Surely he would understand that she wanted to meet, to talk to him.

'An admirable idea, ma'am.'

He appeared to ignore her hint. Pru carried on with determined cheerfulness.

'Allow me to introduce you to the rest of my friends.'

'No need,' he cut in. 'I am acquainted with them all.'

He touched his hat in their direction and received only the chilliest of nods in return. Pru battled on gamely.

'Well, it—it was such a pleasant surprise to see you today, Your Grace. I am sure we shall meet again.'

'I doubt that. I am extremely busy. And I do not go into society.'

*Oh, pray do not be so vexing, you odious creature!*

Pru's smile never wavered, but she hoped he would get the message her angry gaze was trying to convey. She held out her hand to him, daring him to refuse it.

That would be a very public humiliation. To her relief, he did not, but as he bowed over her fingers he muttered, so that only she could hear.

'Enough, madam. Stay away from me. For your own sake!'

Then, with a cold look and a nod, he strode away.

Pru rejoined her party. They were all regarding her with varying degrees of disapproval. Lady Fauls was tapping her foot and looking positively outraged.

'Well, how unfortunate that you should be acquainted with His Grace,' declared Lady Borcaster, two pink spots of indignation on her cheeks. 'Not that you were aware of his reputation, I am sure.'

Aunt Minerva rushed into speech: 'I was just saying, my dear Prudence, that your sense of propriety would not allow you to ignore the duke, however slight the acquaintance.'

'I quite appreciate that Miss Clifford might be a little awed by such a personage,' replied Lady Applecross in repressive accents. 'However, if she will allow me to offer her a word of advice, she would do well not to encourage the Duke of Hartland. Especially after all we have said of the man.'

Pru was silent, but did not look convinced.

'My dear Miss Clifford he is not to be trusted, believe me!' declared Lady Fauls. 'No respectable lady will go near him. Not only is his reputation in tatters, it is well known that his estates are mortgaged to the hilt. He has moved out of Grosvenor Square, you know, and is now living in Dover Street.'

'Yes, he is planning to sell the house, even though his family have been in the Square for generations!' exclaimed Lady Applecross.

'If his affairs are in as sad a state as you say, then that would seem a wise course of action,' argued Pru, refusing to be cowed by these fashionable ladies.

'Most likely he had no choice,' remarked Mrs Johnby. 'But the others are right, my dear Miss Clifford. No good can come of setting your cap at Hartland. Trust me, it won't be marriage he offers any woman without a fortune.'

'And his new bride is unlikely to be uniformly welcomed into the ton, whatever her rank,' added Lady Fauls.

'I have no wish to *marry* His Grace.' Pru laughed, genuinely amused by the idea. 'I would greet any acquaintance in a similar manner.'

Lady Borcaster stared at her. 'After all we have learned about him?'

'It does sound shocking, ma'am, but it is all hearsay. He may turn out to be no worse than any other nobleman. I will not condemn him out of hand.'

'But you cannot continue the acquaintance,' Lady Fauls advised her. 'For a young lady in your situation that would be quite disastrous for your reputation.'

Prudence looked at the shocked faces around her and thought it best not to say anything more. She merely inclined her head and the ladies, taking this for acquiescence, were satisfied. They turned the conversation to the far more agreeable subject of fashion. This lasted until the parties separated, but as soon as they were alone, Lady Borcaster lost no time in expressing her unease at Pru's friendship with the Duke of Hartland.

'Championing such a man is a credit to your good nature, Prudence my dear, but it will not do, you know. Will it, Minerva?'

'No indeed,' Mrs Clifford answered her, although she was distracted. 'But, a *duke*, Prudence! I cannot believe you made the Duke of Hartland's acquaintance and did not tell me!'

'Why, were you aware of the gossip surrounding him?' asked Pru, all wide-eyed innocence.

'No, no. I did not even know he was in Bath! And what Elvira Haddington was thinking of, I do not know, to introduce you to such a man. But then, she is an inveterate matchmaker.' She huffed in exasperation. 'As the countess said, my dear, you must be careful of your reputation.'

'And so I shall, but to cut an acquaintance because of mere tittle-tattle would surely not be right. I shall reserve my judgement until I have the story direct, from one or other of the parties.'

Mrs Clifford squawked in horror. 'Prudence! Pray do not tell me you intend to speak to His Grace about it!'

It was exactly what Pru intended, but she knew better than to admit it.

'I am merely saying I refuse to be swayed by gossip.'

'Happily, there is little chance of our meeting Hartland amongst my circle of friends,' remarked Lady Borcaster, taking a more sanguine view. 'There is the White's Club Fête at Burlington House, of course, but I am told there will be thousands in attendance for that ball, and I distinctly heard the duke say he does not go into society.' She sighed. 'It will be such a crush, and nigh impossible to get near the Prince Regent or his honoured guests, but nevertheless, I am sure we shall enjoy it.'

Mrs Clifford agreed absently. She was still thinking of the recent encounter and said, 'We can only hope Prudence has not offended your friends, Jane.'

'Well, I hope that too, Minerva. Lady Applecross and her sisters are amongst the most influential hostesses in London. I was concerned they might take umbrage at your niece's rather forthright speech, but I think I managed to smooth any ruffled feathers.'

'I beg your pardon, ma'am, for putting you into a difficult situation,' said Pru, sincerely. They had reached their carriage and, as they stopped to wait for the footman to scramble down and open the door, she added, 'I shall endeavour not to do so again. It would be very wrong of me, after all your kindness.'

'Well, well, let us say no more about it, my dear,' said Lady Borcaster, patting her cheek. 'It shows you have a kind heart, does it not, Minerva?'

'Yes, it does, Jane.'

Mrs Clifford was eyeing her niece doubtfully and Prudence gave her a reassuring smile as she followed her into the carriage. However, behind her cheerful expression her mind was working feverishly on how to meet with the duke.

The gossip she had heard did not tally with what she knew of the man. Pru considered herself a good judge of character, and she refused to believe Garrick Chauntry was as black as he was now being painted. She needed to know the truth and there was only one way to find that. However, she knew she would get no help from her aunt or her hostess, and even the duke himself had warned her to keep away from him.

This was going to be far more difficult than she had first thought.

## Chapter Seven

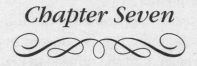

Meeting the Duke of Hartland in Hyde Park caused Lady Borcaster no little dismay. She was still worrying over it at the end of the day and pleaded with her young guest to cut the acquaintance. Pru steadfastly refused to do so, although she agreed it was unlikely they would meet socially and the subject was dropped. Pru did not wish to upset her kind hostess further and decided to say nothing of the note she had penned as soon as they had returned from the park. Nor did she mention the reply she had received by return.

The next morning the subject of the Duke of Hartland appeared to be forgotten. Pru went down to breakfast to find her aunt and her hostess discussing plans to visit Mrs Bell's establishment to buy new gowns. They invited her to join them and she readily agreed, declaring herself eager to meet the celebrated modiste.

The three ladies set off in the carriage for Charlotte Street and spent an enjoyable morning looking at dresses of all styles and colours. Lady Borcaster and

Mrs Clifford both purchased several new gowns and, after some cajoling, Pru allowed her hostess to treat her to an evening gown of apricot blush crepe over a white satin slip. It was impossible not to be tempted by so many delectable creations and Pru also used some of her savings to purchase two new outfits for herself, although she was sorry that Mrs Bell was unable to deliver them until the following week. She would have dearly liked to wear her new walking dress when she sallied forth later that afternoon, rather than her rather dull green kerseymere.

After such a busy time in Charlotte Street the two older ladies retired to their respective bedchambers to rest until it was time to change for dinner. They were a little surprised when Prudence told them she was going out again, but raised no demur when she expressed a desire to visit the British Gallery in Pall Mall.

'To see the paintings,' she explained, observing her aunt's blank look. 'I am told it is very interesting.'

'I am sure it is, although I have never been there myself,' replied Lady Borcaster. 'I will order the carriage to be brought around again.'

'Oh, no, ma'am. Thank you, but there is no need for that. I am very happy to walk. Indeed, I should enjoy the exercise. With the Tsar and the other dignitaries out of town for a few days, the streets will be a little quieter today.'

Lady Borcaster was surprised, but Mrs Clifford,

knowing her niece's energetic nature, merely bade her not to go out alone.

'No, of course not, ma'am,' said Pru cheerfully. 'I thought Meg could come with me. The maid Her Ladyship has so kindly assigned to me for the duration of my visit,' Pru explained to her aunt.

'Yes, an excellent young woman,' nodded Lady Borcaster. 'Bright, too. She is London born and very obliging.'

'She is indeed,' replied Pru, her eyes twinkling in a way that should have made her Aunt Minerva suspicious.

An hour later Prudence had reached number fifty-two Pall Mall, where the British Gallery was situated. However, she did not go in but carried, on, walking past St James's Palace and into Green Park. There were a few people walking in the park, as well as the park's famous milch cows which roamed freely, but Prudence paid no heed to any of them. She saw a small hillock topped with straggling trees and quickly made her way towards the lone figure standing amongst the gnarled trunks. As she drew closer, she could see that the fashionably dressed gentleman was resting on his cane as he gazed out towards the Queen's House.

Pru stopped a short distance from the hillock and turned to the maid.

'Now, Meg, you will wait here for me, if you please,

while I talk to the gentleman. If we move off, you may follow, but at a distance. Is that clear?'

'Yes, ma'am.' The girl bobbed a slight curtsy, her face alight with excitement although she asked no questions. Pru had given her a silver coin for her compliance and there was the promise of more to come, for her discretion.

'The first duty of a lady's maid is loyalty to her mistress,' Pru had told her. 'You are doing nothing unlawful, but I would ask you not to gossip about our little outing today.'

And Meg, who had ambitions to work her way up to become dresser to a fashionable lady, was only too pleased to oblige.

Prudence went on to the top of the rise alone. The gentleman was staring moodily at the ground but as she approached, he looked up, his dark brows drawn together.

'Well, madam, what is so urgent that you must arrange such an improper *tête-à-tête*?'

'And a very good day to you, Your Grace.' She ignored his irritable tone. 'I am very grateful that you agreed to meet with me.'

'I had little choice, since you threatened to come to Dover Street and hammer on my door if I refused! What do you want?'

'To talk to you.'

'You had much better stay away from me.' His

mouth tightened. 'Your friends will have warned you about me.'

'Yes, they did, but I want to hear the truth for myself.' Prudence unfurled her parasol. 'Shall we walk? I think we will look less conspicuous.'

After a brief hesitation the duke nodded and they made their way out of the trees, following the meandering path.

'What happened in Bath?' asked Pru, when she realised her companion was not going to volunteer any information.

'Nothing.'

'When you left my aunt's house you had determined upon a course of action. Did you go ahead with it?' He did not reply and Pru's certainty wavered a little. 'I am curious to know how you fared with Miss Speke.'

'I didn't,' he said shortly.

She stopped and turned to stare at him in dismay.

'I do not understand,' she said at last. 'You told me she was expecting your visit, that her father had given his blessing. Surely you did not...'

He gave a short laugh.

'Oh, I called upon her,' he said, indicating that they should walk on. 'I was determined to put right the injustice I had done, but it seems it was her parents who wanted the match, far more than the lady. When I arrived at the Royal Crescent, she had fled.'

'What! She, she *eloped*?'

'Oh, no. A rival suitor I might have understood.' He

swiped at a thistle with his cane. 'She left Bath. With a Miss Undershaw.'

'Emily Undershaw?'

'Yes, do you know her?'

'I met her when she first came to Bath, although my aunt did not encourage the acquaintance. A strange creature, given to wearing mannish clothes and smoking cigarillos, although her idiosyncrasies are overlooked because of her fortune. Now you mention it, I saw her in company with Miss Speke on several occasions.'

'They are bosom friends, apparently,' said the duke, beheading an errant dandelion with a slash of his cane.

'But how can this be?' demanded Pru, bewildered. 'Miss Speke waited all these years for you...'

'It would appear that it was Lord Tirrill and his wife who were waiting for me, not Annabelle. I gather they had cajoled the poor girl into accepting my offer but when I didn't turn up on the appointed day, her courage failed her. She ran away rather than meet me.'

'Oh, I am so sorry!'

'Are you? I am not.'

Pru looked up, surprised. The shadows had fled from his green eyes and he was smiling. She quickly pushed aside a sudden, alarming jolt of attraction.

'You are not angry?' she ventured. 'The lady has scorned your advances. Many men would be mortified.'

'I am more relieved.'

'But the gossip. Everyone thinks it was your doing.'

'Let them. The family has put it about that it was I who broke the agreement, rather than their daughter.'

Pru stopped.

'That is despicable,' she exclaimed.

'No, it is understandable. There is no denying Annabelle would fare much worse if it was known she had jilted *me*.' He shrugged. 'I have broad shoulders, a little more censure will not hurt me. Besides, I shall not be in town much longer.'

'You are leaving?' she asked, as they walked on.

'Tomorrow. I am going to Hartland. God knows it is time I attended to my business there.'

'And...will you meet with the duchess?'

She waited in silence for him to speak.

'I shall write to her,' he said at last. 'But I shall not call without permission.'

'But if she has heard the rumours...'

His lip curled. 'Oh, I have no doubt some well-meaning friend has already written to inform her of all the new calumnies laid at my door! It will give her even more reason to shun me.'

Pru heard the bitterness in his voice and it tore at her heart.

'But how could any mother not wish to see her son?' she exclaimed.

'Quite easily, it would seem.'

'Surely she will not believe such things without talking to you, as I am doing.'

He exhaled and said impatiently, 'That is just the point, you should *not* be talking with me! You are risking your reputation being here with me, Miss Clifford.'

'There are very few people in the park to see us.'

'It would only take one to gossip.'

'I needed to hear the truth.'

'And you have done so. I rely upon you not to tell anyone else.'

'You have my word, sir.'

'Thank you.' He added, after a pause, 'And thank you for helping me. That night in Bath.'

'I did very little.'

'I really believe you saved my life.' He sighed and glanced about him. 'I should like to kiss your hand, but in such an exposed spot that would not be wise. So I must wish you adieu, Miss Clifford. It is best we do not meet again.'

'You are leaving town tomorrow.' Why did the thought make her feel so empty?

'Yes, that is my intention.'

'And the other rumours?' She hesitated, but this was her last chance to ask him. 'Forgive me, but there is talk that you are a spy for the French...'

'Ah, yes. I had heard that.' His countenance assumed that familiar grim look.

'People think you lived in France for the past ten years, but you said you were in Vienna.'

'And you believe everything you are told?' He threw her a mocking glance. 'What a trusting soul you are!'

She turned and fixed her eyes upon him. 'Not always, but I did believe what you told me in Bath.'

Garrick felt his heart contract when he met the steady gaze of those clear grey eyes. She trusted him and it pleased him more than he could say.

'Hmmph! That night I stumbled into your kitchen I was in no fit state to dissemble, was I? In this instance your trust is not misplaced. I was in Vienna, some of the time. For the past ten years I have been many things, traveller, explorer, wanderer, but never a traitor to my country.'

'But why would anyone spread such a wicked falsehood?' she asked him. 'Could it be the lady's family, trying to blacken your name further?'

'No, I am sure it is not. These rumours began in quite a different quarter.'

'You cannot know that.'

Garrick hesitated. It would be a relief to share his suspicions, but it would not do. He had told this woman far too much already. What was it about Pru Clifford that made him want to confide in her? She was no beauty, her green pelisse was not new and far from fashionable, but he liked her open countenance, the honesty in her steady gaze. He liked *her*.

He said, 'True, I have no proof, but it is not important. There is no foundation to the rumour. Once I have left town it will die down and some other poor soul will become the subject of gossip.'

'But—'

'Enough, madam.' She was looking at him, her eyes full of concern. He said harshly, 'Leave be, Miss Clifford. You must not become embroiled in my affairs.'

'But you need help.'

'Not from you!' He needed to convince her how serious this was. How dangerous it would be for her to become involved. 'If someone really is trying to implicate me in a traitorous plot then the last thing I need is a damned woman getting in my way!'

That did it. She took a step away, her eyes widening in shock at his brutal language. Garrick regretted the necessity of speaking so sharply, but it had worked. He touched his hat and strode away, leaving her standing alone on the path.

# Chapter Eight

'My dear, you are looking decidedly pale this evening, are you sure you are well enough to go out?'

Mrs Clifford peered in concern across the drawing room at Prudence, who straightened her shoulders and forced her lips into a smile.

'I am perfectly well, Aunt, thank you.'

'It is no wonder you are fatigued, my dear, going off again on a jaunt the moment we returned from Mrs Bell's,' declared Lady Borcaster, coming in at that moment. 'And to a picture gallery, too. Nothing could be more tiring! But there, you young people will go your own way. Ah well, a quiet dinner here at Brook Street will perk you up before we set off for Lady Fauls's soirée, I am sure. And here is Cotton now, come to tell us it is ready. Shall we go in?'

Prudence silently followed her hostess into the dining room and took her place at the table. The serious business of eating would preclude any conversation for a while and she was glad of it, because her mind was still going over everything that had occurred in Green Park earlier.

She had been shocked by the duke's language and the way he stormed off but, upon reflection, she was not surprised he was angry with her. The fact that she had fed him when he had stumbled into the basement kitchen did not give Pru the right to pry into his concerns. He was a grown man and quite capable of looking after himself. But Pru could not shake off the nagging anxiety, and even the diversion of the countess's soirée was not enough to banish it completely.

Lady Borcaster had impressed upon Prudence how fortunate she was that the countess had not withdrawn her invitation, following the lamentable scenes in Hyde Park, and as they set of for Fauls House she begged her young guest to be on her best behaviour. Mrs Clifford added her entreaties and Prudence, knowing how much she owed to both ladies, promised to do nothing to draw attention to herself.

Lady Fauls greeted them politely, but their arrival coincided with that of an august group of lords, ladies and visiting foreign diplomats. The countess hurriedly moved off to welcome these important personages, leaving the ladies to make their own way into the elegant salon set up for the evening's entertainment. A pianoforte took pride of place in one corner of the room, with numerous chairs and sofas arranged to face it. However, the entertainment had not yet begun and all the guests were chattering and laughing while silent-footed servants walked between the little groups with trays full of glasses.

Lady Borcaster appeared to be acquainted with nearly everyone present. She moved around the room, assured of her welcome, making Mrs Clifford and her niece known to Lady This and Lord That until Prudence thought her head would burst with so many names to remember. She was quite relieved when Mrs Johnby drew her away to join a party of her own particular friends at the far side of the room. When that little group dispersed, Prudence moved over to the pianoforte, admiring the polished mahogany and rosewood casing with its gleaming brass inlay. It was far grander than the little Pohlman pianoforte that Aunt Minerva owned. Her hand was reaching out to touch the keys when a voice at her shoulder made her jump.

'It is a fine instrument, is it not? A Broadwood, no less.'

Pru look around at the speaker. He was a stranger to her, but fashionably dressed in a dark blue coat over white silk breeches and waistcoat, the whole embellished with a number of fobs and seals hanging about his person.

He went on, 'Will you be delighting us with a recital later, ma'am?'

She shook her head. 'Sadly no, I am too much out of practice, but I should very much like to hear it played by a proficient.'

His appearance was very sleek, the short dark hair was oiled into place and greying at each side of his lean face, while his brows had been carefully plucked into neat arches. The heavy gold ring on his finger suggested a man of means, but she had no idea who he might be.

'Allow me to introduce myself,' he said, as if reading her thoughts. 'I am Sir Joseph Conyers. May I be very forward and ask you to tell me who you are? I know only that you are a guest of Lady Borcaster.' When she hesitated, he said quickly, 'Pray, ma'am, let us not stand upon ceremony! The recital will start soon and there isn't time to find a mutual acquaintance to introduce us.'

The playful look that accompanied his words made Pru laugh.

'Very well. I am Miss Clifford, sir.'

'Miss Clifford. Hmm, then why have we not met? I thought I knew all the pretty young ladies in town.'

Pru felt herself withdrawing slightly. Perhaps he thought he was being avuncular, but his words and tone were not what she had been expecting. Until that moment she had been prepared to be friendly, to overlook the impropriety of a man introducing himself, but now she was on her guard. His smile had not changed, but she could not like the gleam in his hooded eyes and she stepped away a little.

A sudden flurry of activity broke out. Everyone was moving towards the chairs, taking their seats for the recital. Pru quickly excused herself and hurried across to join her hostess and Aunt Minerva.

'My dear Prudence, who was that man talking to you?' asked Mrs Clifford.

'Sir Joseph Conyers,' she said, sitting down with them. 'Do you know him, Lady Borcaster?'

The lady shook her head. 'I am not acquainted with him. Although, I do recall Lady Applecross mentioning him. He has recently come to town with his wife. I am told they hold the most entertaining card parties, and routs full of lively wit and lavish refreshments.'

'Really? How interesting,' remarked Mrs Clifford.

There was no time for more. The audience hushed as Lady Fauls announced the first of the musical entertainments of the evening.

For over an hour Lady Fauls's guests listened to any number of ballads, airs and duets performed with varying degrees of success. Then there was a break for refreshments, a light supper to be taken in the dining room. As Lady Borcaster shepherded her little party out of the room, Pru saw that their hostess was standing near the doorway with Sir Joseph at her side, and as they passed Lady Fauls put out a hand to detain Lady Borcaster.

'I am glad I have caught you, ma'am. Sir Joseph has begged me to make him known to you.'

The gentleman stepped forward.

'I made Miss Clifford's acquaintance earlier and

could not let the opportunity pass to meet her friends,' he said, bowing over their hands in turn.

Pru watched, appreciating the man's elegant manners and address. He charmed her aunt and Lady Borcaster but she thought him a little too polished and was relieved that he did not offer to accompany them downstairs to supper. She said nothing to the others, unwilling to disparage a gentleman upon such little acquaintance. She was unused to society and was probably reading far too much into the situation.

The second part of the soirée was far more informal. Several guests took their turn to sing or play, but only a few hardy souls occupied the chairs around the pianoforte. Wine was flowing freely and most of the guests were now mingling, talking amongst themselves.

Prudence was on the edge of one such group when she heard gasps and stifled laughter coming from the nearby window embrasure. A quick glance showed her that Sir Joseph Conyers was at the centre of a cluster of guests who were hanging on his every word. Across the room, someone was playing a particularly lively sonata but during a short pause in the music, a lady's shocked voice uttered a word that caught her attention.

'...*spying*...'

Pru stepped aside to take a glass of wine from a passing footman and sauntered away, supposedly inspecting the delicate watercolours ranged along the wall but all the time moving closer to the window.

She had reached the final painting, a rather depressing depiction of a ruined castle under a lowering sky, before she could hear anything.

'Shameful!' exclaimed one lady. 'But can we be *sure*, Sir Joseph?'

The gentleman's voice was lower, more muted, and Prudence moved closer until she was able to pick up various words and phrases.

'*...vengeful...villainous duke... Years in exile... Hartland.*'

A chill ran through her at that last word. There could be no doubting the subject of Sir Joseph's disclosures. Pru sipped her wine, straining to hear more.

'He should be exposed,' declared one gentleman with his back to Pru. 'I presume there is proof?'

'Oh, there is, sir, there is.' Sir Joseph replied. 'Naturally, I cannot reveal my sources, but I assure you they are most reliable...'

The silky complaisance in his voice was unmistakable. Others were exclaiming now but Sir Joseph said no more, allowing the gossip to run on without him. Pru moved away, her thoughts racing. This was far more serious than mere tittle-tattle and Sir Joseph Conyers was the source. He was deliberately stoking the fires of speculation and she considered that to be quite wicked behaviour. All pleasure in the evening had been destroyed and she hurried back to her party, eager to be gone. However, Lady Borcaster showed no signs of tiring and Prudence was obliged to curb her impatience as the evening dragged on.

It was approaching two o'clock when at last Pru fell into her bed, but even then, sleep would not come. She did not know quite why it should matter so much to her, but she knew she would not rest until she had seen the duke and told him all she had learned.

'What is it, Stow?' Garrick said, putting the finishing touches to his cravat when his man came in.

'Begging your pardon, Your Grace. There is a visitor for you.'

'At this hour of the morning?' He glanced at the clock. It was not yet seven.

'A female, sir.' Stow allowed a tiny note of disapproval to creep into his usually impassive voice. 'She would not give her name, but said I was to mention Bath to you, sir.'

Garrick frowned. He said brusquely, 'Show her up.'

By the time he had shrugged on his coat Stow had returned, followed by a tall figure enveloped in a red cloak. He nodded to his man to leave them and, as the door clicked shut upon them, two dainty hands came up to push back the hood.

A soft, melodious voice said, 'I beg your pardon for coming so early.'

'Early!' he exploded. 'Miss Clifford, you should not be here at all.'

'But I needed to see you. You told me you were leaving today and I thought it most likely that you would be making an early start.' She glanced down at the red cloak. 'I thought if I wore this I would look like a servant and be less conspicuous.'

'You came here *alone*?' Garrick raked a hand through his hair. 'Of all the hen-witted things to do!'

'No, no, my maid is waiting below. I am not quite lost to all sense of propriety.'

'You are sailing dashed close to the wind, madam!' He glared at her. 'Very well, the sooner you tell me what you have to say the sooner you can be gone.'

Pru took a deep breath. He was very cross with her and it was important he realised she was not here on any trivial matter.

'I heard someone spreading rumours last night. About you being a spy. He said he had proof.' She bit her lip. 'That is far more than mere gossip, Your Grace. I thought, if you could find him, you could make him tell you his sources. Then you could put a stop to it.'

'Who was the man?'

'Sir Joseph Conyers. I met him at Lady Fauls's soirée last night.'

He stared hard at her for a moment. 'Was Lady Conyers with him?'

Pru blinked. 'Why, no, he came alone. It was after midnight that he gathered a little crowd about him and I heard him accusing you of being a French spy. And when someone asked if there was proof, he said yes!' She paused, her brows drawing together in a frown.

'Is Sir Joseph the man you suspected of spreading the rumours?'

'What? Oh, yes.'

'And are you going to stop him?'

'I shall deal with this matter in my own way. For the moment I am more concerned in getting you out of here without causing a scandal.'

'There will be no scandal. Apart from my maid no one knows I am here and it is still very early. We shall be back in Brook Street in plenty of time for breakfast.'

'Then the sooner you leave the better,' he retorted. 'My travelling carriage is due at any moment, and you must go before anyone else sees you.'

She stared at him. 'You are still leaving town?'

'Yes. Put up your hood. My man will show you out.'

Pru did not move. 'Surely you are not going to let Sir Joseph get away with this?'

Garrick gave a growl of impatience. 'My dear Miss Clifford, what I choose to do is no concern of yours.'

She bridled at that. He saw how she drew herself up, that determined little chin rising defiantly. 'My dear duke, it became my concern the moment you confided in me!'

Garrick admired her spirit. He thought idly how tall she was, her eyes level with his chin. Her lips not so very far beneath his own. Two steps closer and he could pull her into his arms. He fought back the sudden jolt of desire, replacing it with anger. How could she be so careless of her good name, of her own safety?

'No! Blast it, woman, this is *not your business*.' She regarded him defiantly and he drew a deep breath. 'Miss Clifford, I am grateful for your help in Bath, but believe me, there is nothing more for you to do. You may safely ignore any rumours you hear. Trust me, they will not last and if you interfere you will regret it.'

Her brows went up, but her clear gaze never wavered from his.

'Are you threatening me, Your Grace?'

'Of course not, but I would not have you drawn unnecessarily into dealings with these unpleasant characters.' He took her arm and led her towards the door. 'Go back to Brook Street and forget all about me. Enjoy the rest of your visit to town.'

He reached over to lift her hood and arrange it over her soft brown hair. Then he rested his hands on her shoulders.

'Well, madam, will you give me your word not to interfere further?'

'If that is what you want, sir.'

'It is.'

She was looking up at him, those clear grey eyes searching his face. Then her chin tilted up a little more, as if in invitation and he could not resist. He lowered his head and kissed her.

Garrick felt the little tremor of surprise run through

her, but she did not pull away. Instead, her hand came up to rest on his shoulder and she returned his kiss. It was a shy, hesitant response. Inexperienced, but that only inflamed him more. His arms ached to hold her. He wanted to deepen the kiss, to enjoy the honeyed taste of her lips beneath his. She smelled of summer flowers, sweet and innocent. Everything he was not.

It took every ounce of willpower to break off and lift his head, his hands tightening on her shoulders as he held her away from him.

'There,' he said roughly. 'If anything should convince you to stay away from me it is that!' He released her, averting his eyes from her startled gaze. He turned to open the door.

'Now go!'

She hurried away down the stairs and Garrick closed the door behind her. He leaned against it, his eyes closed.

'Hell and damnation!'

He had done his best. He had tried to put her off, told her to ignore the rumours but he knew she would not. Prudence Clifford was not a woman to stay quiet in the face of injustice. Left to her own devices she would refute the rumours. She would openly challenge anyone who accused him. And he knew only too well that the perpetrator of these lies was not a man to be crossed.

From the open window came the sounds of a carriage drawing up in the street below. He heard his driver's voice and moments later Stow's feet hurrying up the stairs.

He sighed. One thing was certain, he could not leave town now.

## Chapter Nine

The early morning streets were beginning to fill up with carriages, street vendors and tradesmen going about their business, but Prudence saw and heard nothing as she hurried back to Brook Street. Her thoughts remained in Dover Street, with Garrick Chauntry.

*He kissed me!*

Her lips still tingled. She remembered the soft wool of his coat beneath her hand. The scent of him, that mix of fresh soap and sandalwood, far more enticing than the cloying perfumes that had assailed her senses at Fauls House last night. She should be outraged, shocked at his behaviour, but in truth she had wanted him to kiss her. If he had not stopped she had no idea what might have happened, for she did not think she would have been strong enough to break away.

A little shudder ran through her which should have been shame, but she knew it was not. What she felt was elation. Excitement. And a very strong desire to kiss him again.

'This way, madam.'

Meg's touch on her arm brought her wanton thoughts to an end. She followed the maid into a side turning and through a series of lanes until they reached the back entrance to Lady Borcaster's residence. Thankfully there was no one to see two red-cloaked maids hurrying up the servants' stairs and once they reached Pru's room, she handed her cloak over to Meg to return it to the servants' hall. She also gave the maid another silver coin for her silence, salving her conscience with the fact that she fully intended to employ the maid as her personal dresser when she returned to Bath at the end of the summer.

Prudence sat through breakfast in near silence. The duke would have left town by now and he had told her not to interfere further in his concerns. She had agreed, even though it would be very hard not to speak up when she heard people repeating the gossip about him. She had the distinct feeling there was something he had not disclosed, but why should he tell her anything? Perhaps it was something too shameful to be repeated. She cast about in her mind for possible answers, but her conjectures proved so lurid and outrageous that she scolded herself.

*It is unlikely that I shall ever know the truth*, she thought as she buttered another bread roll. *His Grace the Duke of Hartland has left town and there's an end to it. I have nothing to do now but forget him and enjoy myself.*

* * *

Having made her resolution, Prudence was determined to enter fully into Lady Borcaster's plans for her guests' entertainment, consoling herself with the thought that there was so much interest in the royal visitors there was unlikely to be much gossip about anything else for the next few weeks. Hopefully she would not need to defend the duke.

There was no shortage of diversions during the following week. The crowds were such that Lady Borcaster abandoned plans to see the Tsar riding out in Hyde Park in the early morning or to follow him on his various outings to Woolwich Arsenal or the London docks. Instead they enjoyed a series of carriage outings and card parties with the lady's friends. There was also a delivery of new clothes from the modiste, Mrs Bell, to divert them, and it was in no little excitement that Prudence donned for the first time the evening gown Lady Borcaster had given her.

It was far grander than anything she had owned before, but the apricot crepe enhanced the creamy tones of her skin and highlighted the golden tints in her hair. She had only a simple string of pearls and matching ear drops to wear with it, but when she came down to the drawing room to join the others Lady Borcaster declared that she looked very well indeed.

'Very elegant. There will be so many grand ladies in all their finery at Tarleton House tonight that there is no point trying to compete, my dear Prudence. Simplicity will serve you best.'

Pru was thankful for her advice although when they arrived at Tarleton House, she could not help feeling a little envious of the gorgeously attired creatures who filled the ballroom. Many were even more flamboyant than Lady Borcaster's frock of scarlet gauze heavily trimmed with gold lace. Pru had not been in town very long, but she knew some of the gowns on display cost a great deal more than the year's allowance Aunt Minerva paid her.

Lady Borcaster took great pains to find a partner for her young friend and Prudence was grateful not to be one of the young ladies languishing at the side of the room. After the first dances of the evening she returned to her party in high spirits after her exertions. Aunt Minerva and Lady Borcaster were in conversation with a fashionably dressed couple and as she approached, Lady Borcaster put out her hand to draw her forward.

'Ah, Prudence, my dear. We were just talking of you!'

It was only when the gentleman turned towards her that Pru recognised Sir Joseph Conyers. She schooled her face to a smile and gave a small curtsy.

'My dear Miss Clifford, we meet again.' He made her an elegant bow. 'And now I have the pleasure of introducing you to my wife. Helene, my dear!'

Pru turned her attention to the woman at his side and she was momentarily dazzled. The lady's golden hair was piled high and twinkled with crystals nestled amongst the curls while diamonds glittered at her neck and her ears. Lady Conyers might be on the shady side of thirty but she was undoubtedly beautiful.

She had a straight little nose, delicate brows that arched over a pair of deep blue eyes and rosy lips that were now uttering warm words of greeting. And yet, as she looked into the lady's smiling face, Prudence thought there was something rather cold and calculating about her.

Sir Joseph and Lady Conyers stayed to talk for a few moments and then moved on, leaving Mrs Clifford in raptures.

'Such an obliging gentleman! And his wife, so kind. How generous to invite us to their little party on Monday next.'

'Pity we already have our invitation for the White's Club Ball that evening,' replied Lady Borcaster.

'You are not so enamoured of them, ma'am?' asked Pru, quick to hear the note of reserve in the lady's tone.

'I think his interest is more that I am mama-in-law to Sir Timothy Flowers. I imagine he thinks I can give him entrée into diplomatic circles. He is quite wrong, you know. I have no influence at all.'

'But you have invitations to some of the most prestigious events taking place this summer,' exclaimed Mrs Clifford.

'Yes, the White's Club Ball, for example. Anyone who *is* anyone will be attending Burlington House on Monday night.'

'But not the Conyers,' murmured Prudence, 'if they are holding a party of their own.'

'They would like to be, but clearly did not receive an invitation,' replied Lady Borcaster, her tone dry. She smiled and touched Mrs Clifford's arm. 'My years in London have made me a little sceptical, Minerva. Believe me, I have nothing against the man or his wife. I am sure they are indeed pleasant company, but it is best to have the measure of one's acquaintances, and then you cannot be disappointed in them.'

Prudence was in complete agreement with this worldly-wise view. She was already wary of Sir Joseph, misliking his propensity for mischievous gossip, but she realised now that he had only sought her out to gain favour with Lady Borcaster. It was a lowering thought, but it did not unduly worry her. In fact, she was quite distracted by something else nagging at the back of her mind. At that first meeting with Garrick Chauntry, she recalled him telling her about the duel he had fought over a woman. A beautiful seductress called Helene.

Sir Joseph and Lady Conyers did not speak with Lady Borcaster or her party again that evening, but they were hard to ignore. Lady Borcaster remarked that the lady's dance partners were the most influential persons present, while Pru watched Sir Joseph circling the room, being charming to everyone. She also noticed that Lady Conyers had a herd of young bucks vying for her attention and wondered if she still enjoyed enslaving naive young men with her beauty. Pru tried to dismiss the thought as uncharitable, but could not quite do it.

After Tarleton House, there were only a few days for the Brook Street ladies to recover before the much-vaunted White's Club Ball at Burlington House. Pru was a little dismayed when she heard that upwards of two thousand guests had been invited but Lady Borcaster assured her she would enjoy herself.

'I have enlisted an old friend of mine, General Lechlade, to be our escort, so you may be easy.'

Prudence found it hard to believe that an elderly soldier's presence would add to her comfort, but she said nothing and, shortly after nine o'clock on the appointed evening, their little party joined the crowd slowly making their way into the grand ballroom. She was wearing the apricot crepe again and although part of her would have liked to be showing off a new gown, her sensible side argued that it did not matter what she wore. No one would be looking at plain Miss Clifford when there were so many exalted persons in attendance.

The Allied Sovereigns arrived at midnight, the Tsar delighting the guests by waltzing the night away at the upper end of the ballroom. Pru, who had not yet waltzed in public, preferred to join in the country dances taking place elsewhere.

She had no shortage of dance partners but the rooms were hot, crowded and noisy and Pru was very glad when the signal was given for supper at two o'clock. She dismissed her latest partner with a graceful word of thanks and was about to go off to find her aunt when she heard a deep voice at her shoulder.

'I thought I'd find you here.'

Pru's heart leapt. She turned quickly and found herself facing the powerful figure of Garrick Chauntry, Duke of Hartland. He looked quite magnificent in his evening coat of corbeau-coloured wool. A snowy cravat contrasted strongly with the dark coat and knee breeches and his hair had been brushed back, gleaming like a raven's wing in the candlelight. She thought he could not be called handsome, but those green eyes were certainly arresting.

'What are *you* doing here?' The shock of seeing him threw her quite off balance and she blushed at her own incivility. 'What I mean is, Your Grace, I thought you had left town.'

'And miss all this excitement?' he drawled.

She narrowed her eyes at him. 'I believe you dislike this crush as much as I.'

He grinned. 'I do, but being a duke I received an invitation and thought I might as well use it.' He held out his arm. 'Allow me to take you in to supper.' She hesitated and his brows went up a little. 'Unless you prefer not to acknowledge me…'

'You know that is not the case! I was going to look for my aunt, and Lady Borcaster.'

'You have little chance of finding them in these crowds. Come along.'

She rested her fingers on his sleeve, accepting that it would indeed be difficult to find anyone amongst the thousands crammed into the halls and marquees. The duke guided her unerringly to the supper rooms but made no attempt to follow all those who wanted to dine as close as possible to the royal guests. Instead he carried on until they came to a far less crowded marquee. It was set out more informally than the main rooms and had no musicians secreted in the walls.

'I think we will be more comfortable here,' he said, leading her to an empty table that was positively groaning with food.

'Should I be insulted?' she murmured, teasing him, 'This area is clearly for the lowlier guests.'

'I thought you would prefer this to being deafened.'

She relented and smiled at him. 'You are quite correct. But we must not be ungenerous. White's Club has gone to a great deal of trouble over this fête.'

'Indeed, they have. People will be talking about it for months to come.'

The supper was delicious and the duke proved an entertaining companion. Pru thought he looked very well in the full evening dress. It was a credit to the tailor that his broad shoulders and deep chest did not strain at the seams of his dark coat. He carried himself well and had a natural grace, but he was no courtier, she decided, pushing aside her empty plate. She was a little surprised that he showed no interest in mixing with his peers, but perhaps ten years in exile had embittered him.

'Well?' he demanded, interrupting her thoughts. 'What is your opinion?'

'I beg your pardon?'

'You have been studying me for the duration of the meal.'

He waved to a passing servant to refill their glasses, but his gaze never left her. Those strange holly-green eyes bored into her, challenging her to tell the truth.

'I think you prefer action to doing the pretty at occasions like this,' she said, selecting a sweetmeat from a small dish on the table. 'You would be happier out of doors. Riding or hunting perhaps.'

'Very true. Would not you?'

'I have not ridden since I joined my aunt in Bath.'

'Do I detect a note of regret, there?'

She hesitated. 'A little, perhaps. I used to enjoy riding when I was at home. And country walks. But my life is very full, so I do not repine.'

She remembered the restlessness that had come upon her those last months in Bath and quickly turned the conversation back to the duke.

'But if you would prefer to be elsewhere, why did you come tonight?'

His lip curled in self-derision. 'Can you not guess? Dukes are invited everywhere, whatever the ton might think of them!'

'But that does not answer my question,' she replied. 'You were not obliged to attend. When I last saw you, you were about to set out for Hartland. Why did you change your mind?'

She watched him sip at his wine while he considered his answer.

'I thought…someone might be here.'

'Who?' Pru leaned a little closer, even though there was no one sitting close enough to overhear. 'If you mean Sir Joseph Conyers, he was unable to obtain an invitation.'

'How the devil do you know that?'

'The Conyerses are holding their own little party tonight. He would not have done so if he could have been here instead. He sought my acquaintance in order to get closer to Lady Borcaster, but she is not deceived by him.'

'Ah, yes.' He nodded. 'Her late husband was a diplomat, was he not? And her daughter is married to Sir Timothy Flowers. I see how Conyers might well want to befriend her.'

She looked surprised. 'You are very knowledge-able…how do you know so much about Lady Bor-caster?'

He smiled but did not explain.

'You could be wrong about Sir Joseph,' he said. 'Perhaps you piqued his interest.'

'Do you mean he was smitten by my beauty?' She laughed at that. 'How could anyone think so!'

Garrick frowned. 'Do not disparage yourself, Prudence Clifford. You are a very unusual woman.'

He liked the blush that painted her cheeks. He thought it very becoming and said so, but she only laughed again and shook her head.

'Pray do not tease me. I have seen Lady Conyers— Oh!' Her hand flew to her mouth. 'I beg your pardon. Is she the one who…?'

Garrick froze.

*The one who used me. The one who took advantage of a naive young fool and almost made him a murderer.*

'…the one you spoke of?'

She was watching him closely. The chicken that had tasted so delicious earlier was now like ashes in his mouth. He swallowed it and managed a single word.

'Yes.'

'And Sir Joseph. He was your adversary in the duel.' She nodded, not requiring him to answer. 'I see just how it is. You were the victor and that is why he is spreading such lies.' He heard the note of anxiety in her voice when she continued. 'He said there is proof. Evidence that you are a French agent.'

'He is wrong. Although he might try to fabricate something.'

'What a villain!'

'Do you see now why you should let well alone?'

'No. I am even more convinced that Sir Joseph should be shown for what he is. And for what he has been in the past.' She added vehemently, 'He and his wife should never have been allowed to get away with their wrongdoings.'

'There are many rogues like him in town.'

'That does not make it right.'

He saw the martial light in her eye and leaned forward.

'Miss Clifford. Prudence. Please, be true to your name and ignore any further rumours you hear about me.'

'I cannot. I cannot allow them to spread lies about you. It is *unjust*.'

He shrugged. 'They hurt no one but me.'

'And your family name.'

'My family name has borne much greater slurs in its time. Once I have left town the rumours will die down and soon be forgotten.'

She took another sip of wine, but her mind was clearly still on the injustice.

'So, you intend to walk away.' Two spots of angry colour were flying in her cheeks now. 'I did not think you such a coward.'

She was trying to goad him, and she was succeeding.

'I am no coward,' he ground out, holding on to his temper by a thread.

'Then why will you allow them to get away with this?'

'They won't. The truth will out, eventually. Why are *you* so intent upon me denying the claims?'

Pru sat back. Why *was* she so eager to see him vindicated? What was he to her, after all? Nothing more than a stranger whose story had evoked her sympathy.

'Well?' he demanded, his green eyes hard as granite. 'What is it to you if my name is dragged through the gutter?'

She was silent. She believed he had been treated unjustly in the past. She could understand that he might be able to shrug off Annabelle's rejection. That had been an arranged marriage, with little attraction on either side, but perhaps—something twisted inside her—perhaps he was still in love with the beautiful Helene and did not want her to be punished.

Garrick watched the play of emotion in Pru's countenance. He saw a shadow of reserve cloud those clear grey eyes. A small spark of hope flared that she actually cared for him but he squashed it firmly. He was nothing more than another of her charitable causes, something to amuse her while she was in town until another distraction came along. Women were fickle. No one knew that better than he.

But for all that he liked this woman. He did not want to quarrel with her. He smiled.

'No, no, do not frown at me so, Prudence Clifford.

Here we are, at one of the most prestigious balls of the year and we should be enjoying ourselves.' He rose and held out his hand to her. 'What say you, shall we dance the night away?'

When they returned to the main ballroom couples were already waltzing again, including the Emperor of Russia. Such was the crowd gathered about to watch the Tsar that when the Garrick suggested they should go off and join in with the country dances, Pru readily agreed. She discovered he was an accomplished dancer and excellent partner, as she told him when the second dance came to an end.

'I enjoyed it, too,' he replied. 'Shall we dance again?'

'I really should go and find my aunt...'

Pru was enjoying herself far too much to want this to end and even to her own ears she sounded unsure. Garrick's green eyes rested on her, warm and smiling.

He said, 'You would not leave me just yet.'

There was only a heartbeat's pause before she capitulated. After all, she reasoned, Lady Borcaster's coachman had been ordered not to return before six and it would be far easier to find her party then, when the crowds would be much diminished.

She accompanied Garrick to one of the other marquees and enjoyed a glass of wine while they waited for the next dance to begin. It was a risk, dancing with Garrick again, but she salved her conscience with the knowledge that they had moved to another ballroom and amongst so many dancers, it was unlikely that anyone would recognise them.

'Heavens, that was exhausting,' she exclaimed when the duke led her off the floor after two lively reels. She laughed up at him, exhilarated and not a little light-headed. 'I do not think I can dance again without a rest!'

'Let us step outside to cool down a little.'

She made no demur as he guided her out of the crowded room and they slipped outside through a side door. A grey, cloudy dawn was breaking and Pru closed her eyes as she took in a deep breath.

'How blessedly cool it is out here. I cannot recall ever dancing so much before.'

'Never?'

'Not since I was a child.' She chuckled. 'We keep early hours in Bath, you know. Balls conclude promptly at eleven, even if a dance is in progress.'

'But surely there are private parties?'

'Perhaps, but not the ones I attend with my aunt, where one rarely dances. You must think my life was sadly flat.'

'Do *you* think that?'

She hesitated, then said carefully, 'It is the life I have chosen.'

She was glad to hold on to his arm as they strolled along shadowy paths. She could hear the muted strains of the orchestra coming from the buildings. It sounded magical, unearthly. Glancing up, she could even see the morning star twinkling from a gap in the clouds.

'And have you ever lived anywhere but Bath?' he asked her.

'Why, yes. My parents have a house in Melksham.'

'And you lived there until you became companion to your aunt.'

'Yes, although I am very fortunate. Aunt Minerva treats me more as a daughter than a servant.'

'And yet you are still unmarried.'

She stopped and turned to face him. 'I have had admirers,' she said, with careful dignity. After all, it was not a lie; before Walter's death there had been several of his friends who had shown an interest in her. 'None I wished to marry, however.'

'Really? What dullards they must be, the gentlemen of Bath!'

She laughed. 'No, it is rather that I am too particular in my tastes.' She waved a hand. 'But this is a very dreary subject.'

'I do not think so.' He tucked a wayward curl behind her ear. 'No one could ever call you dreary, Prudence Clifford.'

'How kind of you to say so.'

His own hair was tousled from the dancing, one wayward lock falling over his brow. Without thinking she reached up to brush it aside.

'There.' She smiled up at him. 'That is better.'

He caught her hand and pressed his lips into the

palm. Without thinking Pru leaned closer, turning her face up to him, and when he lowered his head she closed her eyes, giving a little sigh as his mouth closed on hers. Then his arms were around her, crushing her close and he was kissing her with such fervour that her senses reeled.

Pru surrendered to her instincts, her lips parting as she responded to his kiss. Her heart was racing, the blood pounding through her body, and she was tingling, every nerve alive. There was an unfamiliar ache deep inside. Something was unfurling, growing. Possessing her. When at last Garrick lifted his head she leaned against his shoulder and gazed up at him. She felt at peace, languid, and very content.

He cleared his throat. 'We should go and find your friends.'

'Yes.' But she spoke without conviction and when he did not move she whispered, 'Garrick, will you kiss me again?'

His eyes darkened and he captured her lips again. She felt the pull of desire grow even stronger and slipped her arms about his neck, holding him close. She pressed her body against his and kissed him back, eagerly. Their tongues danced and excitement leapt inside Pru, leaving her breathless. Her bones had turned to water and she clung tighter, knowing her limbs would not support her if he released her now.

'Do you really want to dance until dawn?' he murmured, leaving a trail of burning kisses down her neck.

She sighed. 'What else is there?'

'My house. It is only a few minutes' walk from here.'

His house! She wanted to be alone with him, to give in to the urgings of her body. Pru was not ignorant of what went on in the marriage bed and at five-and-twenty she knew she was unlikely ever to find a husband. She had no illusions about her future. After this short season in London she would return to her dull, quiet life.

Suddenly, Pru was consumed by desire and a conviction stronger than anything she had known before. She wanted Garrick. She wanted to feel his body against hers, flesh against flesh. Why not allow herself this one experience of passion? No one had ever made her feel this way before, so full of such happiness and excitement and longing that she thought she might burst into flames.

'Then take me there,' she begged him.

Garrick tried to calm the tumult that raged through his body. It was madness, but this whole night had been folly. As if sensing his hesitation she sought his lips and kissed him.

'Take me, Garrick.'

She was smiling, in the dim morning light he could see her eyes were shining. They held no guile, no fear. Only trust.

Garrick released her and stepped away. 'Go and fetch your wrap. If you are still of the same mind then, come back here. I will be waiting for you.'

She stared at him for another moment then turned and ran off. Garrick drove his fingers through his hair as he paced up and down the path. He thought a few quiet moments of reflection would convince her that it would be folly to run off with him. It would leave her with a lifetime of regret. She would see sense. He hoped, prayed she would see sense.

'Curse it, man, you want nothing of the kind!' he growled to himself. 'You want her to come back and damn the consequences!'

He was still wrestling with his conscience when she returned. He watched her hurrying towards him, looking for some sign of doubt in her face.

There was none. Without hesitation she threw herself into his arms and he kissed her, hard, then he took her wrap and arranged it over her head and shoulders, some small protection against prying eyes. He led her to a wicket gate where a few coins persuaded the lackey standing guard to let them out.

They hurried to Dover Street, half walking, half running, caught up in a fever of excitement such as Garrick had never known. When they reached his door, he ushered her inside, growling to the sleepy lackey as they went in.

'You haven't seen us. Is that understood?'

The house was silent. Pru knew she should be afraid, or at least nervous, but with her hand firmly in Garrick's warm grip she felt perfectly safe. She was strangely light-headed, her body singing with joy. She knew this could not last, but she did not care. She wanted this one night of pleasure.

Garrick ushered her into a chamber where the un-shuttered windows allowed in sufficient light for her to see the magnificent bed with elaborate carvings on the bedposts and the sumptuous red and gold hangings.

'Pru.' She felt Garrick's hands on her shoulders. 'Pru, you do not need to do this. In fact, I am damned sure we should not. Say the word and I will take you back.'

'No.' She turned to him, grasping his coat. 'I want this, Garrick, truly. I am no simpering miss. I know what the consequences may be and I am prepared for that.' She stepped closer, smiling up at him. 'I shall make no demands upon you after this. I have no thoughts of marriage, but I should like to know the pleasures of the marriage state, just once.'

'Pru—'

'No,' she said, resting her fingers on his mouth. 'Make me no promises tonight, Garrick.'

She stretched up and kissed him. He gave a little growl, deep in his throat, and she clung tighter as he teased her lips apart, deepening the kiss. Garrick's arms came around her, pulling her closer and she pressed against him, returning his embrace as fervently as she knew how.

He was a skilful lover, undressing her swiftly and

with an ease that suggested he was well-practised, and all the while he teased her with kisses and caresses that kept her on the edge of swooning. Pru's fingers scrabbled with his clothes, impatient to feel his naked flesh against her own and it was not long before he was tumbling her onto the bed.

The kisses grew more fevered. Garrick wanted to go slower, but she was already trembling at his touch, her body receptive, back arching. He kissed her breasts and fastened his mouth over one hardened peak, his tongue circling it while his fingers teased the other. He delighted in her soft moans of pleasure that sent the blood pounding through his body. He smoothed one hand down over her flat stomach until he was exploring the heat between her thighs.

She gasped, pushed against him before she grabbed his wrist.

'Show me what to do,' she begged, her voice low but not quite steady. 'Show me how to pleasure you, too.'

'Oh, sweeting, just having you here is pleasure enough.'

But all the same he drew back, steadied himself then took her hand and guided it over his aroused body, holding out as long as he could against the demands of desire, then he shifted his weight and covered her. Pru was ready for him. Her hips lifted invitingly and the heat of her almost overpowered him as he entered her. She cried out, a sharp inward gasp quickly followed by a mewl of sheer pleasure as she moved with him, against him.

\* \* \*

Pru's body was out of control. Waves had been rippling through her, building like a spring tide and now they crashed, flooding her body and her mind and then she was falling, falling. It was only later, when silence had descended on them and Garrick was lying with his back to her that she realised he had withdrawn from her before the end.

'Garrick?' She rolled towards him and put a hand on his shoulder. 'What is it? Are you well?'

'More than well,' he murmured turning back and kissing her nose. 'I did not wish to risk giving you a child.'

It was too dark to read his face and she felt a slight chill run over her skin. Was this consideration for her, or himself? Desire sated, she felt less sure of anything now, but her doubts faded when he pulled her into his arms again.

'I wish we could stay here longer, but I must get you back to your aunt.'

His kiss warmed her, she felt another kick of excitement deep inside as she ran one hand over his muscled back. She was hungry for his touch again and snuggled closer.

'Must we go just yet?'

Her hand travelled downwards, cupping his buttock and caressing his hip before slipping between their bodies. The effect upon him was immediate, and very satisfying.

He rolled on top of her. 'I think we can delay a few more minutes!'

\* \* \*

It was gone six o'clock when they slipped back into the grounds of Burlington House. They made their way between the marquees, where the music was still playing, little more than a soft beat on the morning air.

'The last dance is not yet finished,' he said. 'Shall we go back inside?'

'I would prefer to remain out here, with you.'

Pru was still fizzing from all that had happened and wanted to cling onto the memory, cling onto *him*, for just a little longer. She had thrown herself at Garrick, as abandoned as any strumpet. She had asked him to make her no false promises and she was glad she had done that. She would not trap him into marriage, even if she was compromised now beyond redemption.

She knew herself too well to think she would ever be happy as his mistress. She could never live with the distress that would cause her family. Nor could she bear to think that at some point he must take a wife. No. One night was all she could expect. She wanted to savour their time together, knowing it could never again be like this.

As the last strains of the music died away, he pulled her into his arms and kissed her again. Tenderly, a farewell embrace. People were leaving the ballrooms. Voices were coming closer, there were sounds of laughter and reluctantly they moved apart. Garrick slid his hands down Pru's shoulders and caught her hands.

'Well.' She tried to make light of it. 'What an interesting night this has been!'

'I beg your pardon,' he said. 'I should not have imposed on you.'

'No, no, I should beg *yours*,' she told him, squeezing his hands. 'I was lost as soon as you took me in your arms tonight. No one has ever kissed me like that before.'

'I should hope not!' He dragged in a breath. 'There is no time to talk now. I must take you back to your party.'

'Yes.'

He pulled her hand onto his arm and they made their way in silence back towards the house. As they approached the hall where guests were assembling to wait for their carriages, Prudence halted. It was time to live up to her name.

'It would be best if I went on alone. It might be awkward, if we are seen together.' She blushed a little. 'I do not want anyone to, to speculate.'

'Very well. But you will tell me, if there are any… *consequences* of what we have just done?'

She did not pretend to misunderstand him. 'Yes of course. I will inform you if I am with child. You have my word on that. Now, I must go.'

He released her arm and she took a step away, then stopped.

'What has happened, tonight,' she said. 'I want it to be very clear that I do not hold you at all to blame.

It was nothing more than an, an aberration, caused by the excitement of the occasion. You need not call upon me. In fact, it is better if you do not. Please do not think I expect anything more from you. Good night, Your Grace.'

Without another word she hurried away.

# Chapter Ten

*Hell-fire, man, you have compromised a perfectly respectable lady!*

Garrick berated himself as he made his way back to Dover Street. Pru had bewitched him, but that was no excuse. How could he have let himself be carried away like that? And if Pru thought he would allow the matter to end there she was very much mistaken. He was not such a rogue.

Prudence Clifford. He felt light-headed, euphoric just thinking of her. He could not stop smiling. She danced like an angel, made him laugh with her quick wit and having her in his bed had been a revelation. The last few hours were some of the happiest he had spent for years. The touch of her hand set his pulse racing, and when he kissed her—! Even now the thought of it sent desire spiking through his body.

He had believed himself immune to female charms but no, a woman he had met only a couple of times in his life had proved him wrong. Confound it, he had only just left her and already he missed her so badly it was a physical ache. But it should not be, she was not his sort at all. Too tall for one thing and her mouth, by her own admission, was too wide. True, she was intelligent, but she was also stubborn, which was the reason he had remained in town. To prevent her from ruining her reputation in a bid to save his.

*And what a mull you have made of that! You have ruined more than her reputation now, you damned scoundrel. You will have to marry her.*

It might not be what either of them wanted, but he would do his duty by the lady. It would have been better for everyone if he had retired to Hartland and let the ton say what it liked about him. But how could he leave Pru Clifford to stand up for him? If she publicly defended him, she would be ridiculed, perhaps even shunned. It might even be said she had set her cap at him. Or worse, that she was hopelessly in love!

His frown deepened. That was clearly not the case. What had her last words to him been? *'Please do not think I expect anything more from you.'* Did she mean that—would she refuse an offer of marriage from him? He was a duke. Her family would fall on his neck.

But would Pru?

Garrick knew she was angry about the rumours against him. He had told her the truth about Annabelle Speke and he thought she would live with that, if it meant protecting the lady. But he understood Pru now, and he was sure she would never tolerate the slur that he was a traitor.

His sole purpose in coming to the ball tonight had been to reason with her, and possibly to protect her, if Conyers was present. Instead he had made things a hundred times more complicated. But how could he resist, when she had been so close, looking up at him with her eyes shining like stars? He had lost his head like any greenhorn.

Confound it, he knew how fragile a lady's reputation could be and yet his actions this night had compromised her. There was no turning back the clock. Surely that was enough to make her accept an offer.

But the doubt persisted. Garrick decided that if Pru would not accept the protection of his name then he would keep his distance, but he needed to be sure she had no reason to publicly defend him. If she had been a wealthy eccentric she might have been able to set the town on its ears and walk away unscathed, but she was not. If his name was besmirched then hers would be, too. Lady Borcaster might even turn her out. Garrick could not have that on his conscience. He must put a stop to the rumours and if he was going to do that, then he would have to face his nemesis.

He passed a narrow house that he remembered from his time in London, when he had been a young buck with an allowance scorching his pocket. The brass plaque on the wall announced it was still a gentleman's club and, after a slight hesitation, he turned and re-traced his steps. He rapped on the door. All those years ago he had needed someone to introduce him. Now his title ensured that he was admitted immediately.

He ran lightly up the stairs and strolled into one of the elegantly appointed salons. Morning light filtered through the muslin drapes at the windows, but candles still burned in the glittering chandeliers, lighting the small green baize tables that were dotted around the room, where gentlemen hunched over their cards in hushed concentration. For a moment he was nineteen again, a boy in a man's world.

A liveried servant approachcd with a tray and he took a glass of wine and sipped at it as his eyes swept over the players. He was in luck. His quarry was present and playing piquet at a small table on the far side of the room. The man was a little older, a little greyer at the temples but instantly recognisable. He was concentrating on his cards and Garrick moved away. He was in no hurry. He would to wait until the game was concluded.

When the man's opponent threw down his cards and quit the table, Garrick slipped into the vacant seat.

'To the victor the spoils, eh?' he murmured.

Sir Joseph Conyers looked up, his brows lifting in surprise.

'The Duke of Hartland.' There was the hint of a sneer in his greeting. 'How long has it been, ten years?'

'Not long enough,' Garrick retorted.

'What is your pleasure, cards or dice?'

'Cards. Piquet, I think, don't you?' He watched Sir Joseph open a fresh pack and shuffle it. 'I have heard your luck with the bones is, er, extraordinary.'

The sculpted eyebrows snapped together. 'That was never proven.'

Garrick allowed himself a little smile and the older man scowled. 'Be very careful, Duke. I will tolerate no slights against my name.'

'Nor I, Sir Joseph. Which is why I am come to see you.' He smiled. 'Shall we play?'

Garrick cut the lower card and dealt first. The two men played in silence, save for announcing their scores. They were both cautious at first, Garrick taking care over his discards.

'My game,' declared Sir Joseph at the end of the first *partie*. 'But you have improved, Duke. Since we last played.'

'I should hope so.'

His opponent smirked and his tone became a little patronising. 'I am sure you can do better.'

The second game was closer, with scores evenly matched until the sixth deal when Garrick scored a Pique.

'Your victory,' muttered Sir Joseph, clearly rattled. 'I made a foolish discard.' He nodded to the waiter to refill his empty wineglass. 'A beginner's mistake. Shall we play again or are you for your bed, Duke?'

Garrick said, casually, 'One more game, then, if you wish.'

'If *I* wish it? Are you not a gamester, Your Grace?'

'I am not. Cards hold little interest for me.'

Garrick noted with satisfaction the gleam of triumph in Sir Joseph's hooded eyes. Then he closed his mind to everything but the game.

'My dear Prudence, General Lechlade was just about to go looking for you,' exclaimed Lady Borcaster when she saw Pru hurrying towards her.

'I beg your pardon, ma'am,' she said.

'Well, well, I am not at all surprised,' replied my lady, chuckling. 'You young people always like to remain until the very end. And at least the crowd has thinned a little now.'

Mrs Clifford nodded. 'Indeed, we were jostled most unpleasantly on the way down to supper. Thankfully, the dear general was on hand to prevent too much inconvenience.'

'I hope you were not too worried for me, Aunt?' Pru ventured.

Remembering all that had happened to her this evening, she felt sure there must be some evidence of it in her appearance. Garrick had done his best with the buttons and fastenings of her gown, and thankfully her wrap covered up any deficiencies in her dress. As for her hair, several tendrils had escaped but she had seen a number of ladies looking far more dishevelled after just one dance this evening. She could only pray there was nothing in her countenance to give her away.

'Not a bit of it, my love. With the waltzing and country dances all going on at the same time, and the crowds so thick, it would have been impossible to remain together for the whole time. We looked for you at supper, of course, but there was no hope of finding anyone in that crush.'

'I said to Minerva, it was only natural that you should want to be with your young friends,' remarked Lady Borcaster, giving Pru an indulgent smile. 'But I told her you are a sensible puss and would come to no harm.' She broke off, listening to the stentorian tones of a footman announcing the carriages. 'Ah, that is ours now. Are you ready to escort us, General?'

Relieved to have escaped with so little explanation of her absence, Pru settled herself into a corner of the carriage for the short journey back to Brook Street. She felt quite dazed. Her hand crept to her lips and excitement sizzled through her again. How forward of her to ask him to kiss her. How wrong of him to comply! If only it had stopped there. If only she was as sensible as Lady Borcaster thought her.

Pru pulled her cloak a little closer. She had told Garrick she expected nothing more from him, but she had gone willingly to his bed and she might now be carrying his child. If that was the case then they must marry. They were both agreed on that. But what if she had been recognised as she danced half the night away with the duke? That would be scandalous, of course, but not a disaster. Her reputation might be harmed, but she hoped her aunt would not turn her off. If she could return to Bath and her charity work, life would continue as before.

The only problem was, Prudence was no longer sure if that was enough for her.

'Damn you, Hartland. The luck was with you to-night!'

'Not all luck,' Garrick replied, piling up the counters before him. 'I had the advantage of a clear head.'

His opponent gave him a malevolent look. The duke met it steadily.

He said, 'I have learned a great deal in the past ten years, Conyers. Some skill at cards is only one small part of it.'

'Why are you telling me this?'

Garrick sat back, his fingers playing with the stem of his wineglass. 'You have been spreading rumours about me.'

'The devil I have!'

'Do not attempt to deny it. Your bluster is wasted on me and the nearest tables are empty. There is no one to impress with your lies.'

Sir Joseph glowered. 'You cannot prove anything.'

'No, but I am sure in my own mind. I am minded to call you out.'

'You would not dare.'

'Would I not?' Garrick's lip curled. 'I am no callow youth now, Conyers. The first time I bested you it was pure chance. This time, you may be sure I will finish the task.' He scooped the rouleaux at his elbow and rose. 'Take heed of my warning, sir. I am willing to forget what has gone before, but only if it stops now. If you continue to spread your lies, be sure I will destroy you.'

Garrick turned on his heel and walked to the door. He could feel Sir Joseph's eyes boring into him all the way across the room. Garrick knew there was no foundation in the rumours. Conyers had been acting out of spite. He stepped out onto the street and stopped for a moment to take in the fresh morning air.

Hopefully he had done enough to put an end to the rogue's malicious meddling, but it did not fully resolve the situation with Prudence. Now he must steel himself to make everything right with her.

A full week passed and Prudence heard nothing from Garrick. There had been no repercussions from the night of the Burlington House ball. No one mentioned her dancing with the duke, but when her body gave her proof that she was not pregnant, the disappointment was so severe it shocked Pru to the core. Only then did she realise how much she would have welcomed a reason to marry him.

She was still coming to terms with this revelation

when Aunt Minerva came into her bedroom, clearly great with news.

'Oh, my dear Pru, are you not dressed yet?'

She stretched her lips into a smile. 'As you see, Aunt. I thought I might rest another hour and I sent Meg away.'

'Well fetch her back this instant,' cried Mrs Clifford, coming further into the room. 'The Duke of Hartland is downstairs and desirous to speak with you.'

Prudence stared at her. 'W-with me?'

'Yes, yes! It was very fortunate that dear Jane is gone out, because I am sure she would not have admitted him, but when the servant told me the duke was wishful to speak with me, I could not bring myself to refuse.' Aunt Minerva came across to the bed and took her hands. She beamed down at Prudence and said in hushed tones, 'He is going to ask you to marry him.'

'No!'

'It is true, my love. He came in very nervous, and quite properly asked my permission to pay his addresses to you.'

'But he cannot!'

'My dear, why not?' Mrs Clifford blinked at her. 'You were the one who defended him against those vicious rumours.'

'I told you then that I did not wish to marry him!' Pru dragged the sheet up to her chin. 'You must go down and send him away. Tell him. Tell him there is *no reason* for him to marry me.'

'La, my love, I can do nothing of the sort. He is a duke, for heaven's sake. Why would you refuse him?'

'Because...because of his reputation,' said Pru, grasping at straws. 'Lady Borcaster's friends are right, no respectable female would countenance his acquaintance.'

'Have you lost your wits, Prudence love? We are not talking of being *friends*, this is very different. Marriage! You would be a duchess. Think of it. Think how proud your dear father would be.'

'No, he would not,' cried Pru. 'Papa cares more for, for goodness and honesty than titles. Besides, everyone knows Hartland has no fortune.'

'He is hardly a pauper,' retorted her aunt. 'You would be far richer than you are now, that is certain. And a dukedom, too! Do you not realise what an honour he is doing you?'

But it was not honour that Pru was thinking of, it was marrying a man who did not love her. One who was marrying her because he thought it was his duty to do so. He would make her his duchess, but then the long years would stretch ahead of them. Years of polite indifference. Or possibly he would be kind to her, and she thought that would be even more unbearable.

'Please, Aunt, go down and tell him I do not *want* to marry him. Make him understand that our stations are too far removed.'

'My dear, that will not weigh with him if his affections are engaged.'

*They aren't. He feels obliged to wed me.*

But Pru could not say that to her aunt without disclosing the reason for it. She clutched at the sheet and spoke as calmly as she could.

'Aunt Minerva, I cannot marry a man with such a past,' she said. 'Then there are the accusations against him. It is one thing to defend such a man out of, of Christian charity, it is quite another to marry him.'

'Well, I never did!' Mrs Clifford plumped down on the edge of the bed, staring at her niece. 'Are you quite, quite, sure, Prudence, my love? It is a flattering offer, and, at five-and-twenty...'

'I am unlikely to get another. I know that, Aunt, and I am resigned to it. I have enjoyed our holiday, but all I really want is to go back to Bath and return to my charity work at the infirmary.'

Mrs Clifford looked at her in disbelief.

'My dear girl, that is no reason to reject the duke. You could help the poor far more if you were richer.'

'My reason for helping the doctors goes beyond money.'

'Oh, I know, my love. It is guilt that takes you to that wretched place week after week. Regret that you could not save your poor brother—'

'Ah, don't, Aunt!' Her voice cracking, Pru closed her eyes and took a few deep, steadying breaths. She said, quite slowly, 'I pray you will go back to His Grace and give him my answer.'

## Chapter Eleven

London at the end of June was white-hot. The crowds that had thronged the capital for the visit of the Allied Sovereigns had left, but the streets were still busy with traffic, although Garrick barely noticed as he strode along Piccadilly. He had spent the morning with his man of business, signing the papers to dispose of several properties that he did not want and could no longer afford. It was a relief to be free of some of his burden and he planned to drive to Hartland soon and concentrate on improving what was left of his estates. Perhaps that would help him forget Prudence Clifford.

He had not seen her since that fateful night at Burlington House. Nine days ago. Nine long days in which he had thought of her almost constantly, remembering the taste of her, the feel of her in his arms. He had always known he must marry one day. Annabelle's brutal rejection had been a relief but he knew it was his duty to take a wife, so why not Prudence? He could not deny the attraction between them. Besides, he liked her and he had thought she liked him. Which was why he had decided to put it to the touch on Monday. He had called in Brook Street to ask Pru to marry him, but he had been turned away by her aunt. She had not even had the courtesy to tell him in person!

Even now he could not believe she had refused him. He had been convinced she would say yes, but she would not even see him. It was her aunt who had broken the news, laying out gently but with awful clarity the fact that Pru did not consider him respectable enough to accept his offer of marriage. He had argued, explaining to Mrs Clifford that her niece knew all about his protracted betrothal, now at an end, and the scandalous duel that had resulted in his fleeing the country. Her reply was like a blow to the gut:

*'Yes, Your Grace, Prudence told me she is very honoured by your confidences. However, while Christian charity obliges her to defend you to your critics, she says she cannot accept* such a man *as a husband.'*

Even two days on, those words brought him to a stand. He came to an abrupt halt just at the entrance to Albany, his hand tightening on his ebony stick as he tried to suppress the red mist of anger and remorse that enveloped him. Pru did not care for him. She had used him, as Helene Conyers had done. He meant less to her than her damned charities!

'Well, by my stars. Garrick Chauntry! I have been looking for you.'

\* \* \*

The familiar voice snapped Garrick out of his trance. He looked around to see a fair-haired man striding towards him, immaculately attired in a blue coat, snow-white linen, with pale pantaloons disappearing into highly polished and tasselled Hessians.

'Jack! I thought you were in Sussex. What the devil brings you here?'

'You.' Lord John Callater gripped the outstretched hand. 'I told you, I have been looking for you. Where the devil have you been hiding?'

'Nowhere. I have been in London for some months. Since leaving Bath, in fact.'

'When I called at Grosvenor Square all they would tell me was that you no longer lived there.' He glanced back through the entrance to the Albany courtyard. 'Will you come in and take wine with me? I want to know what you have been doing.'

'I am on my way to Dover Street.' Garrick waved his cane roughly in that direction. 'My new house.'

'Then I shall come with you.' Jack tucked his arm in Garrick's and they set off along the street. 'You will not escape me again.'

Garrick smiled. 'I have no wish to escape you,' he said mildly.

'But you have proved mighty elusive. You have not been to any of the usual haunts!'

'I did not come to town to be sociable.'

Jack scoffed at that. 'You were sociable enough

when I met you in Vienna! *Here* you are doing your best to be invisible. And you are selling the Grosvenor Square house?'

'It is sold,' Garrick corrected him. 'I have just signed the final papers.'

'Congratulations. Damned barrack of a place, as I remember, and sadly in need of renovation.'

'Aye, like so much of the Hartland estate.'

'Is that why you have been keeping your head down?' asked Jack bluntly. 'Are you in dun territory?'

'No, no, not as bad as all that. Although if my father had not died when he did, I fear it would be.'

He had seen all the ledgers now. He had pored over the accounts with his man of business and they showed the old duke had not been too ill to travel, or to keep his mistress in luxury. In the years before his death his father had lived extravagantly and run up expenses to throw the estates into even greater debt.

He needed to go to Hartland, to see his mother and discover just how much she knew. Perhaps she was in ignorance of what had been going on. Mayhap she had put her husband on a pedestal. If so, Garrick had no wish to cut him down. It would break her heart, and he had already caused her enough pain.

He felt Jack's grip on his arm tighten for a moment in a gesture of sympathy. They had known one another since their schooldays. Jack Callater knew as much as anyone about his affairs. Almost. Garrick quickly stifled all thoughts of Prudence Clifford and walked on to Dover Street, where he took his friend up the stairs, calling for Stow to bring wine.

'I have not seen you since you quit Bath so precipitously,' said Jack, when they were comfortably seated in the drawing room. 'What happened?'

'I'd prefer not to answer that.'

'Damnation, Garr, we've never had any secrets from one another.'

Garrick waited until Stow had left them with wine and a tray of small fancy cakes before he replied.

'This isn't my secret to share. Suffice it to say I did not offer for Miss Speke.'

'Aye, I have heard the rumours about that, but I don't believe 'em,' said Jack bluntly. 'For God's sake, man, you can tell me the truth. I do not for one moment believe you jilted the girl.'

'I applaud your faith in me.'

'It ain't in your nature,' Jack replied. 'When you didn't turn up at Sally Triscombe's that night some of the others thought you'd got cold feet, but you will remember that I was staying at the Pelican as well as you. When I knocked on your door the following morning your man told me you had gone to Royal Crescent.'

Garrick frowned. 'Stow doesn't know the whole truth.'

'No, I doubt anyone does,' retorted Jack. 'But I am

certain that you did not desert the lady, despite the scurrilous talk.'

'I pray you, leave it there, Jack!' Garrick jumped up and strode over to the window. 'My reputation will survive being labelled a jilt. Miss Speke's would not.'

'Too chivalrous by half, Duke! And if there is no truth to the rumours, why have I not seen you in your usual haunts? Not because some fool has put it about you are a French spy...'

Garrick swung round, frowning. 'I thought I had put paid to that rumour.'

'Oh, I only heard a whisper of it, a couple of weeks since, and I was at pains to knock that back, I can tell you.'

'I suppose I should be grateful to you!'

'Aye, you should, since I have been in an agony of apprehension over you since you left Bath without a word.'

'Your concern was wasted. I have been in London all the time.'

'Playing least in sight and not answering my letters! I knew you hadn't gone to Hartland, so I came posting up to town. And now I am here,' Jack went on, fixing his friend with a determined eye, 'I don't mean to allow you to carry on skulking in the shadows, as if you have something to hide. Time to redeem yourself, Duke.'

'And if I don't want to be, er, redeemed?'

'Well, if you won't defend your good name then I shall be obliged to do so!'

A wry smile tugged at Garrick's mouth.

'Another one,' he murmured.

'What?'

'Nothing.' He shook his head. 'Very well, what do you propose?'

Jack grinned. He carried both their glasses back to the side table to refill them.

'I intend to restore you to your rightful place in society,' he said, handing Garrick his recharged glass. 'Starting tonight, we are going to attend every society event imaginable!'

The ballroom at Shrivenham House was the most magnificent chamber Prudence had ever seen. The ornate plasterwork around the ceiling had been gilded and the walls were covered with green and gold silk which glowed in the light of the chandeliers glittering overhead. Even more sparkling were the jewels bedecking the guests. The room echoed with voices and laughter, but Pru was finding it hard to feel any excitement about the forthcoming evening.

There had been so many parties since she arrived in London and she feared she was growing tired of the constant social whirl. Her spirits had been very low since she had rejected Garrick's offer. Aunt Minerva told her the duke had accepted her decision courteously and even sent her his compliments before leaving the house, but that was little consolation to Pru. His graciousness made her feel even more wretched.

Dancing was already in progress. Lady Borcaster led her little party around the edge of the room, introducing Prudence and her aunt to those she considered would be *useful acquaintances*. She quickly found Pru a dance partner, but immediately sent the gentleman on his way.

'These two dances have a good half hour to run yet,' she told him. 'Come and find Miss Clifford when the next set is forming. There are more people I wish her to meet!'

Pru found it a struggle, constantly smiling and making conversation, and at the first opportunity, she slipped away into the crowd. She made her way across to the long windows that filled one side of the room. She knew they overlooked Green Park, but since Lady Borcaster had declared they should arrive fashionably late, it was quite dark and impossible to see anything save the reflections of the twinkling lights from the ballroom.

How soon could she leave? she wondered. Could she say she was ill, perhaps, and take to her bed for a week? Lady Borcaster had invited them to stay until the end of August and the thought of spending another two months in London weighed heavily upon her spirits.

'You are not dancing, Miss Clifford.'

She gave a little start when she heard Garrick's deep voice and turned quickly.

'Your Grace!'

'You seem surprised.'

'I am.' She gripped her fan, determined to be honest. 'Surprised and embarrassed. I should apologise. For refusing to see you when you called. It was cowardly.'

'Let us not talk of it,' he interrupted her. 'It is forgotten.'

She peeped up at him. He looked quite at his ease, which meant he must be relieved she had refused him. Somehow that thought did not cheer her at all.

She said, 'I thought you had left London.'

'I had business that was not yet concluded. I thought I might as well stay to sign the papers rather than have them sent on to me.'

She nodded. How foolish to think for a moment that he had remained in town for her sake.

'Will you dance with me, later?' Now she was more than surprised. She was astonished. He continued. 'Can you waltz? Since the Tsar's visit it has become quite the rage.'

'Yes.' She felt quite dazed, conversing with Garrick like this, but with so many people around them she could hardly run away. She said, 'It is danced everywhere now, is it not? I *have* learned to waltz, but I have only ever danced it at private parties.'

'Which this is, albeit a very grand affair! So, you will stand up with me?'

Pru looked down at her hands, clasped tightly about her fan. She should not. She *must* not. It would only prolong her agony, since nothing could ever come of it.

*Be sensible, Pru!*

'I am sure there are other ladies you should ask first.'

'I have already danced with my hostess and her daughter. Now I want to stand up with you.' He added, 'We did not waltz together at Burlington House. An omission I now want to repair.'

His green eyes were fixed on her, causing her heart to beat a little faster, and when she finally met his gaze, she knew she was lost.

*Why not? It is only a dance.*

A tremulous smiled hovered. 'I would like that.'

She searched his face, alert for any signs of triumph, but she saw only a faint relaxing in his features. Relief.

'Until the waltz, then,' he said, and with a little bow he was gone.

Pru watched him walk away. She was like a moth, unable to escape the candle's flame. But what of it? It would be another memory to store against the long, lonely nights head of her. But she could not quite think of it like that. Her spirits were rising at the idea of another half hour in his company. With a gasp she suddenly remembered the young man who had claimed her hand for the next dance and she hurried off to find him. Her earlier weariness had evaporated, replaced by a sizzle of anticipation for what the evening might bring.

\* \* \*

Garrick studiously avoided the matrons who were trying to catch his eye. He knew his hostess would think it his duty to choose a partner for every dance, but he was in no humour to do so. He moved to the side of the room and leaned against one of the marbled pillars. His height gave him the distinct advantage of having a clear view of the dancers who were forming a new set. He watched Pru taking her place on the dance floor. She was smiling and chatting as the dancers waited for the music to start, as if she had not a care in the world. She might be taller than her partner and not conventionally pretty, but Garrick could tell the fellow was captivated. Damn him. She might not have fallen in love yet, but it would happen, she was too attractive to remain single. One day she would meet a man who captured her heart. He was surprised to find how much he wished it could have been him.

When he had first seen Pru this evening Garrick had determined to avoid her. It was what his head told him to do, although his body objected strongly. He could not forget how good it was to hold her, to kiss her. To have her in his bed. How *right* that had felt. Although, clearly, she had not thought the same or she would not have refused to become his duchess.

He scowled. Another salutary lesson from a woman. When would he learn? He had agreed to come here tonight, but he was determined not to stay. Perhaps he could leave now, slip away before the waltz. Pru might be angry, even upset, but it would be best for them both. He should go off to Hartland and forget all about Pru Clifford. Leave her to live her own life. Give her the chance to find a better man.

His dark thoughts were interrupted by a hand on his shoulder.

'Don't think you can get away with this, Garrick,' drawled an amused voice. 'Since when have you taken to standing around at parties, glowering like a love-lorn hero?'

He shook off the hand.

'You insisted I come with you, Jack, but you cannot force me to make a cake of myself on the dance floor.'

His friend laughed. 'True, but you could make an effort to be sociable.' He threw up his hands. 'I know, you dislike society with a vengeance—and with good cause!—but refusing to dance will only give people more reason to think ill of you. That is not why I dragged you here.'

It sounded so much like something Pru would say that Garrick smiled, in spite himself.

'I haven't refused. You have seen me dancing.'

'With just two partners!'

'I have a partner for the waltz, too.'

'Ah?' Jack cocked a knowing eyebrow. 'The young lady I saw you talking with earlier? Well, that is something. Any more?'

'Is that not enough?'

'No! By heaven, man, I am beginning to wish I had left you brooding in Dover Street.'

'I wish you had, too!' Garrick glanced over Jack's shoulder. 'I see our hostess is bearing down upon us, her daughters in tow and looking very determined! I am off to enjoy a few moments' peace on the terrace.'

Jack grinned. 'Leaving me to their tender mercies?'

'It's no more than you deserve!' And with that parting shot, Garrick lounged away.

When the music finished, Pru's partner begged he might escort her back to her party.

'Yes of course.'

She accompanied him off the floor, directing his attention to her aunt and Lady Borcaster standing at the side of the room with Sir Joseph Conyers. Her partner slowed.

'Ah, Miss Clifford, pray forgive me, I have just remembered…'

Looking up, Pru saw that his chubby countenance had paled.

'Is anything wrong, Mr Trenchard?'

'No, no, not at all.' His eyes were darting around, anywhere but at her or the little group ahead of them. 'I need to go and talk to…'

By now Pru's mind was seething with conjecture.

'Is it perhaps Sir Joseph that you do not wish to meet?'

His sudden start and the dull flush that mounted

his cheeks confirmed her suspicions, although he was quick to deny it.

'How, how absurd, ma'am. No, it's not that at all! A matter of, of urgent business…'

She pulled him to one side, into a space where they could speak without being overheard.

'Forgive me, sir, but are you…' How could she broach such a delicate business? 'Are you *enamoured* of Lady Conyers?' She fixed him with a steady gaze. The look of alarm in his face gave her the answer and she screwed up her courage to continue. 'Mr Trenchard, pray do not ask me how I know this, but you would be wise to avoid the lady. She has ensnared more than one young man.'

'I beg your pardon, ma'am, I have no idea what you mean!'

His bluster did nothing but convince Pru that her suspicions were correct.

She continued. 'I know it is not usual for single ladies to talk of these matters, sir, but in this case, I believe I must. I know something of the lady and I know that, in the past, she has engineered a compromising situation with her young admirer, where he is discovered by her husband.'

'No, no she wouldn't, I mean…' He broke off, looking alarmed.

Pru put a hand on his arm. 'It is not too late, sir. Give up the lady now. She is not going to leave her husband, whatever she might tell you.'

'You are q-quite wrong, ma'am. It is nothing like that, I assure you.'

He floundered on a little longer then excused himself and hurried away. Pru watched him go. She had done her best, spoken far more plainly than a single lady should and had no idea if her warning would do any good. She abhorred gossips, but in this case she could not stand by and see another young man hurt as Garrick had been.

Sir Joseph was still conversing with Lady Borcaster when Pru came up to the little group. Mrs Clifford saw her approaching and alerted Lady Borcaster, who turned and said in a lively voice, 'Ah, here is dear Prudence now! Not too tired from all your dancing, I hope?'

'Not at all, ma'am.'

'Miss Clifford dances very well,' purred Sir Joseph, giving her a little bow. 'It is a pleasure to watch her.'

Pru kept smiling although she really did not like being discussed as if she was not present. But Sir Joseph had not finished.

'I hope, Mrs Clifford, that you will allow your niece to stand up with me for the next, which is the waltz?'

'Oh, of course, Sir Joseph. I am sure—'

'Alas I regret I cannot,' Pru said quickly. 'I am already engaged. For the waltz.'

'Ah.' She detected a slight annoyance in those hooded eyes. 'A pity. Another time, then, perhaps?'

'Perhaps,' she agreed with cool politeness.

He stepped back, gave a little bow and sauntered off. All three ladies watched him disappear into the card room, then Mrs Clifford turned to her niece, her face alive with curiosity.

'I did not know you had a partner for the waltz, Prudence. Was this Lady Shrivenham's doing?'

'No, ma'am. The gentleman asked me himself.'

'Heavens, how forward of him,' exclaimed Lady Borcaster, mildly reproving. 'He should have requested an introduction from your aunt or your hostess, at the very least.'

'Neither were on hand,' explained Pru. 'But we are already acquainted and as I am not a young debutante, I thought it safe to accept.'

'Yes of course,' agreed Lady Borcaster. 'No lady wants to be sitting out if she can help it. Who is your partner?'

She looked around and Pru saw her stiffen, the smile frozen to her lips when her eyes fixed upon the man approaching them.

'Yes,' murmured Pru, trying hard not to giggle. 'It is His Grace the Duke of Hartland.'

# Chapter Twelve

Garrick observed the older ladies as he approached to claim his dance partner. Mrs Clifford looked stunned and a little discomfited, as well she might after their last meeting, while Lady Borcaster's greeting was positively glacial. Prudence, by contrast was smiling widely, her eyes shining with mischief. Little witch, he thought, his own mouth twitching, she is enjoying this moment. It pleased him. There was nothing like shared amusement to banish constraint.

He said, as Pru took his arm and walked with him to the dance floor, 'I fear we have discomposed your companions.'

'I am very sorry they could not conceal their disapproval.'

'Do they disapprove of the dance, or your partner?'

'A little of both, but you, mostly.' They took their places, ready to begin, and she peeped up at him. 'They disapprove of me, too, for accepting you.'

The music started and Garrick escorted his partner around the room in a slow promenade.

'Then why did you?'

The dancers moved into the *pirouette*. Garrick held Pru's hand in an arch above their heads as they slowly turned.

'Well?' he prompted her.

'I could hardly refuse to dance with a duke.'

'You refused to marry one.' Her eyes flew to his face and Garrick cursed himself silently when he saw the twinkle had faded. He said, 'I beg your pardon, I did not mean to remind you.'

'I need no reminding, Your Grace. The honour you conveyed upon me will last for ever.'

Her words ignited a small spark of hope, but this was no place to discuss such a delicate matter.

'You have not told me why you decided to dance with me,' he prompted her.

'Lady Borcaster was at such pains to find a dancing master for me, that I might perfect the steps. It seems a pity not to put the training into practice.'

She smiled at him and Garrick felt a sudden constriction in his chest. She was entrancing, every touch, every glance inflamed him. He never wanted to let her go.

The tempo changed, became quicker and Pru turned to skip beside him as the circle of dancers progressed around the room in the final movements of the dance. He was hardly aware of the other couples, he had eyes only for his partner as she skipped and twirled beside him in a flurry of silk skirts.

Prudence could not stop smiling. Her feet flew over the floor as the duke guided her expertly around the room. For someone used to looking over her partners' heads, it was a pleasure to dance with a tall man. The duke made her feel dainty, cherished. She would squirrel away these happy memories for the future.

They took their bows and she looked up at him, out of breath but exquisitely happy.

'Thank you, Your Grace,' she said, fanning herself. 'I enjoyed that, very much!'

'But it was warm work. Shall we sit out the next?'

'If we can find somewhere cooler.'

Pru took his arm and they walked across to the wall of long windows. The two doors in the centre had been thrown open to the summer night and she made no demur when he led her out onto the wide iron-railed balcony that ran along the back of the house.

The moon was rising, and once her eyes had adjusted from the glare of the ballroom Pru could see Green Park spreading out into the distance. They were not alone, other couples were on the balcony, taking advantage of the night air, but it still felt very daring to be here with Garrick, in the moonlight.

'I shall be in disgrace,' she murmured.

'Because you have come outside with me?'

He was standing at her shoulder, his voice dark and smooth as velvet.

'Perhaps. Or because I dared to dance with you. Not that I regret it,' she said quickly. 'Where did you learn to dance so well?'

'On the Continent.'

'Vienna?'

'Yes, and in Rome and Paris.'

'But surely those last two were in French hands until recently.'

'They were.'

Pru glanced around quickly. There were only two other couples on the balcony now and they were too far away to overhear the conversation. She turned to Garrick, trying to read his expression in the moonlight. He smiled at her and shook his head slightly.

'You have my word I am no spy,' he murmured.

It took all her willpower not to reach up and put her palm against his rugged cheek. Instead she gazed out over the park again. There was a dreamlike quality to the night and Pru breathed in deeply, content to be standing here with Garrick beside her.

'I am glad,' she said. 'Although I never really doubted your innocence on that matter.'

'I believe it is my reputation as a jilt, a breaker of hearts, that worries you more.'

She smiled into the darkness. 'But I know that is not true.'

'And yet you cannot have *such a man* as a husband.'

Pru turned quickly and her eyes flew to his face. She saw the scornful twist to his mouth. 'Your aunt told me those were your very words.'

'I needed to persuade her that I could not marry you.'

She rubbed her arms, suddenly chilled.

'And yet you do not doubt my innocence! That makes no sense. Tell me the true reason you will not marry me.' He said roughly, 'Is it because I killed my father?'

'No! You did *not* kill him. I do not believe that.'

'My mother does.'

'But you said your father was in ill health.'

'He was. For years, but my youthful follies were too much for him.'

'Your father sent you away,' she persisted. 'He banished you, when it was you who was the victim. The duel was forced upon you.'

'Yes. But my actions hastened his demise.'

'No. He lived for years after you left England. Whatever else you have done, you did not kill him.'

'But his death still haunts me.' He fixed his eyes on the moon and sucked in a breath. 'You cannot know what that is like.'

Pru reached out and took his hands. 'Yes, I can. I do.'

She said slowly, 'My brother, Walter, had a riding accident five years ago. He fell and hit his head. He never regained consciousness, although he lived on for more than a week. My father was distraught and

Mama had to look after him as well as the house and Home Farm. My younger sisters, too, depended upon her, so I took on the task of nursing Walter. We tried everything suggested by the doctors and the apothecary. I even consulted the local midwife. I could not save him.'

'Oh, Pru, I am so very sorry.' Garrick squeezed her fingers, his gentle touch warm and comforting. 'But if the doctors could not cure him, it was not your fault.'

'No, I know that, but it does not stop me feeling guilty. If I had only known more, acted sooner! Since moving to Bath I been working at the infirmary, helping the doctors to look after such injuries. Somehow, that helps with the pain of losing Walter.'

Garrick heard the wistful note in her voice and his heart lurched. He wanted to take her in his arms and kiss away her pain, but even if she wanted his attentions, even if she had not rejected his offer of marriage, there were too many people around them.

'Thank you for telling me,' he said gently. 'It could not have been easy, sharing your confidences.'

'You honoured me with yours, that night in Bath.' She smiled up at him. 'We are friends, are we not?'

Friends! Her trust in him was humbling. He was suddenly aware of how much that meant to him. It did not matter if she would not be his duchess. After all, what had he to offer, save a tarnished reputation and a lifetime of debt?

He said abruptly, 'We should go in.'

'What?' she teased him. 'Are you tired of my company already?'

'You must go back to your aunt before you are missed.'

Pru was surprised by this sudden change. One moment Garrick was smiling at her, kind, compassionate. Now he had withdrawn and he was scowling as if his thoughts were very dark. He must be impatient to be rid of her. He did not offer his arm so she slipped her hand onto his sleeve. Whatever demons he was fighting she did not believe his anger was directed against her.

They stepped back into the noisy glare of the ballroom. Little had changed, the candles still burned brightly and the dancing continued, but suddenly Pru felt exhausted. Desolate, too. Garrick was tired of her company, that much was clear. If she could not remain with him then she would rather go back to Brook Street immediately.

She was wondering if she could broach the subject to Lady Borcaster when a cold, disdainful voice cut through her thoughts.

'Well, well, it is the Duke of Hartland.'

She looked up quickly to see Sir Joseph Conyers and his beautiful wife blocking their way.

# Chapter Thirteen

Garrick tensed. Pru felt his muscled arm harden beneath the sleeve of his coat.

'Sir Joseph.' He nodded, his voice cool. 'Lady Conyers.'

'Have you been enjoying the moonlight?' Helene glanced past them towards the open doors. 'How romantic.'

Her knowing smile brought the blood rushing to Pru's cheeks, but the duke replied calmly enough.

'After the exertions of the waltz we needed a little fresh air.'

'And the lady caught herself a duke for her partner.' Sir Joseph's cold smile turned into a sneer. 'I trust he did not disappoint you, Miss Clifford.'

'Not at all.' She lifted her chin. 'His Grace is a most accomplished dancer.'

She noted that Lady Conyers was studying her, as if she scented a rival.

'Something perfected during your years abroad, perhaps, Your Grace,' murmured Sir Joseph. 'I believe the waltz is very popular in France.'

'That I wouldn't know,' retorted Garrick.

A soft laugh came from Lady Conyers. 'I believe I am considered to be moderately accomplished at the waltz myself,' she purred. 'I should very much like to dance with you, Duke, and have your opinion on the matter.'

The duke inclined his head. 'One day, madam, perhaps you shall. But not tonight.'

They moved on, but not before Pru saw the look Lady Conyers threw at Garrick as she passed. It was blatantly inviting. It angered Pru to think any lady would flirt with another man when she was with her husband.

She was even more unnerved by the jealous rage that ripped through her.

Garrick escorted Prudence back to her friends and went in search of Jack Callater. He had had enough of society for one night. What ill luck to bump into Conyers while he had Prudence on his arm. He wouldn't put it past the rogue to try and do her a mischief, if he thought Garrick might suffer for it.

He found Jack in the card room, but when it was clear that he would be engaged for some time yet, Garrick went away again. He rarely played at cards these days, although he knew he had a talent for it. In his darker moments he considered playing deep as a way to restore the family fortunes, but the idea of fleecing some fool and leaving him destitute did not appeal.

He returned to the ballroom where the cotillion had just commenced. He spotted Sir Joseph dancing with the eldest Miss Shrivenham. Worming his way into respectable society, he thought sourly. But to what end?

A light touch on his arm put an end to his musings. He looked down to find Helene Conyers beside him.

'Escaped from your Long Meg at last, Your Grace?'

She was so close he could smell her perfume, a heavy, cloying scent. It had once turned his head, but not now.

'Miss Clifford honoured me with a dance,' he replied, keeping his tone indifferent.

'I think she would like to honour you with much more than that,' she purred. 'I saw the way she looked at you.'

Garrick was in no mood to play games. 'What do you want, Lady Conyers?'

'Lady?' she moved closer still. 'You used to call me Helene.' When he did not reply she went on. 'I wanted to warn you that Joseph is planning mischief.'

'What is there new in that?'

'Mischief against *you*, Garrick.' She put a hand on his arm, the jewels winking on her thin fingers. 'I could help you.'

His lip curled. 'No thank you. I have some experience of your help.'

'Ah, Garrick, surely you feel *something* for me, for old times' sake?'

Her red lips pouted and she peeped up at him from beneath her lashes. He remembered that look. Alluring, sensual. Full of promise. Once it had driven him wild, now he was surprised that he felt nothing, not even anger for her betrayal.

'You are wasting your time, Helene, your tricks will not work with me now.'

She raised her finely pencilled brows, as if to imply she did not believe him. Relieved that he was no longer in thrall to the woman, Garrick plucked her hand from his sleeve and carried it to his lips. A brief, final salute, for old times' sake.

'Go back to your husband, madam. You deserve one another.'

He saw the flash of anger in her eyes and thought for a moment that perhaps it was not wise to snub her. But he could not regret it. She had hurt him too much as a boy. It was good to know she no longer held any power over him.

Pru was standing with her aunt, watching the dancing when Garrick emerged from the card room. Not that she had been looking out for him. Of course not. It was merely that his tall, impressive figure was hard to miss. Her eyes followed him, admiring his lithe movements and remembering how well he danced. He was a large man but he had the natural grace of a sportsman.

The crowd had thinned a little and there was no one obscuring Pru's view. She saw Lady Conyers approach the duke, precious stones glistening from her golden curls. They were talking, the lady standing very close, her hand on the duke's arm. Every movement was designed to attract, thought Pru, unable to drag her eyes away. Garrick kissed the lady's hand and she noted how his eyes followed Lady Conyers as she moved off. A shiver ran down her spine. He was still in love with the beautiful Helene.

Garrick was hoping to find Jack and make his escape when he was waylaid by Lady Shrivenham. She was not about to allow a duke to slip away when there were ladies in need of dance partners. Resigning himself to his fate, Garrick gave in to the blandishments of his hostess. He fulfilled his obligations for the rest of the evening, smiling, dancing and saying all that was necessary to his partners. An exemplary guest, as he told Jack Callater when they finally made their way down the grand staircase at the end of the night.

'I hope you are satisfied!'

'It's a start, Garr.' Jack laughed as they stepped into the hall, where the guests were milling around, waiting for their carriages. 'Admit it, man, you enjoyed yourself! You always liked dancing.'

'I wish now I had spent the last few hours in the card room, as you did.'

'But *I* had already done my duty and danced with all the prettiest young ladies.'

Not all of them, thought Garrick, his eyes resting on a willowy lady in a rose silk cloak. She was standing at the foot of the stairs and, as if aware of his gaze, she turned and looked up, her grey eyes widening and a faint blush staining her cheeks. They were so close there was no avoiding her, even if he had wished to.

'Miss Clifford.'

'Your Grace. I am waiting for my aunt and Lady Borcaster...'

Garrick felt Jack's sharp nudge in his ribs and said, 'Will you allow me to present to you my good friend, Lord John Callater?'

He watched as Jack made an elegant bow and exchanged a few words with Prudence, drawing a shy smile from her with something he said. Curse it, the fellow was always so charming! Handsome, too. And the eldest son of a marquess. Was it any wonder he had ladies throwing themselves at his feet?

Not that Jack ever did more than indulge in a little flirtation with any lady, but that was enough to have some of them sinking into a decline once his interest had waned. Garrick did not want that to happen to Pru.

At last they moved on. Jack took his arm as they strolled in the direction of Dover Street, making their way past the string of carriages waiting at the side of the road.

'So that is Miss Prudence Clifford.'

'What of it?' Garrick was on the defensive.

'She was your waltz partner. I hope she appreciates the honour you have done her.'

'She is far too sensible for that!'

'But you like her, I think. Have you known her long?'

'We met in Bath.'

The moment the words were out, Garrick knew he had made an error.

'Really? When you went there to propose to Miss Speke? Or have you made another visit since?'

'Damn you, Jack, you know I have only been to the cursed place once! We met there by chance.'

'And you met again in town. How, may I ask, when you did not come here *to be sociable*?'

'She accosted me in Green Park,' Garrick admitted. 'She is a most resourceful lady.'

The memory evoked a smile, but it disappeared at Jack's next words.

'She has set her cap at you, then?'

'No! The truth is, she is an interfering wench who wants to help me.'

'Is that so?' Jack's brows rose. 'There is something you are not telling me, my friend.'

Garrick realised he was going to have to explain at least some of the story.

'Miss Clifford knows about Miss Speke. When I was in Bath I was obliged to tell her what had occurred.

Her sense of justice objected to Lady Tirrill's version of events, which has been circulating in town.'

'What!' Jack stopped and because of their linked arms, Garrick was obliged to halt, too. 'Do you mean she knows everything you have refused to share with me? Just how close a friend is she, Garr?'

'For heaven's sake let us walk on,' Garrick urged him. 'We cannot talk here!'

'Very well, we are nearly at Dover Street. I shall come in with you. Be sure, Garr, I shall not leave until I have had the truth of this matter!'

An hour and several glasses of brandy later, Garrick has given his friend the whole story.

Jack shook his head. 'I find it hard to believe you divulged everything to a complete stranger. And a female, at that!'

'I was very drunk and feeling incredibly sorry for myself.'

'I daresay, but even so, that is unlike you, Garr.' Jack grinned. 'And the sensible Miss Clifford wants to be your champion.'

'She *did*. Hopefully I have nipped that in the bud now.'

'Sounds like a case to me. I saw the way you looked at her, my friend. By heaven, I think you are in love!'

'Don't be so damned foolish.'

'I knew it!' Jack cried, triumphant. 'And from what

you have told me of the lady, I suspect she must return your regard. So, are you going to offer for her?'

Garrick pushed himself out of the chair and took both glasses to the side table to recharge them while he considered how best to answer.

'That is out of the question.'

Jack accepted his full glass and stretched his long legs out in front of him.

'Why? Do you intend to marry an heiress?'

'You know I don't.'

'Then why not put it to the touch?'

Garrick sat down and sipped at his brandy. Jack was his oldest friend; he could not lie to him.

'I can offer her a title, but there is no fortune to go with it.'

'Would that worry the lady?'

'It would worry *me*.' He realised he meant it. 'I want to give her all the pomp and ceremony that should go with the title.'

'By heaven, Garr, you really do love her!'

Garrick threw him a fulminating glance but did not deny it. Jack sat forward.

'Make Miss Clifford an offer and let her decide. You said yourself she is a sensible lady.'

'She is. Too sensible to marry a man with my reputation, however she may defend me in public. Then there is my mother. It is impossible to take any bride to Hartland until I have made my peace with her. She could turn the whole county against us. And I need to live at Hartland if I am going to turn our fortunes around,' he added, anticipating his friend's next suggestion. 'I have neglected my duties there for too long.'

'And you prefer to do so as a lonely bachelor.'

'Hell and damnation, Jack, do you think I enjoy being pointed out to everyone as the man who drove his father to the grave?'

'No, that I will not allow,' exclaimed Jack. 'We both know that is not true. The old duke had a weak heart, caused by a life of excess. Everyone who knew him is aware of it. The duchess too, only she prefers not to acknowledge it.' He emptied his glass and rose. 'I must go—no don't get up, old friend. I will see myself out.' He put a hand on Garrick's shoulder. 'You have done ten years of penance, Garr. Time now to live your own life. Propose to Miss Clifford, if you think she is the one for you. What's the worst she can do?'

He went out then and Garrick was left alone to consider his words. The worst? His hands closed tighter around his brandy glass.

She had not laughed him as Helene had done, when he had been a mere stripling in the throes of his first love affair. Neither had she run away like Annabelle Speke, who preferred to leave her home and everything she had known rather than be his wife.

Pru's rejection had been kindly meant, he knew that, but it had hurt him far more than the others.

## *Chapter Fourteen*

Following the Shrivenham Ball, Lady Borcaster developed a slight chill and did not leave her house for several days. Mrs Clifford and Pru kept her company, not wishing to attend any of the various entertainments without their hostess. Pru was grateful for a quiet period of reflection, because the attentions of the Duke of Hartland at the ball had left her confused and perplexed.

She had thought her rejection of his proposal had put an end to their friendship, but the interlude on the balcony proved that was not the case. The bond between them seemed as strong as ever. Yet the feelings that had raged through Pru when she saw him with Helene Conyers proved that friendship was not enough for her. She concluded it would be better to avoid his company altogether.

She hoped that being confined to Brook Street would help her to forget about Garrick Chauntry, but alas, a week after the ball, the duke was once more thrust into her thoughts. She was quietly engaged with the other ladies in the morning room when the butler came in, asking if Her Ladyship was at home to visitors.

'Lady Applecross is here to see you, ma'am.'

'Yes, yes, Cotton. I am quite recovered now,' said Lady Borcaster. 'Send her up. I am sure we could all do with a little amusement after being cooped up for so long.'

But then Lady Applecross hurried in and her news was not in the least amusing. She barely waited for the butler to withdraw before bursting into speech.

'My dear Lady Borcaster, have you heard the news? I had it from my sister Mrs Johnby this very morning and came directly to see you. And to warn Miss Clifford.'

Lady Borcaster stared at her visitor. 'News? Warn Prudence? My dear ma'am, pray sit down and tell us what on earth is the matter.'

'I can hardly credit it myself,' said Lady Applecross, sinking onto a chair. 'I know there have been rumours, but nothing prepares one for it...'

'For what, ma'am?' Lady Borcaster pressed her.

'The Duke of Hartland. Spying for the French! A witness has come forward.'

Pru clutched the arms of her chair. 'I do not believe it.'

'Alas, there can be no doubt now, Miss Clifford.' Lady Applecross gave her a pitying look. 'I know you want to think well of His Grace, but I understand there can be no doubting the evidence. Letters, papers, a sworn statement...his accuser was a junior official in Bonaparte's cabinet. He saw Hartland in Paris, and in the company of the monster's most loyal ministers.'

'And where did you learn this, ma'am?' enquired Aunt Minerva.

'Applecross himself heard it at his club. Everyone is talking of it.'

'But has anyone spoken to the duke?' asked Pru.

Lady Applecross fluttered one hand. 'Oh, he has denied it, of course, although one sees very little of him these days. What else can he do? And he has his supporters, but this does appear to confirm all the rumours that have been flying about concerning him.'

'Good heavens, a spy!' exclaimed Lady Borcaster, 'Surely the man should be locked up.'

Another pitying look, but not this time at Pru.

'He is a *duke*, ma'am,' Lady Applecross replied. 'He cannot be clapped in gaol without very good reason.'

'And the evidence might yet prove to be false,' put in Mrs Clifford, with an anxious look at her niece.

Lady Applecross gave a little shrug. 'That is unlikely. My lord tells me the witness is in hiding, fearing for his safety. Which is why I came directly to see you all this morning, and to caution Miss Clifford.'

Lady Borcaster fell back in her chair and closed her eyes in dismay. 'I *knew* she should not have danced with him at the Shrivenhams. The waltz, too! Oh, my dear Prudence, I am sorry now I insisted you take lessons.'

'Quite.' Lady Applecross nodded. 'It will do her no good at all to be too closely associated with the Duke of Hartland at the present time.' She hesitated again. 'It would also reflect badly upon her relatives and friends.'

While the three older ladies continued to speculate over the matter, Prudence was silent. Indeed, what could she say? The duke had told her he was no spy and she believed him, but how could she defend him, when the evidence was so strong, and Lady Applecross had pointed out that her actions might rebound upon her aunt and Lady Borcaster. Galling as it was for her to sit idly by, Pru would have to wait until she knew more.

Lady Borcaster's recovery meant the resumption of a busy social round of balls, routs and breakfasts, to say nothing of visiting the most fashionable shops and silk warehouses. Prudence saw nothing of Garrick and she did not know whether to be reassured or worried that he had withdrawn from society again.

Then came the news Pru was dreading. She was engaged in mending a flounce on her walking dress when her aunt came in, clutching a folded newspaper.

'Oh, my dear Prudence, the accusations against the Duke of Hartland,' she cried. 'They are all too true!'

'Indeed they are,' added Lady Borcaster, following

her friend into the room. 'Lady Applecross sent word early this morning, telling me to look out for it in to-day's *Morning Post*. It is all there, reports of the letters, the accusations, even details from the witness's statement.'

Prudence took the folded newspaper and scanned the page. She wanted to argue that they did not accuse Garrick by name, but that would be foolish. Who else could they mean by *the D— of H—*?

'I thought he had been in Vienna,' was all she could think to say.

'He was abroad for some years and it is very likely he visited many places,' replied Aunt Minerva. 'But you will see, there is evidence he was in Paris on the dates his accuser mentions.' She sighed. 'It looks very bad for the poor man, I have to say.'

Pru ran her tongue over her dry lips. 'Has he been arrested?'

'Not yet,' said Lady Borcaster. 'Lady Applecross says he has been questioned, but nothing more. If Sir Timothy were in England, I would ask him to look into it. As it is, we must rely upon my friends and the newspapers for information. I am only thankful we have kept a proper distance.'

A proper distance! Pru fought down a slightly hysterical laugh at that.

Lady Borcaster went on, 'He only called here the once, when I was out, and you sent him away, did you not, Minerva?'

'Why, yes,' replied Mrs Clifford, with a quick, guilty look of apology towards her niece. 'Yes, I did.'

Prudence was well aware her aunt had not disclosed the reason for the duke's visit to their hostess and guessed she must now be profoundly thankful for it. She sat down beside Pru and laid a hand on her arm.

'I am so very sorry for this, my love.'

'If he is cleared, of course, then I should be happy to welcome him here to Brook Street,' declared Lady Borcaster. 'Until then, I would advise that you have nothing more to do with the man, Prudence.'

'No, of course. I understand.'

My lady smiled, clearly relieved at Pru's quiet acquiescence, but after a moment she threw up her hands, exclaiming, 'Goodness, what a to-do! I have no doubt it will be the main subject of conversation at Carlton House tonight.'

The idea of listening to everyone gossiping and gloating over the subject made Pru feel slightly sick.

'Must I go, ma'am?'

Aunt Minerva stared at her. 'Of course you must go, my dear. The Prince Regent's ball! We shall never have such an opportunity again.'

'Yes, yes, you must go, Prudence,' declared her hostess. 'Why, it will be the grandest event of the season and it would be a great shame for you to cry off now, especially when Sir Timothy went to such lengths to procure the invitation. Heaven knows whom he had to impress to add my name to the list! My dear, Field

Marshall the Duke of Wellington himself will be present. Think of how much you will have to tell your friends, when you return to Bath!'

Pru realised she was in danger of offending her hostess and she quickly tried to repair the damage.

'Then of course I shall go. It was very thoughtful of Sir Timothy to ask his friends to arrange this for you while he was away and I do not want to see his efforts wasted.'

'Indeed, it was. My Susan was very lucky to find such a husband.'

She stopped, looking a little guiltily at Prudence, as if regretting her young friend's misfortune in not being similarly blessed. There was an awkward silence and Aunt Minerva stepped into the breach.

'Well, well, I am sure it is a very great honour, Jane, and we are very grateful you wish us to go with you. We must make sure we are all looking our best this evening. Prudence, my love, I shall lend you my diamonds!'

And that, thought Prudence ruefully, was all that appeared to matter. The Duke of Hartland was forgotten as the two older ladies decided upon what jewels they would wear for the ball.


Myriad lamps were already twinkling at Carlton House when Lady Borcaster's party arrived. They moved slowly forward with the crowd and for once the colourful gowns of the ladies were overshadowed

by the magnificence of the uniforms on display. Even
Lady Borcaster was impressed.

'My dears, the assembly bears a strong resemblance to a military fête,' she remarked, her bright
eyes sweeping over the crowd. 'And I see several old
friends here, including General Lechlade!'

She sailed off to accost her elderly admirer, leaving
Pru and her aunt to follow in her wake.

'Well, this is such a crush I am sure there will be
no room for dancing,' declared Aunt Minerva as they
moved into yet another lavish reception room. 'I—'
She broke off suddenly and gripped Pru's arm. 'My
dear, look who is here! I suppose, given his rank, I
should have expected it, but how he has the nerve to
show his face I do not know.'

But Pru had already seen the Duke of Hartland
walking towards them.

Garrick had come early to Carlton House. He might
curse Castlereagh for insisting he be included in these
events, but for once the invitation was useful, since it
allowed him to meet with several persons he needed
to see, rather than going through the official channels,
where it could take weeks to grant an appointment.
However, it would be best not to stay. With the current accusations about him flying around, his presence
might prove embarrassing to the royal family.

As soon as his business was concluded, Garrick
made his way back through the rooms to the entrance.

He was halfway across the chamber celebrating the country's military triumphs when he saw Pru. She was wearing a gown of kingfisher blue trimmed with cream lace and a diaphanous spangled scarf draped over her arms. Diamonds winked at her throat and ears, and her hair was piled up on her head with only a few soft curls framing her face. Garrick's breath caught in his chest. He had seen many beautiful ladies this evening, most of them far more lavishly dressed than Prudence Clifford, but she was the one who held his attention.

He thought she looked glorious.

Even if he had wished to avoid a meeting, he could not do it without turning back. Mrs Clifford and her niece were standing just inside the double doors that marked his exit. A few more steps and he was standing before them. He bowed and received the smallest of curtsies in return. One look at Pru's face told him she had heard the rumours.

'Come, my dear,' said Mrs Clifford, clutching her niece's arm. 'We dare not lose sight of Lady Borcaster. Your Grace, if you will excuse us?'

'Of course.'

He stepped aside, keeping his eyes on Prudence and willing her to look at him, but she stared resolutely ahead. Nothing could be clearer. She believed those damning stories about him. The sudden pain he felt took his breath away and at that moment he realised just how much he cared for her good opinion.

Garrick turned and continued on his way until he was out of the building and on his way back to Dover Street. As soon as he had learned of the accusations, he had fired off several letters and his efforts tonight had resulted in promises of support, but those who could help him most were out of the country, and their replies could take weeks. In the meantime, details of the accusations were appearing everywhere. Garrick knew he would be exonerated eventually, but for now there was nothing he could do to prove his innocence or prevent a scandal bigger than any other clouding the Hartland name.

## Chapter Fifteen

Pru accompanied her aunt through the crowded rooms, seeing nothing of the elegant decorations or the military trophies on display. Garrick's rugged countenance was imprinted on her mind. Their brief meeting had only increased her confusion.

He had looked grim and drawn, the eyes shuttered against expression, but he had none of the swagger of a man attempting to cover his guilt. She wondered if she was merely trying to convince herself of his innocence, but the conviction remained stubbornly in place, even when they reached the tented ballroom.

Lady Borcaster was in her element. As the widow of a prominent diplomat, she was well acquainted with many of the guests and able to recognise most of the important figures present. She performed numerous introductions and Pru could only nod when her aunt whispered that they would never remember the half of them.

There was no shortage of dance partners for Prudence, who obligingly stood up for several dances without pause. It was as she was leaving the dance floor after a particularly energetic reel that she glimpsed a familiar face. It was Lord John Callater, the man Garrick had introduced to her as they were leaving the Shrivenham Ball.

Pru quickly dismissed her escort and slipped through the crowd to follow her quarry.

'Good evening, Lord John.'

'Miss Clifford.' He gave a smile of recognition. 'Quite a crush is it not?'

'Yes.' She clasped her hands together. 'I saw Sir Garrick here earlier.'

'Why yes, but he did not stay.'

The smile remained in place but she saw the wary look in his eyes. She must take her chance.

'Is he quite well, my lord?'

'As well as one can expect.'

It was a cautious reply and Pru hesitated. This was really none of her business. Garrick would not thank her for it, yet she could not turn back now.

'You are his friend, I believe,' she said, keeping her eyes on his face. 'His *good* friend, he called you. I have heard. That is…'

She was floundering and Lord John held out his arm. 'Let us go to one of the supper tents. There will be only the servants there at this hour, and they will not disturb us. We shall tell them you were feeling faint and then we will be able to talk privately.'

Amazed at her own temerity, Prudence accompanied him. She was very sorry for the gentleman who would look in vain for his next dance partner, but it could not be helped.

A short time later she was sitting at one end of a long supper table with Lord John beside her.

'You should make use of your fan,' he suggested, smiling. 'Swiftly, as if you are overcome with the heat.'

'Yes, of course.'

'Now.' He swung his quizzing glass idly but his gaze remained watchful. 'How much do you know?'

'Only gossip, and what I have read in the newspapers.'

'Well, there is some truth to the allegations.'

She raised her eyes to his in alarm and after a moment he gave a little nod.

'Garrick trusts you, so I will, too, and tell you what the duke has discovered so far. His accuser, Albert Vence, had some minor role in Bonaparte's government. His statement is in most respects correct. Garrick was in Paris at that time and he did have meetings with some of Bonaparte's ministers, but not the ones mentioned by Vence. The duke is not, nor ever was, a *French* spy.'

Relief flood through her. Lord John leaned closer.

'I tell you this in confidence, Miss Clifford, because I believe you have the duke's interests at heart.'

'I do. He thinks me interfering but...'

'You care for him.'

She felt the tell-tale blush warming her face. 'As I would for anyone wrongly accused!'

'Of course.' He spoke gravely, but Pru wondered if he believed her. How much had Garrick told him about her? He went on, 'The thing is, Miss Clifford, Lord Castlereagh is the only one who can vouch for Garrick. But he is out of the country and it will be some time before we can expect a response from him.'

Pru plied the fan more quickly, trying to hide the sudden fear that gripped her, but Lord John was not fooled. He smiled slightly.

'It is not quite so bad. Two witnesses would be required to testify in order to gain a conviction, but whoever is doing this either has no idea of the law, or has merely set this particular hare running to cast more slurs upon Garrick's good name.'

'And the longer it goes on, the more damage it will do,' she added bitterly. 'I observed for myself how society gloated over the earlier rumours. It made me so angry!'

'Aye, Garr told me you had tried to be his champion.'

'Champion!' She flushed at that. 'I doubt that was the word he used for me.'

He grinned. 'Well, no. The duke has never been one to accept help easily, but he needs it now. If you are willing.'

'Me?' she looked at him in surprise. 'No, no, Lord John. You are far better placed to help him than I.'

'Alas, ma'am, I have the reputation of being a frippery fellow, whose only interest is fashion. I should be looked upon with suspicion if I begin asking questions. Also, everyone knows Hartland and I have been friends since childhood.'

Pru looked at him. 'Why should that be a hindrance? Surely everyone will understand your wish to discover the truth?'

'Not everyone, Miss Clifford. The person who instigated this mischief will not wish for it to be concluded too soon.'

'And you know who that is?'

'No. My first thought was that Lady Tirrill had started it, out of spite, but Garrick says not.' He gave a sigh of exasperation. 'The duke can be damned tight-lipped when he chooses! I will be frank with you, Miss Clifford. He wants me to leave well alone. He insists the truth will out in due course.'

'He is trying to protect you.'

'From what?' Lord John frowned at her. 'What is it that you are not telling me, ma'am?'

Pru hesitated. What did she know of this man, after all?

She said at last, 'If you are indeed the duke's close friend, you will know about the, the duel that caused him to leave England?'

'Aye, it was a dashed hum! Garr was bamboozled by a woman. It hit him very hard…but never mind that. Go on, ma'am.'

'The duke's opponent in that duel is in town now.

Earlier this summer I overheard him spreading rumours about the duke being a French agent. I told His Grace, but he refused to act. He said the gossip would die down of its own accord and that I should leave well alone, which I did. Then, a week ago, the allegations appeared in the *Morning Post...*'

'And you think it is the sneaking husband that Garrick wounded in the duel? Damnation, if only I could remember the doxy's name...'

Prudence swallowed, unable to speak the lady's name. Then she gave herself a mental shake. This was no time for missish hysterics.

'Conyers,' she said. 'He is now Sir Joseph Conyers, and the last time I saw him was at the Shrivenham Ball, three weeks since. It was very clear there is no love lost between him and the duke.'

'I can imagine, after the dastardly trick he and his lady played upon Garrick.' Lord John frowned. 'It is possible he is involved, I suppose, although after all this time—'

Pru felt the knot of anxiety tighten inside. Perhaps Sir Joseph was merely passing on tittle-tattle he had heard, and if that were the case then how were they ever to discover the culprit?

'Very well,' declared Lord John, 'I will make enquiries, and I would be grateful for anything you can discover, Miss Clifford. Lady Borcaster has acquaintances in government circles—I hope they might be able to tell you more about this Frenchman.'

'I believe there is a charitable society set up to support the émigrés,' said Pru, frowning a little. 'I have read reports of it. A scandal like this will certainly be of interest to them. They may even know who the man may be.'

'Good. How does one find them, talk to them?'

This was familiar territory for Pru. She said, 'I have some knowledge of charitable work, Lord John. Leave that to me.'

'Thank you, I shall. Let us agree to meet again. Shall we say Wednesday next, in Green Park?'

Pru recalled her meeting there with Garrick. How long ago that seemed now. How much had happened since.

'What is it, Miss Clifford?' Lord John interrupted her thoughts. 'Do you not think the park a suitable place for a rendezvous?'

'I think the circulating library would be better,' she suggested. 'My aunt and I are regular subscribers to Hatchards, in Piccadilly.'

'Then we shall meet there. If you need to contact me in the meantime, you can send a message to Albany, where I have rooms.'

'Pray do not be too hopeful of my helping, sir. I am not sure I can be of any use at all.'

'Garr confided in you, Miss Clifford. He also told me you are a very resourceful lady. That is a high compliment coming from the duke, I assure you. His experience of your sex has not been the happiest.' He rose. 'I had best get you back to the ballroom before we are missed.'

'Yes, indeed.' She smiled, trying to be as resourceful as Garrick thought her. 'Let me go in first. It will not do to have anyone think we are plotting.'

The rest of the evening was a trial for Pru. She was on the alert now for any whisper regarding the duke. Not that there was any lack of gossip, but it was the sort of tittle-tattle she had heard many times and from people who could have little knowledge of the facts. The more she considered the matter, the more she was convinced that Sir Joseph Conyers was behind this latest scurrilous attack.

When the ladies finally climbed into their carriage, Pru sat quietly in her corner, going over her conversation with Lord John Callater. They were almost at Brook Street when her attention was caught. Lady Borcaster was discussing with Aunt Minerva the evening party she was planning for early the following week.

'I shall be delighted to help with the arrangements, Jane,' declared Minerva. 'It is very kind of you to put on this little party for us. Do you not agree, Pru?'

'I do indeed, Aunt. Who is invited, ma'am?'

'Oh, it will be a quiet affair, my dear. A dozen or so close friends whose company I think you might enjoy. And perhaps we may have a few country dances for the younger ones, if we remove some of the furniture.'

Pru brushed a speck of dust from her skirts, saying casually, 'Are Sir Joseph and Lady Conyers invited?'

'They are not,' replied my lady. 'I did not take to the man, although I hear he is quite the favourite now, and invited everywhere.'

'I have heard that, too,' replied Pru. 'I wonder, then if perhaps you should include him?'

Lady Borcaster chuckled. 'Oh, that is a relief! I was very much afraid you were going to suggest I should invite the Duke of Hartland! Given his present circumstances, I should have had to refuse you, my dear.'

'I understand that,' said Pru. 'But going back to Sir Joseph, I think perhaps it would not do to be backwards in any attention.'

'Goodness, Prudence, you are becoming quite at home in town, these days,' declared her aunt, impressed.

'But she is quite right, Minerva. If the man is a rising star, then Sir Timothy would wish me to further the acquaintance. Although, my dear Prudence, I was under the opinion that *you* did not care for him.'

'No, ma'am, my first impression was not favourable, but I think that was because I am not accustomed to society manners.'

Her explanation appeared to satisfy Lady Borcaster. Nothing more was said, and when Prudence climbed into bed that night, she realised the die was cast. She would do what she could to discover if Sir Joseph was behind the accusations against the Duke of Hartland.

## Chapter Sixteen

Lady Borcaster's reception rooms were transformed. Furniture had been rearranged or removed to make space and the hostess had the satisfaction of knowing that apart from one elderly dowager, who was indisposed, not one of her invitations had been refused.

Pru was already acquainted with most of the guests, but there were a number of government ministers whom she did not know. She did her best to be polite and charming to all of them; if the duke was arrested, it might be useful to have such contacts. When Sir Joseph arrived with his beautiful wife, Pru was in no hurry to approach them. She was not sure what she would say, or even what she expected from the evening.

In the event it was Sir Joseph who made the first move. Lady Conyers was on the far side of the room, flirting with one of the government ministers, when her husband came up to Pru. They exchanged civilities and a passing waiter afforded Sir Joseph the opportunity to procure two glasses of wine.

He handed one to Prudence, remarking, 'I see your favourite is not here tonight, Miss Clifford.'

'Oh, who had you in mind, sir?' Her look was all innocent enquiry.

'Hartland.'

She frowned, as if having difficulty placing the name. 'Ah, the Duke of Hartland. I remember him now. I have not seen him since the Shrivenham Ball.'

'You danced the waltz with him.' Sir Joseph was smiling, but his hooded eyes were watching her closely. 'Some might think that dance a bold choice for a single lady.'

Pru's eyes widened. 'But since the Tsar's visit *everyone* is dancing the waltz.'

'You refused to waltz with *me*, if my memory serves.'

'Because I was already engaged.' She added, hoping to stop him asking her to dance again, 'To be honest, Sir Joseph, I did not really enjoy the experience.'

'Perhaps it was the choice of partner that was at fault,' he purred. There was a lascivious glint in those hooded eyes and she was obliged to suppress a shudder.

'Perhaps it was.'

He laughed softly. 'And His Grace is quite out of favour now, is he not? I suppose that is why he is not present.'

'This is Lady Borcaster's party, sir. She and my aunt

wrote the invitations. But I am quite content with the company, I assure you.'

Pru could not replicate his lady's flirtatious glances, but she gave him her sunniest smile, and there was no mistaking Sir Joseph's satisfaction with her response. He remained at her side, conversing on unexceptional topics until Lady Conyers came up to them.

'There you are, Joseph. I should have known I would find you with a pretty young lady.'

Her friendly smile should have robbed the words of any offence, but Prudence felt a chill of apprehension. She knew her opinion was coloured by what Garrick had told her of the beautiful Helene, but she could not like the woman. She sincerely hoped the duke was no longer in thrall to her.

'Miss Clifford and I have been having the most interesting coze, my sweet.'

'Indeed?' She turned those limpid blue eyes back to Pru, who wondered if she was being assessed as useful, or a rival.

'Yes, most interesting. Have you invited Lady Borcaster to join us tomorrow, Helene? I hope you made it clear that her guests are invited, too.'

'Why, of course, although I am not sure our little party will be quite to Miss Clifford's taste. There will be no music, no entertainment.' She pursed her mouth into a comical moue. 'I fear the conversation will be all politics.'

'I should be delighted to attend,' cried Prudence.

'This is my first, possibly my only visit to London, and I am anxious to enjoy everything I can!'

Her enthusiastic response appeared to please Sir Joseph, if not his wife, although Helene did her best to appear gracious when she replied.

'Then we look forward to welcoming you tomorrow evening, Miss Clifford. Your aunt, too.' She slipped her hand onto her husband's arm. 'Come, my love. Let us seek out Lady Borcaster now and make sure there is no misunderstanding.'

They moved away and Prudence felt the tension easing in her shoulders. Dissimulation was abhorrent to her but she had an invitation into the Conyerses' inner circle, and she must make the most of it. For Garrick's sake.

Sir Joseph had rented a house for the season, not far from Brook Street, and Lady Borcaster decided they should take chairs, rather than call out her carriage for such a short journey. They arrived to find the house glittering with light and the reception rooms already full.

'There is no denying he has done very well for himself,' muttered Lady Borcaster, casting an approving glance around the assembly. 'Two government ministers, a former treasury minister, as well as Lord and Lady Fauls. Sir Joseph has ambitions in a political direction, I suspect.'

'Is that a bad thing?' Pru asked her.

'No, no, although I suspect his politics will shift with the prevailing wind.'

On this cryptic statement Lady Borcaster carried off Mrs Clifford to greet a bejewelled matron, leaving Prudence to her own devices. She did not object; she had several acquaintances amongst the guests and went off to sit down with a little cluster of ladies who welcomed her in a very friendly way.

The wine flowed freely and the conversation became much more relaxed as the evening wore on. Prudence tried to circulate, never stopping too long with any one group. As she expected, she soon heard mention of the Duke of Hartland. Some people were shocked by the revelations concerning him, others gloated over his misfortunes. One matron was particularly scathing in her comments and Prudence was surprised when Sir Joseph, who was passing, stopped and wagged a playful finger at the speaker.

'Now, now, Lady Slocombe, we must not be hasty in our judgements.'

'Hasty!' scoffed the lady. 'The man's a rogue. I have heard nothing but scandal attached to his name this season. *And* I am old enough to remember the grief he caused his sainted father when he first came to town all those years ago. What *I* say, Sir Joseph, is that a leopard does not change his spots!'

Her host laughed gently. 'Perhaps not, but one should not judge a fellow on his youthful peccadillos.

We must be charitable and believe the best of a man until it is proven otherwise.'

Listening to this interchange, Pru felt a slight quiver of uncertainty at his words. Perhaps she was wrong about the man. Then he turned away from the group and she saw the smirk of satisfaction on his face as he walked off. Her doubts vanished like smoke.

By midnight, Pru had seen and heard enough. She was ready to leave, but Lady Borcaster and her aunt were enjoying themselves and she resigned herself to staying for another hour at least. She moved away from the chattering groups and amused herself by looking at the various paintings that adorned the walls. Most were copies of famous landscapes or scenes from the classical world, but on one wall she found a pleasant little watercolour. It was so different from everything else that she stepped closer to examine it.

'Had enough of politics, Miss Clifford?'

She turned to find the Earl of Fauls at her shoulder, smiling at her in his good-natured way.

'I am very ignorant of such matters, my lord, and fear I have little to offer,' she said, ruefully. 'Is it very bad of me not to join in?'

'No, no, not a bit of it! But if you are hoping to improve your knowledge of art you won't do so here.' He stepped a little closer to the wall, raising his quizzing glass to inspect a gaudy landscape. 'Copies, all of 'em, and not the best, either.'

She acknowledged this with a smile. 'I thought as much. But this is not a copy, surely?'

She indicated the watercolour.

'No, that is a depiction of Alder Grove. Somewhere near Dartford, I believe. It used to be the Conyerses' family seat, although Sir Joseph has recently vacated it and bought himself a new property in Buckinghamshire. Much more in keeping with his ambition.'

She detected the slight disapproval in the Earl's tone and ventured to comment.

'That is the second time I have heard the word *ambition* used in connection with our host,' she remarked. 'Is he planning on entering politics?'

'If he was offered a sinecure, perhaps. Something to advance his own fortunes.'

The Earl stopped. He looked a little uncomfortable, as if he had been caught out in an indiscretion and changed the subject. Pru made no attempt to question him further but when she finally climbed into her chair for the journey back to Brook Street she felt sadly deflated. She had learned nothing that might help Garrick. Nothing at all.

Wednesday dawned wet, and the rain had barely ceased when Prudence set off with her maid for her meeting with Lord John Callater. She decided to wear the walking dress of flax-blue muslin with the sarsnet pelisse that she had purchased from Mrs Bell. The pelisse was trimmed *à la Russe*, and had a matching bonnet *à la militaire* and, regarding herself in the long glass, Pru was quite pleased with the result. She thought that at last she might be acquiring what Lady Borcaster termed *town bronze.*

Hatchards bookshop and circulating library in Piccadilly was Pru's destination, a reasonable walk but Pru enjoyed the exercise. When they reached the door, she handed her umbrella to Meg and left the maid to wait outside the bow windows while she stepped into the shop. She politely waved aside the assistant who hurried towards her and made her way over to the bookshelves, where she had spotted Lord John Callater.

It was only when he turned to greet her that Pru noticed Garrick Chauntry standing in the alcove behind him.

Lord John touched his hat to her. 'Miss Clifford, good morning to you.'

She heard the note of warning in his voice and schooled her face to one of surprise.

'Why, Lord John, good day to you. And to you, Your Grace.'

The duke was glaring at her but not by the flicker of an eyelid would she betray any agitation at seeing him.

'My aunt asked me to collect a book for her,' she explained, adding with a twinkle, 'However, I can never enter a bookshop without taking a moment to browse their stock.'

'Exactly, ma'am,' replied Lord John. 'That was just

my intention this morning, then Hartland arrived and decided to accompany me.'

Garrick uttered a small growl of annoyance.

'There is no need to carry on with this charade, Jack,' he said bluntly. 'I knew from the outset that you were up to something.'

'Now, Garr...'

'Don't *now Garr* me! What is going on?'

Pru interrupted them, aware of the helpful assistant hovering nearby.

'I thought I might look at those books over there, on the next counter.'

She moved across to a more deserted area of the shop and the two gentlemen followed her.

'Have you read this one, Your Grace?' She picked up a book and glanced through it. 'I thought it might interest my aunt.'

'Byron's *Corsair*. A courageous choice.' His eyes glinted at her. 'I do believe you are heading into dangerous waters, Miss Clifford.'

She did not pretend to misunderstand him, but before she could reply Lord John cut in, keeping his voice low.

'Enough, Garr. Miss Clifford and I want to help you!'

Garrick was doing his best to keep his temper. To discover that the two people he trusted most were conspiring against him was almost too much! He selected a book at random and inspected the cover.

'I have told you,' he ground out. 'I neither want nor need help.'

'You really have no choice in the matter,' retorted Prudence. 'If you insist on being obstinate then I suggest you go away and leave Lord John and I to handle the whole.'

'And allow you both to put yourselves in peril?'

His friend pounced on that. 'Aha, you admit your situation is dangerous!'

'No, Jack. My situation will resolve itself, in time.'

'And meanwhile your good name is sullied. Dash it, Garr, what sort of friend would I be if I allowed that?'

'Quite right, my lord,' Prudence agreed, smiling her approval.

Garrick scowled. He recognised that stubborn tilt to Pru's chin and Jack was staring at him, challenging him to argue. Damned fools, both of them!

He sighed, his anger fading. He did not deserve friends like this.

'Very well,' he muttered. 'Tell me what you have discovered.'

Jack's frown was telling.

'To be truthful, nothing that can advance our cause. The Frenchman is in London, but I could not find out where, nor who brought him here. Perhaps Miss Clifford has had more luck?'

'Alas, no. I attended the Conyerses' soirée last night and, from what I learned, Sir Joseph is clearly intent upon gaining favour at Whitehall.'

Garrick met her eyes. She was expecting him to say I told you so, but he refrained. He had no wish to tease her. He wanted to drag her into his arms and cover her face with kisses. Or carry her back to Dover Street and take her to his bed. What he would give to hear her moan with pleasure again...

Damnation he must stop thinking about that!

'I see.' Quickly, he turned away. 'And is that all, ma'am?'

'Well, I am taking tea with Lady Elsdon later today,' she said. 'She has established the Philanthropic Society for the Relief of French Émigrés and is raising funds for them. I am hoping I might learn something there.'

Garrick nodded, forcing himself to think about charitable causes rather than the delights of the flesh. It worked, for now, and he was able to concentrate on what she was proposing. He could not see how visiting Lady Elsdon would help his cause and a glance at Jack's face told him his friend thought very much the same. However, he did not wish to dampen Pru's spirits and it seemed an innocent enough activity for her. He nodded.

'Good idea, that might be useful.'

The pleasure in her face caught at his heart. He reached out towards her, only to snatch his hand back again immediately. But he was not quick enough, she had seen the gesture and understood it. He knew that from the way her grey eyes softened and warmed. She believed in him, which made his spirits rise. If only she did not think of him as an object of pity!

Garrick fixed his eyes on the book in his hands and said gruffly, 'You should go, Miss Clifford. The less time we spend together the better for you.'

'Of course.'

He was surprised that she did not argue with him. Disappointed, too, because he could not deny he wanted her to stay. Grasping her copy of Byron's latest tale, she walked away. He pretended to flick through the book he was holding, but all the time he was watching her, the proud tilt of her head and straight back, the way she seemed to glide across the floor.

Beside him, Jack gave a low whistle. 'Damn my eyes, Duke, if ever I saw two people more in—!'

'Enough!' barked Garrick. 'I wish to heaven you had not involved her in this damned tangle.'

Jack shrugged. 'She is unlikely to come to any harm at a tea party.' He took out his watch. 'What do you do now? I have an appointment with my tailor shortly, do you want to come with me?'

'Thank you, but no. I have another engagement.'

'Then dine with me later.'

'I do not know when I shall be back.'

Jack's eyes narrowed. 'And may one enquire where you are going?'

'No, one may not!' Aware of heads turning towards them, Garrick lowered his voice. 'I wish you would leave me to my own business.'

'Let me come with you.'

'And miss your appointment with your tailor?' he grinned. 'I assure you, Jack, it is not worth that sacrifice. Now, we have been here long enough. Let us be gone.'

'We can hardly leave without purchasing something.'

'If you recall, this was your suggestion, so you must pay. Here, take these.' He thrust a pile of books into Jack's hands.

'What is it? Oh, a novel in three volumes.'

'Aye,' said Garrick. *'Pride and Prejudice.* High time you read something other than the *Gentleman's Magazine*!'

# Chapter Seventeen

Garrick and Jack parted ways at the bookshop door. Jack making his way to Jermyn Street to visit the fashionable tailor who enjoyed his patronage while Garrick raised his ebony cane to hail a passing cab. He gave the driver an address in Somers Town and settled himself back against the squabs. Then he reached into his pocket and pulled out the note he had received that morning.

It was very short, the language formal.

If His Grace wishes to present himself at the sign of the Golden Cockerel, Somers Town, today at two o'clock in the afternoon, he will find his Accuser in residence and enjoying the benefits of the Private Parlour. Alone.

A Well-Wisher

'But *is* it someone who wishes me well?' Garrick mused.

He did not recognise the hand, although the neat, precise writing suggested a man of letters. A clerk perhaps. It might well be a trap, but he was prepared for that. His grip tightened on the handle of his cane. The trusty sword stick had helped him escape far more dangerous situations during his time abroad.

It was not long before the carriage was making its way through a semi-rural area with several streets of shabby-genteel houses leading off the main highway. There were signs of recent development, but the building work appeared to have ceased, leaving unfinished shells of houses lining the road. The cab lumbered on and eventually stopped outside a small inn where a sign with a gaudily painted cockerel swung above the door.

Garrick jumped out of the cab. Everything was peaceful. The sky had cleared and a skylark trilled joyously over a nearby field. He threw a coin up to the driver, ordered him to wait and walked into the inn.

There was no sign of the landlord, but a tap boy directed Garrick to the private parlour and received sixpence for his pains. Garrick hesitated for a heartbeat in the passage before going in. There was only one occupant in the room, a small man in the plain black coat and knee breeches of a clerk. As he heard the door open, the man jumped up. He looked frightened, but not startled. As if he had been expecting a visitor, which put Garrick on his guard.

'Good day to you,' he said pleasantly, closing the door behind him. 'Monsieur Albert Vence, is it not?'

'*Oui, Excellence.*' The man had backed away a little, towards a door at the side of the room.

'You know who I am?'

'*Oui.* The Duke of 'artland.'

Garrick studied the man, taking in the slightly shabby clothes and thin face. He could not remember seeing him before.

He said, 'Forgive me, monsieur, but have we met?'

'I know you, Your Grace. I saw you in Paris.'

'Did you indeed?' drawled Garrick, leaning on his cane. 'Do remind me, when was that?'

'Three years ago. I was a clerk in the office of the Comte de Montalivet.'

'The French minister of the interior?'

'*Oui, Excellence.* You came to see him.' Vence licked his lips, nervously. '*Mais*, you were not the Duc then.'

'We both know you are lying. I never met with Montalivet. Who is paying you?'

'I—I do not know what you mean.' The man was visibly shaking now.

'I think you do,' said Garrick. 'Tell me—'

Vence turned and hammered on the door beside him. '*M'aidez! Viens!*'

Almost immediately two men appeared and stepped in front of Vence.

'This is a private parlour,' barked one, a tall spare man with a balding head. 'What is your business here?'

'He is the Duke of 'artland,' shrieked Vence, cowering against the wall. 'He is come t-to k-kill me.'

Garrick frowned. 'Nonsense.'

The men looked uneasily at one another.

'Is it true?' asked the tall man.

'It is true I am Hartland,' said Garrick, 'but I only came here to talk—'

'He attacked me!' cried Vence.

The second man stepped forward and cleared his throat. 'If it please, Your Grace, you should not be here. We have been instructed that Monsieur Vence is to see no one.'

'Instructed by whom?' Garrick demanded.

'The home secretary, Lord Sidmouth.'

Garrick considered this. Both men were dressed neatly in dark tailcoats and cream trousers. Not servants, he thought, but quite possibly Whitehall aides.

The balding one edged over to the door and opened it. 'Please leave, Your Grace. We cannot allow you to stay here.'

Garrick knew he would get nothing more from the Frenchman now and he nodded.

'Very well, I'll go. But you will have to answer my questions in court, Monsieur Vence, under oath!'

On that parting shot he went out. The door closed behind him and he heard the key scrape in the lock.

Aye, let them keep the fellow safe. Vence would not hold out long under questioning.

Garrick climbed into the waiting cab and set off back to town. Whoever had found the Frenchman was playing a dirty game. Garrick could not remember Vence, but it was possible the fellow had seen him in Paris, although not with Bonaparte's loyal ministers. Far from it. But why would the fellow perjure himself, unless someone was paying him well for his false testimony?

He pondered the idea as the carriage rumbled back towards town, slowing down to pick its way through the derelict area at the edge of Swallow Street. Garrick thought nothing of it until the cab came to a stand and the door was wrenched open. He found himself looking down the barrel of a pistol.

'Now, what have we here?' cried a rough voice. 'Step out, good sir, and let's have a look at ye.'

The owner of the pistol had a muffler wound around the lower part of his face, and his hat was so low over his eyes it was impossible to see his face. Glancing past him Garrick saw several burly individuals standing close by. One of them was levelling a pistol at the cab driver.

'No need for that,' he said, calmly. 'I have little of value, save my purse.'

'I said get out, and hurry up about it.'

Shrugging, Garrick picked up his cane and jumped out of the cab. Although he looked at ease, every nerve was on the alert. A quick glance showed that the houses here were empty ruins, the only people around would be beggars or scavengers. No help to be had there. The man with the pistol took a few steps back.

'Come along, sir, over here and give us your purse.'

As Garrick stepped away from the coach he heard someone bark an order to the driver, who whipped up his horses and clattered off. Surprised, Garrick swung around, but before he could shout out, he was stunned by a blow to the head.

The ground was still damp from the earlier rain but the dust and dirt cushioned his fall. As he tried to get up a boot smashed into his body and he fell back, winded. Another blow, this time to his head, left his senses reeling and he lost consciousness.

When Prudence left Lady Elsdon's elegant town-house she was tempted to walk the two miles back to Brook Street. There was plenty of time to change for dinner and she wanted to think over all she had learned. However, Lady Borcaster had insisted she should go by cab and, remembering the rather dilapidated areas she had passed through on her way to Russell Square, she allowed her hostess to summon a hackney carriage for her return journey.

Pru had much to occupy her mind and she stared, unseeing, out of the window as the hired vehicle rumbled through the unfamiliar streets, until the sight of a figure clinging to the railings of an empty house caused her to rap sharply on the roof and order the driver to stop.

Even before the carriage came to a halt, she opened the door and jumped out with no thought for decorum.

'Garrick! What has happened to you?' She ran up to him, shocked by his bloodied face and dirty clothes.

'Footpads,' he muttered, before collapsing to the ground.

## Chapter Eighteen

Garrick was regaining consciousness. He had a split-
ting headache and it was difficult to think. Carefully
opening his eyes, he stared at the yellow-stained ceiling and the walls with their dark wainscotting. He was
propped up against a bank of pillows but this was not
his bedchamber, nor was the lumpy mattress beneath
him anything like his own featherbed. And apart from
his coat and boots, he was fully clothed. He heard a
movement in the room and shifted his gaze.

'Prudence.'

She was busy placing a bowl on a table beside the
bed but when he spoke her name she looked up.

'You are awake, thank heaven!' Her face lit up with
relief. For a moment she looked as if she might cry,
but the shadow passed and she smiled at him. 'How
are you?'

He really wasn't sure, and some instinct told him
he did not want to move and find out.

'What happened?' Just speaking was painful; his lip was swollen.

'You told me footpads attacked you.'

'Ah, yes.' Some memory was returning, but so was the pain. His ribs in particular were on fire, hurting with every breath. His face, too felt odd. Stiff. He lifted a hand to his throbbing cheek but she caught it.

'No, don't touch. We have yet to clean you up.'

It was easier to comply than argue and he allowed her to push his hand back gently to his side.

'Where am I?' he mumbled. 'And what are you doing here?'

She dipped a cloth in the bowl of water and began to wipe his face, very gently.

'We are in a tavern called The Dun Cow,' she said.

'That does not explain your presence.' He winced at the initial sting of the water.

'I was on my way back from Lady Elsdon's house when I saw you. You have a cut on your head and from the marks on your clothes, you have taken blows to your ribs. Consistent with a beating,' she added, her face clouding again with anxiety. 'I did not want to risk further injury by bundling you into a cab and jolting you over the cobbles all the way to Dover Street.'

'Then how did you get me here?'

'I enlisted the help of the builders working nearby. They lifted you onto an old door and carried you.'

She continued to clean the dirt and blood from his

face and Garrick concentrated on breathing, trying not to move his ribs more than necessary.

'There.' Finally, she stepped back, satisfied. 'You have a bump on your head and cuts on your face, but nothing too serious, I hope.' She pulled a fresh cloth from a jug and wrung it out. 'There is no ice to be had, but the water is cold and it might help with the swelling.'

She placed the cool rag gently against his temple then lifted his hand up to hold it in place.

'You are very sure of yourself,' he observed.

'I have some experience of caring for victims of attacks such as these. From my charity work with paupers and vagrants, in Bath.' A shadow of pain crossed her face. 'And you know I nursed my brother.'

'But you should not be nursing *me*.'

'There is no one else,' she said simply. 'Before you passed out, you were most insistent that I should not summon a doctor.' She began to unbutton his waistcoat. 'You took quite a beating and I need to ascertain what other injuries you may have.'

'Only my ribs, I think. I remember one of the rogues kicking me.'

Her brow darkened, she looked angry but said nothing as she continued loosening his clothes. When she began to unbutton the waist of his pantaloons his free hand shot up and closed over hers.

'Enough!'

'Why? I have seen your bare chest before.'

Her eyes widened when she realised what she had said. The faint blush colouring her cheek was telling and despite his pain, Garrick felt a rush of satisfaction. The attraction between them was as strong as ever. If only he was fit enough to take advantage of it! He kept a firm hold of her hand, reluctant to allow her to see his injuries. He hated feeling so helpless. He should be protecting *her*, not the other way around.

She said, 'I need to pull out your shirt in order to examine your ribs.'

'It is not fitting,' he told her. 'You are not married.'

'But neither am I a child. As you are well aware.' She met his eyes then, and something sparked between them. A flash of recognition that they were equals. Friends.

Gently, she pulled her hand out of his grasp. 'Trust me, it is not the first time I have examined a man,' she told him, calm, in control. 'Although, never a duke, I admit.'

Her riposte made him want to smile, but she was easing his shirt free and despite her care, he had to brace himself against the pain.

'You are a constant surprise to me, Miss Clifford,' he muttered, between clenched teeth.

'Thank you. Now, I am told one can sometimes hear broken ribs creaking on an inbreath, so I must listen. Just stay silent and relax, sir.'

But that was the one thing he could not do. It was not merely the agony of his cracked or broken ribs every time he breathed, nor the throbbing of the cut on his cheek. He closed his eyes but was still agonisingly aware of her gentle fingers on his skin and the faint citrus smell of her perfume as she leaned over his chest. Did she not realise how tantalising it was, to have her mouth so close to his bare skin?

In truth, he was glad of the pain, otherwise he was afraid his body would have given him away.

She filled his senses. He clenched his fists at his sides, but he could not prevent his mind racing off into highly inappropriate scenarios involving tangled sheets and moonlight…

'I am sorry, did I hurt you?' Her soft voice brought his thoughts back with a jolt. He opened his eyes and found her watching him anxiously.

'You groaned. I am afraid you might have sustained some injury to your internal organs.' When her fingers slid over his abdomen, he caught her hand again and she said crisply, 'I have no time for your stubborn male pride, Your Grace!'

'There is nothing wrong with my organs, internal or external, Miss Clifford.' She tried to free herself, but he tightened his grip. He said softly, 'I would prove it to you, if I were not in so much pain.'

She blushed furiously at that and he grinned, which turned to a wince as it stretched the cuts on his face. Immediately she was all concern.

'Hush now, you need to rest. I could not hear anything to indicate your ribs are broken, which may be good news, but you will need to be careful.'

'Aye, dash it. I feel as weak as a cat.'

She smoothed his hair back from his brow with her free hand. She was gazing at him so tenderly that his pain faded. Something shifted inside him.

'Pru, are you sure you cannot marry me, even though I am *such* a man?' He smiled as far as his split lip would allow. 'Will you not allow me to make an honest woman of you?'

She froze and stood, motionless, looking down at him. She had not recoiled and he thought he saw a wistfulness in her grey eyes. He was about to press home his advantage when the door burst open, shattering the silence and the moment.

'Here we are, ma'am, more hot water. And I have the laudanum you asked for, too.'

There was no mistaking Pru's relief. She freed her hand from his gasp and turned away from him to greet the newcomer.

'Ah, our landlady. Thank you, Mrs Hayes.'

'Is there anything else I can do?' asked the woman, putting the jug down on the table. 'P'raps I can help you undress your man and get him into bed.'

'Yes, thank you, that would be very helpful, but not until after I have administered the opium and it has taken effect. I fear it will cause him a deal of discomfort to be moved.'

'In that case, ma'am, I'll come back and help in a

while. And shall I bring you up something to drink? I've put another kettle on to boil.' She added, with a hint of pride, 'I can offer you both tea and coffee.'

'Coffee would be very welcome, thank you,' said Pru.

'Very well, Mrs Garrick, and I'll bring a jug of ale for your husband, in case he's thirsty.'

With a curtsy she bustled out again but Garrick knew better than to return to the subject of marriage. Instead he risked the pain of raising his brows and teased Prudence.

'Well, *Mrs Garrick*?'

'I think you should take the laudanum now.'

'That is not what I meant.'

'She naturally assumed that you...that I.' She eyed him resentfully. 'I judged it best, in the circumstances, to allow her to think you were plain Mr Garrick. You were so dishevelled I doubted anyone would believe your true identity.'

'You are right about that,' he replied, becoming serious. 'However, you have done your duty and can leave me now. Go back to your aunt. You will be missed.'

She shook her head. 'I paid the driver to take a message to Brook Street, informing them I am dining in Russell Square with Lady Elsdon. Thankfully I was using a hackney, Lady Borcaster and my aunt having an engagement this evening and needing their carriage. If it had been my lady's coachman, I would have been in trouble.'

'You are in trouble in any event,' he retorted. 'You really should not be here, Pru.'

'And who else could look after you? Mrs Hayes and her daughter run this tavern alone, they do not have time to tend you as well.'

'You should send for Stow.'

'And so I will, later,' she replied, a stubborn look in her eye. 'My work at the infirmary has taught me that I cannot leave you until I have ascertained there are no lasting injuries.'

'Ah yes. I am one of your charitable causes.' He tried to laugh, but it ended in a grimace.

'Nothing of the sort.' She picked up a small phial and brought it across to him. 'And pray do not try to tell me you are not in pain. Take this.'

He tipped the medicine down his throat and handed her back the bottle. 'There, are you satisfied now?'

'Not quite.' She sat down beside the bed. 'I wish you would be honest with me.'

'When have I been otherwise?'

'You said you were set upon by footpads.'

'I was. Too many for me to defend myself. Which reminds me, did you pick up my cane?'

'No, although I looked for it. I concluded you did not have it with you.'

'I had it when they attacked me. The rogues must have stolen it.'

'Strange that they should take your cane but leave

your purse. I found it in your pocket when I removed your coat.'

She looked around as the landlady returned.

'I brought you up your coffee and the ale, ma'am, and some of my plum cake, too, which I thought you and the master might like.'

When she had gone away again Prudence poured some of the small beer into a tankard.

'Can you hold it, or shall I?' she asked Garrick.

He took the tankard and sipped gingerly while Prudence sat beside the bed, watching him. The liquid stung his split lip, but it soothed his parched throat and was soon finished.

'Thank you.' He handed her the empty tankard, hoping he had distracted her from their discussion, but when she had returned it to the tray, she fetched a cup of coffee for herself and sat down again at his bedside.

'Now perhaps you will tell me truthfully how you came to be attacked, Your Grace.'

'I have told you. Footpads.' She narrowed her eyes at him and he knew that would not do. He sighed. 'My cab was stopped by a group of men armed with pistols. I was ordered to step out and the driver was sent on his way. Then one of the rogues clubbed me from behind.'

'And continued to beat you when you were on the floor.' Her grey eyes were dark with anger.

'Yes. Hence the sore ribs.'

The laudanum was having an effect. The pain in his chest was easing and he could watch Pru in more comfort. She was sipping her coffee and he thought how beautiful she was. He would very much like to kiss those ruby lips again. Not that she would allow it. She had made that very clear.

'It is very unusual for such an attack to take place in daylight,' she said slowly. 'Could they have been lying in wait for you?'

'I am almost certain of it.'

'Perhaps they were hired by the same person who wants to see you arrested.'

'That thought had occurred to me,' he said sleepily. 'The only question is, why did they not kill me?'

'Because whoever is behind this does not want you dead.' She added ominously, 'Yet.'

Garrick fought against the drowsiness. He had said too much. Pru should not be worrying about such matters.

'What a devious mind you have, Miss Clifford,' he murmured.

She smiled but was not distracted. 'It begins to make sense, I think.'

'What does?' Her silence made him suspicious. 'Pru?'

She looked up quickly, as if she had forgotten he was there, and shook her head.

'Nothing that cannot wait until you are feeling better,' she said briskly. She rose to her feet. 'Mrs Hayes and I will undress you and then you must rest.'

'Pru.' He reached out and took her hand. She gave him a tight little smile.

'You need not be anxious, sir. While you sleep I shall send a note to Dover Street and summon Stow to attend you.'

'No, no that's not it!' He gave her hand a little shake. 'You must not leave while I am sleeping. Promise me.'

His touch and the intense look in his green eyes sparked a sudden excitement in Pru, but it was outweighed by concern. Fear for Garrick was uppermost in her mind. Everything else must wait. If he was not lucid the next time he woke up then she would summon his doctor, despite his objections.

'Promise me!' he insisted.

She tried to speak calmly, as she would to any patient. 'No, I shall not leave just yet, you have my word.'

He gave a slight nod of satisfaction and closed his eyes as the laudanum began to take effect. Pru's fingers tingled in his grasp and she reluctantly eased her hand free. She was in danger of losing her heart to the duke but she must not lose her head. He needed her nursing skills now, nothing else.

Slowly Pru carried the empty coffee cup back to the tray, taking her time, not rushing back to the bedside. She must not to fuss around him like a mother hen. The man had enough troubles without having a lovesick female fawning over him.

And yet.

Pru resumed her seat at his bedside. He had asked

her again to marry him. He might be delirious, that would account for it, but she thought it far more likely that he was trying to protect her. Why would he do that if he did not like her?

A ragged, derisive laugh clogged her throat.

'There is a vast difference between liking and love,' she told herself sternly. 'What would the Duke of Hartland see in a lanky, plain Jane like me?'

But even this was not enough to kill the tiny seed of hope that had taken root inside her.

When Garrick woke again, night had fallen. A few lighted candles had been placed around the room and their dim light showed him he was alone. He was in the bed now, clad in a nightshirt and with a thin cotton sheet pulled up across his chest. His ears caught the sound of someone on the stairs. The next moment the door opened and Prudence came in. He glared at her.

'Who undressed me?'

She gave him a wicked look. 'Perhaps it is best that you do not ask that.'

An angry retort sprang to his lips, but before he could utter it she laughed and shook her head at him.

'No, no, I am teasing you,' she said, the candlelight dancing in her eyes. 'It was Stow, with the landlady's help. I was not even in the room.'

'Stow is here?'

'Yes. He has taken your clothes away to do what

he can with them. Most are ruined but he hopes your coat may be saved.' She came closer and straightened the sheet. 'How do you feel now?'

'Sore.'

'That is to be expected.'

'The headache has eased,' he admitted. 'What time is it?'

'Gone midnight.'

'Confound it, you should not still be here! Why did you not wake me?'

'I was about to do so, had you still been sleeping,' she replied, laying a cool hand on his brow. 'I told you I wanted to ascertain there has been no damage to your brain. There is no fever, and you appear to be your usual curmudgeonly self, so I think I may safely leave you now.'

'Witch!'

She laughed. Garrick watched her put on her pelisse, thinking how much he liked having her with him.

'How will you get back to Brook Street at this late hour?'

'Stow came here in your carriage. Your driver is even now waiting for me. I shall be quite safe.'

'But how will you explain yourself?'

'They know I was visiting Lady Elsdon.' She smiled again. 'I shall say, quite truthfully, that I have been engaged upon charitable work.'

A black cloud descended on his spirits. There was that word again, he thought bitterly. She might as well say outright that she pitied him! His man came into the room and she turned to speak to him.

'I shall leave His Grace in your capable hands now, Mr Stow. I rely upon you to send me word at Brook Street of how he goes on.'

'You may be sure I will, ma'am, and thank you.'

She picked up her reticule and went out, pausing at the door to cast one final glance towards the bed before closing the door. Garrick listened to her footsteps on the stairs, then there was only silence and a strange hollow feeling inside him.

## Chapter Nineteen

Pru arrived in Brook Street before the other ladies returned from their supper party and she slipped quickly up to her room. There would be time enough for evasions and explanations in the morning. There might be no need for her aunt or her hostess to know that she had not dined with Lady Elsdon. Neither was particularly interested in her charity work and she hoped that she might be able to deflect their questions without telling a direct lie.

The events of the past few hours had taken their toll and she felt exhausted, but when she finally blew out the candle, she found her mind would not be still. She went back over everything that had happened after finding Garrick, the sickening fear that had gripped her as he had been carried to the inn. She was haunted by the memory of Walter being brought home in just such a condition, from which he had never recovered.

Being able to nurse Garrick, albeit for such a short time, was a bittersweet comfort. She had been glad to be busy, tending his wounds and bathing his face, but sitting beside him as he slept was a trial, unable to do anything for his unseen injuries and afraid she might lose him. It did no good to tell herself he was not hers to lose.

Pru was confident Stow would look after his master equally well. He might even persuade Garrick to be examined by a doctor, although she doubted it. Proud, obstinate man! She resolutely turned her thoughts away from the duke to consider the other interesting event of the day: taking tea with Lady Elsdon.

It had started very much as expected; Pru had been introduced to Lady Elsdon's guests, all of whom were a little surprised to find a young and unmarried lady so intent upon helping the émigrés, but Pru's experience in Bath stood her in good stead.

After an hour of talking, Lady Elsdon declared Miss Clifford would be a very valuable member of the group. Not, perhaps, in financial terms, but full of useful suggestions for setting up a refuge and raising funds. However, as the afternoon wore on Pru began to think she had learned nothing of any use to Garrick. Then, just as she was about to make her excuses and leave, another guest hurried in, gushing apologies.

'My dear ma'am, I beg your pardon for arriving so late! I trust I have not missed anything of importance?'

'No, no, Lady Conyers. We have barely begun.'

Prudence was sitting with her back to the door when

Lady Elsdon welcomed the latecomer, but that soft, melodious voice was unmistakable. Removing all trace of shock or surprise from her countenance, she fixed a smile in place and turned.

Pru smiled again now, in the darkness, but this time with genuine amusement as she recalled the astonishment on the beautiful Helene's face when she saw her. Lady Conyers had been suspicious at first, but Prudence greeted her calmly enough and gave such a good account of herself in the following discussions that there could be no doubting her extensive knowledge of charitable work. The meeting had given Pru much to think about, but when at last she drifted off to sleep, her thoughts returned to Garrick and her dreams were troubled by concern for him.

Garrick was back in Dover Street shortly after noon the following day. Ignoring his man's suggestion that he should go to bed, he insisted on taking a bath before changing into a fresh suit of clothes. He was standing before the mirror in the drawing room, tying his neckcloth, when Jack Callater burst in.

'So you *are* here, Garr! What the devil has been going on?'

'And a good day to you, Jack.' Garrick tried not to wince as he moved away from the looking glass. 'I'd be grateful if you could moderate your language. I have a shocking headache, you know.'

'From what I've heard you have a damned sight

worse than that,' retorted Jack. 'I have just spoken with Miss Clifford—'

Garrick made no effort to moderate his own language and cursed roundly.

'Damned interfering woman.'

'She rescued you, confound it!'

'I did not need rescuing,' he said, lowering himself gently into an armchair.

'No?' Jack threw himself down onto the sofa and looked at him, his brows raised. 'God knows what would have happened to you if she had not come upon you when she did.'

'Someone else would have found me.'

'Aye, thieving rascals who would have stripped you clean!'

'Not everyone is a villain, Jack.'

'Perhaps not. In any event you could have lain in the dirt for hours.' He paused as Stow came in carrying a tray.

'I didn't order wine,' barked Garrick, glaring at his man.

'No, Your Grace, but Lord John is partial to a glass of claret in the afternoons,' Stow replied, unmoved by his master's anger. 'And I thought one glass would do you no harm, Your Grace, if you would care for it. Or would you prefer the laudanum the apothecary has sent round?'

Garrick's look left his man in no doubt of the answer to that.

Jack laughed and Garrick bade Stow put the tray down on a side table, saying, once the man had withdrawn, 'I take it your meeting with Miss Clifford was not by chance?'

'No, she sent me word and we met in Green Park this morning,' said Jack. 'After that, I went directly to The Dun Cow only to be told you had left. Against Miss Clifford's advice, I am sure.'

'Aye, if she had been nursing me I should be there still.' A smile tugged at Garrick's mouth. 'A most redoubtable woman. But her concern and yours is misplaced. I am perfectly well now.'

'Do not try to gammon me! Your face looks as if it's taken a battering from Gentleman Jackson.'

'It will heal.'

'And your ribs? Pru said they kicked you while you were down.'

'Pru?' Garrick's brows snapped together. 'Getting might friendly with the lady, ain't you, Jack?'

'Don't change the subject...or do I detect a hint of jealousy there, old friend?'

Garrick almost ground his teeth when he saw the amused glint in Jack's eye, but he was too wise to argue.

He said, 'It's possible the ribs are cracked. But it could have been much worse.'

'So, who do you think was behind it?'

'I am not sure yet, but I think it was connected to my appointment yesterday.' Garrick described his visit to Albert Vence, ending, 'It seems too much of a co-incidence that I should be attacked on my way back from Somers Town.'

Jack frowned. 'Aye, damned suspicious, if you ask me.'

There was a knock at the door and Stow came in again.

He said woodenly, 'Viscount Sidmouth is down-stairs and wishes to see Your Grace.'

Garrick met Jack's eyes. 'Is he, by Gad. I wonder what the home secretary wants with me?' With an effort he levered himself out of his chair. 'Send His Lordship up.'

'Good of him not to barge straight in,' muttered Jack, also rising.

There was no time for more. Stow ushered the visi-tor into the room and Garrick managed to incline his head in greeting without wincing with the pain.

'Lord Sidmouth. To what do I owe the pleasure of your call?'

'I did not know you had a visitor, Your Grace.' His Lordship bowed to Jack. 'Lord John.'

'Oh, Jack and I are old friends,' said Garrick cheer-fully. 'We have no secrets from one another. Shall we sit down?'

Lord Sidmouth indicated he would rather stand.

'This concerns the charges that have been made against you, Your Grace,' he said. 'You are aware of them?'

'Of course.'

The home secretary was looking a little uncomfortable and Garrick decided to help him out.

'I presume you know I called to see Monsieur Vence yesterday.'

'Yes.' Lord Sidmouth frowned. He said heavily, 'I was informed you attacked him.'

'I did not,' Garrick retorted. 'The fellow panicked and shouted for his guards. They will tell you that I left when they asked me to do so.'

'And you did not go back?'

'Of course not.' It was Garrick's turn to frown. 'What is this about?'

'Last night someone tried to murder Albert Vence.'

## Chapter Twenty

Garrick stared in silence at the home secretary.

He said, slowly, 'It was not I.'

'Your Grace, can you prove you did not return to the Golden Cockerel, can anyone vouch for you?'

Jack shifted and Garrick threw him a warning glance.

'No.'

'And the bruises on your face?'

'Footpads. I was attacked on my way back to Dover Street.'

Lord Sidmouth's eyes narrowed suspiciously but Garrick did not look away.

'Perhaps, Lord Sidmouth, you should tell me what happened last night. That is, I should like to have the account of what your men saw or heard.'

'Monsieur Vence was distressed by your, ah, visit, Your Grace, and he retired early, as soon as it grew dark. Someone broke into his bedchamber shortly after and attacked him. Fortunately, my men were on guard in the next room, and heard the commotion.'

'The Frenchman seems particularly nervous,' observed Jack. 'Can you be sure he was not having a nightmare?'

Lord Sidmouth threw him a disdainful glance. 'It was no dream, sir. My men saw a figure climbing out of the window, but by the time they ran downstairs he had vanished.'

'Was Vence seriously hurt?' demanded Garrick.

'A blow to the head. He is convinced it was you, Your Grace.'

'It was not. You have my word for it.'

'Then why was your sword stick found in his room? The coat of arms on the silver handle is unmistakable.'

Jack stifled a curse.

'I lost in when *I* was attacked.' Garrick looked Lord Sidmouth in the eye. 'Are you here to arrest me?'

With an oath Jack took a step forward. 'On what grounds? Did anyone actually *recognise* the intruder as the duke?'

'Sit down man,' growled Lord Sidmouth, waving him away. 'This is a very delicate situation. If His Grace will give me his word that he will not leave town, I will accept that. For now.'

'Then you have it,' said Garrick promptly. 'What about Vence—has he been moved?'

'He has gone into hiding in the country. He has friends with whom he feels safe.'

Garrick nodded. 'Believe me, Lord Sidmouth, Vence poses no threat to me. I told you to ask Castlereagh about my actions in France. Once you have his testimony, and the reports from my fellow agents at the time, it will become clear that Vence is lying, and I am innocent of the charges brought against me.'

'As to that, we shall see,' replied His Lordship, unconvinced. 'But it will go ill with you, Your Grace, if people think you tried to murder your accuser.'

With a brisk nod to both men, Lord Sidmouth departed and Garrick sank thankfully, but carefully, back into his chair.

'So now we know why those rogues took your cane,' said Jack.

'Aye. Someone is trying to make me look guilty. I have my suspicions who it may be, but no proof, as yet.'

'I think I might be able to help you there,' said Jack. 'Pru told me about her visit to Russell Square yesterday. Lady Elsdon's charitable work for French émigrés,' he added, when Garrick looked blank. 'We both thought it a waste of time, but now I am not so sure. Lady Conyers was there.'

Garrick was suddenly alert. 'Go on.'

'She turned up shortly after Pru arrived.'

'Another coincidence? I cannot believe it.'

'Nor I,' Jack replied. 'The point is, she is one of the charity's most ardent supporters.'

'Is she, by Gad? That is the first I have heard of Helene doing anything for anyone other than herself.'

Garrick shook his head. 'But Pru should not have gone there. I don't want her caught up in all this.'

Jack grinned. 'Not sure you could stop her, my friend. The lady knows her own mind.'

'She's damned obstinate.' Garrick glanced at his friend's face and he sighed. 'I know, I owe her a great deal, but you must keep her away from me, Jack. She is far too careless of her reputation.'

'You could change that. Marry her.'

Garrick's hands clenched into fists. He could not bring himself to admit she had rejected him, even to his friend.

He said, 'You know I cannot do it while this, this cloud is hanging over me.'

'She does not care for that.'

'But *I* do! Prudence Clifford is not of my world. Pray do not look at me like that—I am not saying she is beneath me. On the contrary, she is too good, too kind. She would be honouring *me* if she agreed to be my duchess.

'No. I mean the scandal that surrounds me would embarrass her family, her friends and the charities she cares so much for. That would cause her distress. Even if she can overlook my past demeanours, these current, unfounded accusations are far more serious and must be refuted. Only then can I ask a woman such as Pru Clifford to marry me.'

'I suppose you would not believe me if I said I thought you were wrong about that.'

'You may think what you like, Jack, but you must keep Pru from behaving rashly.'

'I will do my best, my friend, but she is her own mistress. And you have yet to hear what she learned about Lady Conyers. It appears that the beautiful Helene joined Lady Elsdon's committee in early March, working with the émigrés.'

'It is highly likely, then, that Helene knows Vence. Or at least knows *of* him.'

'Yes. I think she may have passed the information to her husband.'

'And out of spite, they persuaded the fellow to make the accusations against me.' Garrick waved a hand, suddenly too exhausted to talk. 'It matters not, Jack. Once Castlereagh sends word I shall be cleared.'

'But a reply could take weeks, months to come back. Until then do you want to stay in London, kicking your heels while your name is bandied about by everyone? If Conyers is trying to smear you then the longer it goes on, the more mud will stick.'

Garrick knew he was right. He wanted to be free of this latest slur so he could set about courting Prudence in earnest. He wanted to prove himself worthy of her, and of his name.

He looked up as Stow came in.

'Miss Clifford to see you, Your Grace.'

Garrick muttered under his breath. What sorcery had conjured her? He closed his eyes and ordered his man to send her away.

'I knew you would say that,' replied Pru from the doorway. 'Just as I guessed you would return here as soon as my back was turned. I needed to know how you are recovering.'

She was again wearing the cherry-red cloak in the mistaken belief that it made her look like a servant. In Garrick's opinion nothing could disguise the lady's quality. His concern for her made his reply sound rough and ungrateful, even to his own ears.

'You did not need to do anything of the kind. Jack would have informed you.'

'But I wanted to see for myself. No, don't get up.'

He had tried to rise and was glad to slump back in the chair, but this sign of weakness did nothing for his temper.

'By God, woman, do you not understand?' he said irritably. 'The home secretary was just here. If he had seen you—'

'But he did not. I waited until his carriage had turned out of sight before I approached the house.'

Jack laughed. 'By Gad, ma'am, you're a cool one!'

Garrick ground his teeth, hating to agree. He had never known anyone like Pru Clifford. He watched her remove the cloak and drape it over a chair-back. Annabelle Speke had always been such a timid little creature and his sharp tongue would have had her in tears, or going off in a dead faint. Helene would have raged at him, possibly hurling anything that was to hand in his direction.

No, this woman's calm, unflappable demeanour reminded him most closely of the duchess. The old duke had been profligate and unfaithful, but Mama had loved him deeply and without question. Yet she had not railed at Garrick in her letters, even though she blamed him for his father's death. Her missives were always cool, considered. The language had been temperate but unyielding and when she told him she never wanted to see him again he had known there was no arguing with her.

'You are as stubborn as my mother,' he muttered. 'I pray to heaven the two of you never meet!'

Pru flinched at his words but she gave a little shrug. 'It is very unlikely we ever shall, so let us waste no time on futile conjecture. Tell me instead what Lord Sidmouth wanted.'

'Garrick's head,' Jack interjected.

She stared at him, the blood draining from her face. 'What has happened?'

'It's to do with the fellow Garr went to see yesterday.'

'What fellow?' Pru looked from one to the other.

'The Frenchman. Did Garr not tell you?'

'I was in no state to tell anyone anything,' snapped Garrick. 'Besides, it is none of her business.'

'I believe it is, Your Grace.' She sat down and folded her hands in her lap and addressed Jack. 'Pray tell me everything.'

Pru listened in growing horror as Lord John explained about Garrick's meeting with Monsieur Vence and the home secretary's visit. When he had finished, she turned to Garrick.

'They think you tried to kill him.'

'But you know I did not. You were with me until midnight.'

'Did you tell Lord Sidmouth that?'

'How could I, without implicating you?'

Pru bit down her annoyance. 'You will have to tell him, if they decide to put you on trial.'

'It will not come to that. Castlereagh's evidence will prove Vence is lying.'

'Where is the Frenchman now?'

'Sidmouth said he is in hiding.'

'Where?'

'With a friend. Someone he trusts.'

'That could be the man who put him up to this in the first place,' she reasoned.

'Very likely. Now what is it that makes you frown?'

'I saw Lady Conyers yesterday.' She stopped, looking uncertain. Garrick nodded.

'Jack told me about that.'

'Yes, of course. I heard her say Sir Joseph was going out of town today.' She raised her eyes to his face again. 'What if *he* has taken the poor man away? What if he murders him and blames you for it?'

'Even he wouldn't be such a villain!' exclaimed Jack.

'Quite,' said Garrick, frowning. 'You are being fanciful, Pru.'

'Am I? Lord Sidmouth already thinks you are responsible for one attempt upon the man's life.'

'Only because I refused to give him your name as a witness.'

'But Sir Joseph could not have known I would find you,' she persisted. 'He may have hired the henchmen who beat you unconscious and stole your cane. You said yourself the attack took place in a deserted area. If I had not come across you, who knows how long you might have lain there? And you would have had no one to vouch for you at the time that Vence was killed.

'We know Sir Joseph hates you,' she went on. 'I have no doubt now that it is he who started the rumours about your loyalty to the Crown. Then there is Lady Conyers. I cannot believe it is pure chance that she is part of Lady Elsdon's charitable group.'

'No, neither can I,' Jack agreed. 'Doesn't it strike you as odd, Garr, that she began helping Lady Elsdon shortly after you returned to this country?'

'Perhaps, but what can we do?' said Garrick. 'If it is Sir Joseph who has hidden the fellow away, how are we to find him?'

'We could go to Lord Sidmouth, tell him what we suspect,' Jack suggested.

The duke shook his head. 'No, he would not act against one of his own on mere suspicion. On the other hand, he is not a man to take a risk. He must be very sure of Vence's protector.'

'Even if it is Conyers?' said Jack.

'The fellow is extremely plausible.'

'Which makes him particularly dangerous,' Pru insisted. 'What if he arranges for the poor man's death and then fabricates more evidence of your guilt? Lord Castlereagh cannot vouch for your actions here in England, can he?'

'She's right,' said Jack. 'It could be difficult for you if the fellow should die now. We need to find him.'

'Aye, but where do we start?'

'I think I know.' Pru found two pairs of eyes fixed upon her. She said, 'I attended a party at Sir Joseph's townhouse and saw a watercolour on the wall. A painting of Alder Grove, in Kent. Lord Fauls told me it is Sir Joseph's old home. He said the house was empty now, Sir Joseph having bought a larger property, more fitted to his station.' She frowned trying to recall details of the little painting. 'The house looked to be in a very rural landscape. It is surrounded by woodland, but near Dartford which is not, I think, too far from town.'

'A perfect hideaway then,' declared Jack. 'Well, Duke, what do you think, could Vence be there?'

Garrick shrugged. 'It is worth a try. We have nothing else to work on. We could ride there tomorrow.'

'*You* cannot,' Pru declared. 'You are already under suspicion, besides being unwell. I could—'

'No!' exclaimed Garrick. 'I will not have you involved further in this!'

'No need for anyone to accompany me,' said Jack hurriedly. 'Sidmouth expressly forbade you to leave town, Garr, but I can go.' He pulled out his watch. 'I will ride to Dartford tonight and make enquiries as to the location of Alder Grove. If Vence is there I will try to persuade him to come with me and put himself back into Lord Sidmouth's protection.'

'*Can* you persuade him?'

Garrick heard the doubtful note in Pru's voice.

'I shall do my best. The first thing is to locate the fellow.' Jack grinned. 'Don't look so anxious, Pru, my dear. We will come through this.'

'Pray, my lord, be careful.'

'I shall, no need to fret.'

Pru received a reassuring smile from Jack—damned charming fellow that he was—who then picked up his hat and gloves and went out. His footsteps could be heard running down the stairs and Garrick shifted restlessly in his chair.

'Don't worry,' he said. 'Jack can take care of himself.'

'But he is a stranger to Monsieur Vence, why should the man trust him?'

'If he refuses to budge then I will take my suspicions to Lord Sidmouth and let him deal with it. At least he will have been warned.'

'I should go with you. I could tell him I was with you until midnight yesterday.'

'No.'

'Garrick—'

'No!' He drew a breath. 'Don't you see, you have

already done enough. I cannot involve you further in this.' She was still looking stubborn and he raked one hand through his hair. 'Hell and damnation, Pru, I expect a visit from your aunt at any moment, *insisting* that I marry you!'

'And neither of us want that!' she retorted.

Garrick bit his tongue and glared at her. Why did she insist on putting words into his mouth?

'No one knows I am here,' she said, turning away from him. 'I kept the hood pulled up to disguise me from any inquisitive glances.'

'By God, madam, you are too reckless. I would like to pick you up and *shake* you!'

No, he admitted, but only to himself. He wanted to pick her up and carry her to his bed, only he was too damned weak to do so. His head was beginning to throb again. He sighed and rubbed a hand across his eyes.

'You must go now. There is nothing more you can do here.'

'Very well.'

She threw her cloak about her shoulders and fastened it.

'Prudence.' He reached out and caught her hand as she passed him. 'For heaven's sake act up to your name for once. Go home and stay there until you hear from me.'

'As you wish.'

There was a note in her voice he had not heard before. She sounded weary, defeated. It flayed him.

'It is not that I am ungrateful, believe me. I owe you a great deal already, but you must not call here again.' His grip tightened and he said roughly, 'Do you understand? I shall give Stow instructions that you are not to be admitted.'

Pru felt suddenly close to tears.

'I thought we were friends,' she said, her voice low.

'Friends!' He gave a bark of laughter but it lacked any humour and merely grated on her nerves. 'How the devil can we be that, after all that has occurred?'

Feeling sick at heart, she nodded. 'You are quite right. I shall wait to hear from you, or Lord John. You will keep me informed, will you not?'

'Of course.' He released her. 'Now get you gone, madam. I need to rest.'

# Chapter Twenty-One

Keeping her head high, Pru walked slowly down the stairs. Stow was waiting to let her out of the house.

'Thank you for calling, madam.' He gave her a little bow. 'A few days' rest and His Grace will be back to his old self, I am sure.'

There was no mistaking the sympathy in his eyes.

'Of course.' She answered him calmly enough and pulled her hood up as she stepped out of the building into the rain.

Garrick was afraid for her. That should have been a comfort, but his comments cut deep. She remembered the night they had met in Bath, when he had told her of Lady Speke's letter and that he was obliged to marry Annabelle. There had been a bleakness in his eyes that night and she had seen it again today. It was also in his voice, when he said he anticipated Aunt Minerva calling upon him. If he married her at all it would be from a sense of duty. Pru felt a hot tear slip down her cheek. And now he had said they could not even be friends.

Stow was right, of course. The duke was not himself, but his current malaise had merely stripped away
prevarication. He had told her nothing but the truth,
and it hurt.

What a fool she was to lose her heart to a man who
did not want her help or her friendship.

Friday passed in Brook Street with no word from
either Garrick or Lord John. Pru was not surprised.
She knew it might take Jack some time to locate Alder
Grove and even longer to discover if the Frenchman
was in hiding there. She did not want to believe that
Garrick was deliberately keeping her in the dark, but
she could not quite suppress the suspicion. However,
the next day an unexpected morning visit gave her
thoughts quite another turn.

All three ladies were in the morning room when
Lady Conyers was announced. She sailed in, resplen-
dent in a powder blue promenade dress and a delightful French hat of blue and white satin. There was a
flurry of activity as polite greetings were exchanged
and refreshments brought in, but as soon as they were
all settled Pru found herself the object of Lady Conyers's attention.

'My dear Prudence—I may call you that, I hope? I
feel we are such good friends now! It was quite a surprise to see you in Russell Square the other day. I had
no idea you were interested in our little cause.'

'Oh, my niece is a great one for charitable works,' declared Aunt Minerva. 'She is quite renowned for it in Bath. The Widows and Orphans, Relief of the Poor or nursing the sick at the infirmary! Prudence has such a kind heart.'

'Indeed?' Helene's beautiful smile never wavered but Pru detected a hint of contempt in those blue eyes. 'Miss Clifford is a veritable saint, then.'

'That is too kind of you, my lady, I am no saint,' replied Pru, giving the lady a smile every bit as false as her own. 'But I do find great satisfaction in helping those less fortunate. Which is why I was so pleased to support Lady Elsdon's efforts on behalf of the French émigrés.' She paused. 'You mentioned yesterday Sir Joseph had been obliged to go out of town. I hope he has returned safely?'

'No, he is still away.' Lady Conyers gave a little trill of laughter. 'He may be waiting for me when I get home but, in truth, I have no idea when he means to return.'

'Was he called away on business, ma'am?' asked Aunt Minerva. 'I do hope he will not miss the Grand Jubilee on Monday. It promises to be a great spectacle.'

'It does indeed, but my husband is not one for these celebrations, you know. Are you planning to attend, Lady Borcaster?'

'Why yes, it is not to be missed, if the reports are to be believed.'

'Oh, quite so, ma'am, quite so. It will be a very grand affair. I wonder—' She paused, as if hesitant to make her request. 'I wonder if I might steal away your young guest for the day?' Her charmingly diffident smile swept over all three ladies. 'That is the reason for my call today. I am come to invite Miss Clifford to join me on Monday. You see, I promised to help Lady Elsdon at the fair and would welcome a little company. She has hired a booth from which the committee will sell the little pieces of art that the poor émigrés have been making. You will know the sort of thing, ma'am, fancy boxes and reticules, purses and pincushions made from scraps of silk or velvet, painted notebooks, toys...' She laughed. 'French rags, we call it, but those sympathetic to their plight will buy them as gifts or keepsakes, I am sure.'

'What an admirable cause,' declared Lady Borcaster. 'Although, sadly, I do not intend to visit the fair booths. The crowds there will be fearsome.' She turned to Mrs Clifford. 'I thought we would take in Green Park, and perhaps even St James's Park, if it is not too busy.'

'That sounds delightful, and I am sure we will manage without Prudence, if she wishes to be elsewhere,' replied Aunt Minerva. 'I certainly have no objection to her joining you, Lady Conyers, but it really is up to Prudence.'

With the eyes of the three ladies upon her, Pru was obliged to think quickly. She had no idea what had prompted the invitation and was a little suspicious. Yet it was a perfectly reasonable request.

'I do remember Lady Elsdon mentioning the fair,' she said now. 'However, I thought all the arrangements were in place for the ladies of the committee to take their turn in the booth.'

'They are, but my lady expressed the hope that I might find someone to assist me for an hour or two. An extra pair of hands and eyes would be most helpful.' Lady Conyers leaned forward, saying earnestly, 'Oh, do say you will come, Prudence. Sir Joseph is very impatient of my good works, as he calls them, and is not minded to come with me, even if he is returned by then. And after we have performed our duties, as it were, we may go off and explore the rest of the entertainments.'

'I should like to see as much as possible of the celebrations,' Pru admitted.

'Excellent! Then it is settled.' Lady Conyers smiled broadly and clapped her hands. 'I shall send my carriage to call for you. Oh, we shall have such a splendid day, my dear!'

The conversation moved on and Pru sat back to drink her tea. She had no idea what had prompted Lady Conyers to invite her, although it was possible Helene had no close female friends willing to go with her. In fact, she thought uncharitably, that was very likely. And spending a few hours with Lady Conyers might be advantageous.

Lord John might return with Vence today or tomorrow and if so, Pru could always cry off from joining

Helene at the fair. However, if there was no sign of the Frenchman, she would be well placed to learn something more about Lady Conyers and her husband. And working in the booth would also be an ideal opportunity for her to discover if any of the committee knew where the Frenchman might be.

Whatever Garrick might say, thought Pru, rebelliously, she could still be useful.

Garrick slept most of Friday, which prevented him fretting too much over how Jack was faring in Kent. By Saturday, although his ribs still hurt, he felt physically much recovered. However, he could not settle to anything and raged inwardly against his enforced inactivity. It was not merely Jack's mission to Alder Grove that preyed upon his mind. He had been less than kind to Pru.

He knew his weakened state and anxiety for her had made him more irritable than usual. He was unable to shake off the black depression that clouded his thoughts, but that was no excuse. He wanted to go to Brook Street immediately and apologise, but Jack might return at any time and he needed to be here when he called. Garrick considered writing a note to Pru, begging her pardon for his boorish behaviour, but after several aborted attempts he gave up. What he wanted to say, what he *needed* to say, could not be written in a letter.

If she was angry with him so much the better, it

might keep her from calling in Dover Street again. He wanted to see her so badly that it hurt quite as much as his bruised ribs, but he did not want her good name dragged through the mud. She did not deserve to be vilified for her association with him. However, when this damned business was over, he would find her. He would prove to her how much he loved her, even if it took him a lifetime.

Jack arrived in Dover Street at noon, still dressed for riding.

'Forgive me for coming in all my dirt,' he said, tossing his hat, gloves and riding crop on the table. 'I did not want to waste time changing my clothes.'

Garrick waved away his apology. 'What news?'

'Not good, I'm afraid. Vence is at Alder Grove—I saw him for myself—but he never leaves the grounds. He is as good as a prisoner there.' He took a brimming tankard of ale from Stow and drank deep before continuing. 'I did talk to him, though.'

'Oh, how did you manage that?'

'I, er, persuaded one of the maids to take a message to him.' Jack's wicked grin appeared, briefly, then he was serious again. 'The fellow came out to take the air this morning and we exchanged a few words, over the wall. I tried to convince him to come back to town with me, but to no avail.'

'Confound it!'

'I told him he has nothing to fear from you, Garr. I

said we would both give him our protection and support him if he tells the truth, but he will not budge. I gained the impression he is more afraid of Conyers than anything you or the court can do to him.'

'Damned fool.' Garrick stared into his own tankard, frowning. 'Then our only hope is to lay the whole before the home secretary. Perhaps Vence will trust Sidmouth enough to put himself back under his protection before it is too late. I must speak to him.'

'Now?'

'If he is to be found. The longer we wait the more chance there is that something will happen to Vence.'

'Very well. Give me time to go to Albany and change my clothes and I will come with you. We'll try Whitehall first, then his house in Richmond Park.'

It was dark by the time the two friends arrived back in Dover Street, and Garrick's bruised ribs were making it plain they did not appreciate being bounced around in a travelling chaise, albeit a luxurious one. He let out another hiss of pain as he climbed out of the carriage.

'You should have let me go alone,' complained Jack.

'This is my problem and I must deal with it, although I admit your father being a friend of Lord Sidmouth is an advantage when talking to the man.'

'Very magnanimous of you!'

'Aye, and I shall repay your assistance by inviting you to dine with me tonight.'

'I would rather you took to your bed and rested. You have been in agony all day.'

'You are exaggerating. I have had a little discomfort, nothing more.' Garrick caught his friend's eye and exclaimed, 'Damn it, Jack, I ain't an invalid, and I need a good meal, even if you don't!'

'Very well, let us eat together, since it is pointless arguing with you,' Jack retorted. 'How soon, do you think, before we hear from Lord Sidmouth?'

'Not before tomorrow night at the earliest.'

'You really believe he intends to travel to Alder Grove on a Sunday?'

'Aye, he said he would do so. Sidmouth's no fool. He knows better than to ignore our warning. I only hope he is not too late already.'

'And Prudence,' said Jack, following him up the stairs. 'Will you write and tell her about Vence?'

Garrick did not reply immediately. She was never far from his thoughts, but he was strangely loath to contact her. Everything might yet come to nought and, if that were the case, what was the point? She would be better off without him.

'She will want to know what is happening,' Jack persisted. 'I could send her a message—'

Garrick hissed out a curse. 'Let it be, Jack! I will write, once we are sure of Vence.'

It was in fact late Sunday night when Garrick received word from the home secretary. Jack had once again dined in Dover Street and was about to take his leave when Stow came in with a note. Garrick tore it open and quickly perused the contents.

'Well?' Jack demanded.

'All is well. Vence is now at White Lodge with Lord Sidmouth. He expects the fellow to make a full confession in the morning.' Garrick held out the letter. 'Once that is done, Sidmouth will be able to use his evidence to indict Conyers for perverting justice.'

'But Vence will still be guilty of making false accusations against you.'

'Aye, poor devil, but at least he will be alive. When the truth finally comes out, that he was coerced into this, I hope he will be shown some mercy.'

'And you have promised to give the fellow your support, which should count for something.' Jack handed back the paper and rose from his chair. 'Well, a good day's work, my friend. It is time I was going.'

He took his leave, but at the door he stopped and turned back.

'And you will send word to Prudence?'

Garrick sighed, causing his ribs to protest again. He waved a hand.

'I will write in the morning. She will be sleeping now.'

He felt Jack's gaze upon him and glared across the room, daring him to argue, but there was only understanding in his friend's eyes.

Jack nodded and smiled. 'Aye, get some sleep, Garr. You look spent.'

\* \* \*

Garrick slept late the next morning but woke up much refreshed. The black melancholy that had dulled his spirits since the attack had lifted and he was eager to get about his business. His ribs hurt a lot less as he climbed out of bed and he decided he would go and see Prudence. He would apologise for his boorish behaviour and tell her the news about Vence.

And perhaps, if the moment seemed propitious, he would tell her how much he loved her.

However, when he looked at his face in the mirror, the bruising on his cheek had spread to cover almost half his face in varying shades, from red to an ugly dark purple.

'Curse it, that is no sight to inflict upon a lady!'

'If I might say, Your Grace,' said Stow, pulling a clean shirt from the linen press, 'I do not think you need worry that your appearance will shock Miss Clifford. She has seen Your Grace in a far worse state.'

Garrick knew it and that grated on him, too. He knew it was mere vanity on his part. Stubborn male pride, as she had called it. Whatever it might be, he did not want her to see him like this.

'I shall write to her,' he decided. 'Fetch me pen and paper, Stow, and you can take a message to Brook Street for me.'

The morning was well advanced by the time Garrick was dressed and ready to sit down and write his letter. Then the words would not come. How did he explain his temper, or admit he did not feel worthy of her? After several false starts he penned a simple apology, vowing to explain everything when they next met. He followed this with the news about Monsieur Vence and ended with a promise to call in Brook Street as soon as he was fit to be seen.

Garrick put down his pen and read the letter through again before sealing it and addressing it to Miss Prudence Clifford. Then he summoned his man.

'There,' he said, handing it over. 'Not the most eloquent prose I have ever written, but it will have to do. I would be obliged if you would take it in person, Stow. I do not expect a reply, but if you should see Miss Clifford, if she should have a message for me...'

'I understand, Your Grace.'

With a bow, Stow took the letter and went out. Garrick sat back in his chair, knowing full well he would not rest until his man returned.


When he heard a hasty step on the stairs, Garrick threw aside the book he had not been reading.

'Well?' He frowned when he saw Stow's face and said urgently, 'What is it, what has occurred?'

'Miss Clifford was not at home, Your Grace,' he said, between panting breaths. 'She is gone to Hyde Park. To the Great Fair.'

'Ah yes. I had forgotten about the Jubilee celebrations today. That explains the unusual amount of noise coming in from the street.'

'Aye, Your Grace. There are so many people abroad that London has almost come to a stand. That is why I ran back rather than taking a cab.' He put a hand to his heaving chest and gasped out, 'She has gone with Lady Conyers!'

## Chapter Twenty-Two

Garrick ignored the screaming pain of ribs as he hurried to Hyde Park, weaving through the crowds that thronged each street. Stow had learned at Brook Street that Lady Conyers had taken Pru off to help in Lady Elsdon's booth, raising money for the émigrés. He had no reason to believe Helene meant any mischief, but the doubts would not go away.

He remembered the speculative look she had given him at Shrivenham House, when he had come in from the terrace with Pru on his arm. If she thought his affections were engaged, that alone might be enough for her to wish Pru harm, but if she thought the lady was actively helping to thwart her husband's plans…

The doubt hardened into certainty. His fingers tightened on the Malacca cane, wishing it was his sword stick, but that was still in Lord Sidmouth's possession. He lengthened his stride, praying that his quarry was indeed in Hyde Park.

\* \* \*

Lady Conyers's note arrived as Pru was drinking her morning hot chocolate. It informed her that my lady would call at ten o'clock, which meant Pru had to rush her breakfast and scramble into her walking dress. Once they reached the booth she made herself useful, helping to unpack the items made by the French men and women who needed support in a strange land.

Pru would have been happy to work with the other ladies for much longer, but after an hour Helene suggested they go off and look around the fair.

'It will be a sad crush, I fear, but we have Ronald in attendance,' Helene told her, glancing towards her liveried footman. 'We will be perfectly safe.'

Pru's kind heart suggested that the lady might be lonely and in need of a companion, so she readily agreed and they set off into the throng.

Several hundred tents and booths had been erected selling everything from trinkets and ribbons, small pots and fancywork to all manner of food and drink. Printing presses had been set up, offering engraved views of the Temple and Chinese Pagoda for a few pence.

Helene was going out of her way to be charming and Pru could not deny she was enjoying herself. After they had tried several of the little delicacies on offer in the food tents, Helene suggested they should walk to Green Park.

'There is to be a re-enactment of the Battle of the

Nile here, but that does not start until six o'clock and we can easily come back later, if you wish to watch it.'

Prudence had seen enough of the stalls and hawkers and readily agreed to move on. They strolled away from the bustling fairground and Pru was glad of her straw bonnet with its wide brim to protect her face from the sun. Green Park was just as busy. Lady Conyers took Pru's arm and guided her towards the large wooden edifice that had been erected, chattering all the while.

'That is the Fortress,' she explained. 'It was fashioned by builders from the Theatre Royal, I believe, and is cleverly designed to transform into a Temple of Concord later this evening, which I think will be very exciting.' Helene's fingers tightened on Pru's sleeve and she gave a little cry of delight. 'Look, my *caro sposo* is come to join us. Over here, my dear!'

Pru's spirits sank when she saw Sir Joseph coming towards them. Not that there was anything to fear, she told herself. They were amongst so many people, she was perfectly safe. All the same she was suddenly on her guard and her greeting was civil, but not warm.

The gentleman laughed gently as he bowed to her.

'Oh, dear, I fear Miss Clifford is angry with me for interrupting your *tête-à-tête*, Helene. I must be on my best behaviour to regain her favour.'

Pru smiled politely but did not respond. She was relieved that Sir Joseph took his wife's arm and left her free to walk beside them. Gradually her tension eased. The gentleman's behaviour was polite enough, he made no attempt to flirt with Pru or to tease her and he was well enough informed on all the exhibits to keep the ladies well entertained. All the same, she wished now that she had not accepted Lady Conyers's invitation. She would have been much more comfortable with her aunt and Lady Borcaster.

Garrick had been searching for two hours and still he had not found Prudence. He sent word to Albany, asking Lord John to join him at Stanhope Gate and made his way there, waiting impatiently until he saw two familiar figures coming towards him.

'I fetched Stow along with me,' said Jack by way of greeting. 'I thought he might be useful.'

'I'd like to help, if I can, Your Grace.'

Garrick put his hand briefly on the man's shoulder to convey his gratitude. 'Thank you, Stow.'

'You say Pru is here somewhere with Lady Conyers?' asked Jack.

'Yes. They were both at Lady Elsdon's booth this morning, but then they went off and are not expected to return. I have no idea where they are heading, and the crowds are such I have not seen them yet.'

'Well, three of us will stand a better chance,' said Jack.

'Aye.' Garrick felt a little of his anxiety easing. He explained his plan for searching the three parks where the Jubilee celebrations were taking place and they agreed various points to meet throughout the day. As they prepared to move off Jack gripped the duke's arm.

'Don't worry, Garr. This could be nothing more than an innocent outing for two friends.'

'You do not believe that any more than I,' Garrick retorted.

Jack held his eyes for a moment, then he shook his head. 'No, sadly I don't. We had best get searching.'

Sir Joseph accompanied the ladies back to Hyde Park to watch the naval re-enactment and after that he announced that he had hired a supper booth for them all in St James's Park.

'How clever of you, my love. You think of everything,' sighed his wife, admiring. 'Is that not wonderful, Prudence dear?'

But Pru had had enough. She said, 'You are both very kind but you must forgive me if I do not stay. I have been out all day and I should be getting back to Brook Street.'

'Oh, but we have not seen the Chinese Pagoda!' exclaimed Helene. 'Surely you would like to see that. It has the new gas lighting, too, which will look splendid now it is growing dark.'

'And my carriage waits on the Mall, on the other side of St James's Park,' added Sir Joseph. 'We may see the Pagoda on the way.'

'I am happy to find a cab to take me back to Brook

Street,' said Pru. 'I would by no means curtail your enjoyment.'

'I would not hear of it,' exclaimed Helene. 'You are my guest. What would your aunt say if I allowed you to go home unattended?' She sighed. 'What a pity we sent Ronald away when Sir Joseph arrived. He might have accompanied you. But I do not think it would be wise for you to go off alone, and in the dark, too.'

'I agree.' Sir Joseph nodded. 'I fear some of the spectators have been drinking too freely.'

A sudden roar of raucous laughter added weight to his words and Prudence bit her lip. Sir Joseph had done nothing so far to arouse her suspicion and she could not deny that the crowd was becoming unruly. Helene took her arm again.

'I am sure your aunt will not expect you to leave before you have seen the fireworks, my dear. We will take you home directly after that, if you wish to go.'

'An excellent idea, my dear,' purred Sir Joseph. 'Well, Miss Clifford, will that do for you?'

Prudence could not deny she had been looking forward to the firework display, which promised to be a magnificent spectacle. It had been a long day, but she had seen nothing in the behaviour of Helene or her husband to suggest they had any motive for this outing, other than to enjoy themselves.

'Very well,' she said last. 'I will leave directly after the fireworks.'

* * *

Garrick walked to the toll gate at the corner of Hyde Park for the next rendezvous. The area was well lighted with oil lamps and he looked at his watch. Ten o'clock. And there was Jack, coming towards him.

'Anything?' he asked, although one look at his friend's face told him no.

'It is hopeless, Garr. The crowds are constantly moving. We would need the devil's own luck to find anyone here tonight.'

His final words were drowned out by the sudden thunder of artillery.

'The fireworks in St James's Park,' said Garrick. 'We will go there. It is my last hope. After that we should go to Brook Street. Prudence might have returned there by now.'

Brave words, but he could not bring himself to believe them.

'Your Grace!'

Stow's voice made him spin around, his hopes rising once more. 'You have found her?'

'No, Your Grace, but I did notice Sir Joseph's carriage standing in the Mall. I got talking with the driver and he told me he had orders from his master to wait there for him.'

'That's better,' exclaimed Jack. 'News at last!'

'It is, although you say the man mentioned his master. Does that mean Sir Joseph is here somewhere, too?'

'Aye, sir.' Stow nodded at him. 'The driver said he

had brought his mistress and her friend to Hyde Park early this morning and had to make the same journey again, some hours later, with Sir Joseph.'

'It is likely they are all together in one of the parks, then,' said Garrick, his spirits reviving.

'And that ain't all, Your Grace,' Stow went on. 'Since we was none of us in a hurry to move on, I treated the driver and the footman to a pie from a passing hawker. After which we fell into quite a conversation. It seems the footman had been following the ladies around the parks all morning, until Sir Joseph turned up. Then he was sent back to wait at the carriage, but he did mention that his master had booked a supper booth for the evening. To watch the fireworks.'

'Excellent work, man. Remind me to increase your salary when we get to Hartland!'

Stow grinned. 'Thank you, Your Grace.'

'Come along, we'll get to the Mall.' Garrick put a hand to his aching ribs. 'If Sir Joseph's carriage is still there then Stow and I will keep a watch on it while you, Jack, take a look around the supper booths, to see if you can find the Conyerses.'

The plan agreed, they set off, accompanied by the noisy woosh and bang of the firework display, which lit up the night sky. When they reached the Mall, they soon spotted the Conyerses' carriage. Keeping to the shadows, Garrick and Stow strolled under the trees that divided St James's Park from the thoroughfare while Jack went off to search the hired booths.

'This is as far as we can go,' muttered Garrick, when they drew level with Sir Joseph's coach. He led Stow further into the shadows. 'All we can do now is wait.'

When they reached the supper booth Sir Joseph had reserved Lady Conyers insisted upon Pru having first choice of the dishes. The food looked delicious, but she merely picked at it. She was growing increasingly uneasy, although she could not say why.

'Lost your appetite, Miss Clifford?' remarked Sir Joseph.

He offered to top up her glass, which was still half full, but she refused politely.

She said, 'It has been a long day, sir. I fear I am too tired to be much company now. I really think it would be best if I left.'

Lady Conyers cried out immediately at that.

'Oh, my dear, but the fireworks have just started. Will you not stay until the end?'

'I think not,' said Pru, having made up her mind. 'In fact, I think it is just the time to go, for the display is lighting up the whole park as bright as day. Pray do not get up—it is but a short walk to the Mall, where I am sure I can find a cab to convey me back to Brook Street.'

'No, no I will not let you go alone,' exclaimed Lady Conyers, pushing aside her plate. 'Mrs Clifford would never forgive me! We shall come with you.'

Nothing Pru could say would dissuade them and as they stepped out of the booth Helene took her arm.

'I should hate us to be separated by the mob,' she said with a theatrical shudder.

'No indeed,' said Sir Joseph, walking close on the other side of Pru. 'We might never find each other again.'

Pru made no reply. Perhaps she was being over-anxious, even melodramatic, but it was clear that any attempt to escape would be instantly foiled.

The fireworks lighting the skies overhead had brought even more people into St James's Park and Prudence quite lost her bearings as they wove their way through the crowd. She felt very tired and a little light-headed when at last they emerged onto the Mall. The road was lined with stationary carriages including, Pru noticed, a number of vehicles for hire.

'There really is no need for you to accompany me further,' she said. She was so fatigued now that her words were slurring. 'I can easily find a cab here to take me home.'

'Nonsense, my dear.' Lady Helene's hold on her arm tightened. 'It is not far out of our way, and our carriage will be far more comfortable.'

Sir Joseph lifted his cane and pointed. 'Look, it is but a step away.' He caught Pru's free arm. 'You look very pale, Miss Clifford. Let me help you.'

She did indeed feel a little unwell now, but when

Sir Joseph put his hand beneath her elbow, she was overcome by panic. She began to struggle against the hands holding her.

'No. No. Let me go! Let me *go*!

But Sir Joseph's arm came around her like a vice, squeezing her so tightly against him that she could scarce breathe, let alone scream for help. Her head felt very heavy and it was difficult to think clearly.

'There, there, ma'am, do not take on so.' Sir Joseph turned his head to address a concerned passer-by, saying ruefully. 'Wife's sister, having one of her turns. We should not have brought her out.'

'The wine,' she mumbled. 'You poisoned the wine!'

Pru struggled to cry for help but could not catch her breath and the straw bonnet, which had served her so well during the heat of the day, now cast a deep shadow over her countenance. Even if they should pass someone she knew, there was little chance of them recognising the struggling, confused woman as Miss Prudence Clifford.

'Nearly there,' declared Helene, holding Pru's arm tightly. 'You will soon be at home, my dear, safe in your own room.'

They were approaching the carriage now and Sir Joseph shouted to the footman at the back.

'Ronald, open the door. Quickly now, the lady is not well!'

The driver was gathering up the reins and Pru forced

her numbed limbs to struggle. She made a last feeble attempt to cry out, to no avail. She was lost.

Garrick and Stow were in the shadow of the trees, watching the crowds spilling out from the park. Men, women and children were strolling along the Mall, bumping into one another as they looked up and exclaimed at the spectacle in the sky above them.

'Where are they?' muttered Garrick, shifting his weight to relieve his aching body. Then his heart contracted. He saw Sir Joseph and Helene, half dragging, half carrying a drooping figure between them.

'There they are. Come on!'

He pushed his way through the press of spectators, shouting as he went.

'Stop! Abduction!'

But his words merely added to the noisy confusion of the crowd and he was obliged to barge past the last few people to reach his quarry.

'Conyers, stop!'

Sir Joseph had just reached the carriage. He released his hold of Pru and turned to face Garrick.

'Hartland.' He spat out the name; his face was contorted with rage. 'I have not finished with you yet!'

'Oh, I think you have. Sidmouth has the Frenchman safe. He knows of your plans.'

'No matter, I shall be in France by tomorrow, but I shall still make you pay before I leave!' He swung around to address his wife and the footman, who were bundling Pru towards the coach. 'Get her away. I will follow you.'

With an oath Garrick made for the carriage but Sir Joseph barred his way, the gleaming point of a sharp blade between them.

'You may have lost your sword stick, Hartland, but I still have mine.'

'I'm with you, Your Grace!' declared Stow, stepping up, but Garrick threw out an arm to stop him.

'No, you are unarmed.'

'But I am not!' Jack appeared, a sword in his own hand. 'Leave this to me, Garr.'

Sensing a drama, the crowd had moved away, but only to form a circle at a safe distance. They were very ready to be entertained by the anticipated brawl. With a snarl Sir Joseph turned to face the new threat.

'Ronald, to me, to me!' He shouted over his shoulder to his footman, who was closing the carriage door upon the ladies.

Garrick ran towards the coach. The lackey was in his path but Stow charged forward, knocking the man out of the way.

'Go on, Your Grace, I'll deal with this!'

The driver was whipping up the horses, the wheels were turning. Garrick sprinted onto the road and made a desperate leap for the back of the coach.

# Chapter Twenty-Three

Pru's head was spinning. She was thrust roughly into the carriage and had not gathered her wits before Helene was behind her, one arm around her neck in a choking hold. Despite her diminutive form, Lady Conyers was strong and Pru scrabbled to loosen the suffocating grip as the coach lurched into motion.

'Interfering jade!' Helene screamed at her. 'Do you think Garrick Chauntry could ever be yours?'

'I don't think that,' was all Pru could manage. She was gasping for air.

'But you have been spying for him! Well, you will regret it now, and so will he! You will both be ruined by the time we have finished with you.'

From the corner of her eye, Pru saw Helene raise her free hand and the sudden flare of a streetlamp glinted on the small glass phial she was holding. It smelled sweet, very like the laudanum Pru had given to Garrick, and she pressed her lips together, determined not to swallow it. The carriage was swaying wildly now and it was difficult to keep her balance as her hands clawed at the arm around her neck.

'But it's not only the duke, is it?' Helene hissed in her ear. 'Remember young Trenchard? I saw you dancing with him at the Shrivenham Ball. He was ready to fall into my hands like a ripe plum before you warned him off. You must pay for that, too!'

A sudden lurch threw them onto the seat and Pru broke free from the stranglehold. She thrust Helene away and saw the phial fly from her hand, but Pru barely had chance to draw a breath. With a shriek of rage, Helene launched herself at Pru again, kicking, biting and spitting.

Garrick clung on to the back of the coach, fighting down a sudden bout of dizziness. He couldn't faint off now, he needed to help Pru. At last his head cleared. He climbed up and scrambled across the roof to the box. He wrestled the reins from the driver, but in the ensuing struggle the man lost his balance and fell. Garrick was still untangling the reins but he glanced back and was relieved to see the fellow climbing to his feet. He appeared to be unharmed, and Garrick turned his attention back to the task of controlling the horses. Now all he had to do was find somewhere to stop. And stop soon, judging by the noise from inside the coach. The screeches and thuds suggested that the two women were fighting like wildcats.

\* \* \*

Garrick drove away from the parks, looking for a quiet street into which he might turn and stop the carriage. His ribs were sore from the exertion, which was also making his head swim, but finally he found what he was looking for. He drew up and called to a man walking towards him.

'You, fellow, would you like to earn yourself a shilling?'

'What, me? Earn a shilling?' The man stopped and looked up. He did not sound quite sober, but he looked respectable enough, and Garrick had little choice. He could not leave the restive team unattended while he jumped down.

'Two shillings then, if you will hold the horses' heads for a while.'

'Aye, sir. Gladly.'

The man took up his position and Garrick scrambled down from the box. He snatched open the door, half afraid of what he might discover, but it was Pru's voice that came from the darkness.

'Thank goodness, it is you,' she exclaimed. 'I thought we would never stop.'

'Did you follow us, Your Grace?'

Pru sounded unhurt and Garrick felt some of the tension ease from his body.

'No. I, er, ejected the driver.'

His eyes were adjusting to the dark interior. He could see she had lost her bonnet and her hair was hanging loose about her shoulders. She seemed to be crouching on the floor, but a closer look showed that she was in fact sitting upon her adversary.

He glanced back towards the horses. They were standing quietly with their minder and he turned his attention back to the ladies.

'Perhaps you should let Lady Conyers get up now.'

Prudence moved back onto the seat and Helene climbed up from the floor. In the dim light she looked even more dishevelled than her opponent.

'Thank heaven you are here, Garrick,' she said, her voice shaking with rage. 'This, this *harpy* tried to kill me!'

'Indeed, I did not,' Pru retorted. 'You were going to drug me! Laudanum,' she said, when Garrick smothered an oath. 'I think they had put some in the wine they served with supper. Thankfully I did not drink too much of it.'

'Thank God for that,' he muttered, climbing into the coach and sitting down. His head was hammering fearfully.

'What do we do now?' Pru asked him.

'Not too sure.' The pain had shifted to his eyes, his vision seemed to be narrowing. He tried to make his spinning brain concentrate. 'I think…'

The blackness closed over him.

\* \* \*

'Garrick!' Pru flew across the small space between them. 'Garrick!'

He was slumped in the corner and she tapped his cheek. There was nothing, not even the slightest flicker of life. But he was breathing. That gave her some comfort.

Lady Conyers jumped up, but Pru turned on her, fierce as a lioness.

'Sit back down!'

Helene subsided, eyeing her warily. 'What do you propose to do now? You cannot keep me here and tend the duke at the same time.'

She was right, Pru acceded as she eased the unconscious duke down onto the bench seat. Garrick was far more important to her.

'Very well,' she said, 'Take yourself off. I am sure Lord Sidmouth will find you soon enough.'

For the first time Lady Conyers looked uneasy. 'You cannot steal my coach!'

'I will do whatever is necessary to save the duke!'

Prudence climbed out and went to have a word with the young man holding the horses. He looked terrified when she suggested he should drive the carriage to Dover Street.

'I could run for a surgeon,' he suggested.

Pru shook her head. She had no idea what sort of man he might bring back with him and she knew that a bad doctor could do more harm than good. Biting her lip in frustration, she ran back to check on Garrick, who was still stretched out on the bench seat. She put her fingers gently on his neck. It was a relief to feel a faint pulse. It was erratic, but definitely there.

'What are you doing?' Helene demanded. 'What is happening?'

'We must get him back to Dover Street with all speed.'

'And what about me?'

Pru was very tempted to say she neither knew nor cared. Instead, she said, 'Can you drive this carriage?'

'Of course not!'

'Then you are no use to me.'

Spotting her reticule lying on the carriage floor, Pru snatched it up and jumped out, ordering Helene to follow her. Gently closing the carriage door upon Garrick's unconscious form, she went up to the young man at the horses' heads.

'Keep them steady while I gather up the reins.' She handed him her purse. 'Then I would be obliged if you would find a cab and escort this lady to her house.'

'Y-yes, ma'am.'

Ignoring Helene's continued protests Prudence walked back to the carriage. She glanced up at the box seat, high above her head. She was accustomed to driving a gig and had occasionally handled the reins of the waggon, when everyone was needed to help with the harvest on Home Farm, but she'd never driven such a vehicle as this. However, there was no one else to do it.

Swallowing hard, Pru hitched her skirts and climbed up. She gathered up the reins and, heart thudding, she called to the man to release the horses.

Somehow, Pru managed to drive the team to Dover Street without mishap. Lights shone from Garrick's house and Stow and Jack Callater rushed out as soon as she drew up. While Stow took care of his master, Jack helped Pru to descend from the perilously high box seat. He wanted to carry her off to the drawing room, but Pru would have none of it. The danger was not over yet and she knew she must remain in charge, at least for a while.

Once Stow and the servants had carefully undressed the duke and put him into his bed, Prudence insisted on staying beside him. Calmly, she gave orders to his servants and sat beside his bed, bathing his forehead with lavender water. Only when the duke's own doctor arrived did she join Jack in the drawing room.

'Ah, the sawbones is here, then,' said Lord John, pouring a glass of brandy for her.

'Yes. I have asked him to report to us once he has finished his examination.'

'Good. Now, sit down and drink this. You are looking alarmingly pale.'

He settled her into a chair, pressing the glass into her hand, and it was a measure of how frail she felt that Prudence did not refuse. She took a sip, trying not to gasp as the fiery liquid burned her throat.

'I was very glad you came out to meet me,' she told him. 'I was trembling so much I could not have climbed down to knock on the door.'

He said, 'We were keeping watch, although, frankly, we had little expectation of seeing either of you before morning.'

'How did you know what had happened?'

'Stow called at Brook Street with Garrick's note, telling you that Sidmouth had been to Alder Grove and taken Vence away to safety. He reported that you had gone to the fair with Lady Conyers and Garr set off immediately to look for you. Stow and I joined him later, and it was fortunate that Stow spotted the Conyerses' coach or we would never have found you.' He grinned. 'Garr was quite the hero, leaping onto the carriage as it drove off.'

'He did that, to rescue me?' She felt suddenly quite tearful.

'Yes. Stow and I saw Garr hanging on the back but there was nothing we could do until we had dealt with Conyers and his servant.'

'Oh, dear, I appear to have caused you a great deal of trouble.'

'Devil a bit,' declared Jack cheerfully. 'But how came you to be driving it back?'

'There was no one else,' she said simply. 'Garrick had overpowered the driver and pushed him off. When we stopped, he climbed into the carriage to see if I was safe and, and collapsed, unconscious. All I could think of was to bring him here to Dover Street, with all speed.'

'I see.' Lord John went over to the side table to refill his brandy glass. 'What happened to the belle Helene?'

'I was obliged to let her go.'

'Stow and I failed to apprehend Sir Joseph, too. He and his footman ran off. Ah well, it hardly matters. We sent word to Lord Sidmouth as soon as we got back. With our testimony and Vence safe in his keeping, he will deal with the matter now.'

He went on to tell her that the Frenchman had withdrawn his accusations against Garrick. Pru was relieved, but even that seemed of little importance, compared to Garrick's present predicament. When the doctor came in she looked up hopefully, but he could give them little cheer. There was nothing he could do until the duke regained consciousness.

'*If* he does,' he concluded. 'You said he was attacked recently, Miss Clifford? Well, it is very likely that the exertion of this evening was too much too soon. Now all we can do is wait.'

It was then that Jack voiced the questions Pru was afraid to ask.

'But will he recover, Doctor, and will his brain be damaged?'

'As to that, only time will tell. Call me again once he shows signs of consciousness.'

The doctor departed, leaving behind him an atmosphere of gloom. Pru refused to give in to melancholy and turned her thoughts to practical matters.

'The duke will need someone at his bedside constantly, in case he becomes fractious. I suggest Mr Stow and I do that between us.'

'That is impossible,' declared Jack. 'You cannot stay unchaperoned in a bachelor's house.'

'I can and I will,' Pru retorted. 'I have more experience with head wounds than anyone else here.'

Lord John looked mutinous, but Pru found an ally in the duke's man, who had come in at that moment.

'Miss Clifford is right,' Stow concurred. 'She is by far the best person to care for His Grace.'

Jack continued to argue, but Pru would not be moved and at last he went back to Albany, leaving Stow to keep watch over his master for the next four hours, while Prudence was shown to the guest room, where she soon fell into a deep sleep of sheer exhaustion.

The first flush of dawn was creeping into the bedroom when Pru opened her eyes. She stared up at the unfamiliar canopy for a moment as the events of the previous day flooded back, then she pushed back the covers and sprang out of bed, eager to be up and doing something. It had been agreed she would relieve Stow at six o'clock and she hoped Mrs Almond, the duke's housekeeper had not forgotten to send a maid up, for she judged it must be nearly that time now.

She had no wrap with her and was grateful for the

shift she had borrowed from Mrs Almond. It was a little short, but roomy and warm enough for her to sit down at the little table and finish writing the letter for Aunt Minerva that she had started last night.

She had just added a carriage clock to the list of items she wanted sent over from Brook Street when a maid came bustling in.

'Good morning, ma'am, I'm Betty. Mrs Almond sent me up to wait on you.' She nodded towards the clothes over her arm. 'She says to tell you she's cleaned up your gown as best she can, and mended a torn flounce on the skirt, but there's nothing she can do for the stain on the sleeve of your pelisse.'

'No matter, Betty, I shall not need that today.'

She was dressed in a matter of minutes then asked Betty to wait while she finished her letter.

'It will only take me a moment and then you may go downstairs and ask Mrs Almond if she would kindly have someone carry it to Brook Street for me.'

'Very well, ma'am. And shall I show you to the breakfast room?'

But this offer Pru politely declined. In truth, she was too anxious to eat anything until she had seen Garrick for herself.

The duke's bedchamber was much as she had left it last night except for the tell-tale smoky haze hanging in the air where the candles had recently been snuffed out. Stow looked up as she came in and answered her unspoken question.

'He has not stirred, ma'am.'

Stifling her fears, Pru came across to the bed and laid a hand on Garrick's forehead.

'At least there is no fever. Thank you, Mr Stow. I will sit with him now while you get some sleep.'

'Aye, ma'am, thank you. Is there anything I can fetch you?'

'Thank you, no. Mrs Almond is sending up tea and bread and butter for me. And she has agreed to make some lemonade for the duke. She says he was very fond of it as a boy.'

'Aye, he was.'

Her brows rose. 'You knew him then?'

'I did, Miss Clifford. I was footman at Hartland in those days, and training up to serve as valet to the old duke when Sykes, his own man, was growing too old to do everything. Then Lord Garrick, as he was then, went off to France and asked me to go with him, as his valet. We've seen some hard times together, His Grace and me.' A shadow passed over his face and for a moment Pru was afraid he might break down, but he shook it off and gave her a cheerful look. 'But we came through them all and we shall do so again.'

With that he went out and Prudence turned back to the figure lying in the great bed. If it had not been for the steady rise and fall of his chest beneath the snowy nightshirt, she might have thought him lifeless. His face was still badly bruised, but this did not worry her so much as his immobility. She had no idea how deeply unconscious he might be. Despite that, she knew what she must do.

'Good morning, Garrick.' She bent and gently kissed his cheek, feeling the rasp of stubble against her skin.

He did not respond. There was no miraculous recovery, not even the flutter of an eyelid to show he was aware of her.

*Perfectly natural. No need to lose heart yet.*

'I hope you do not mind me making you a little tidier,' she said, gently straightening the bedcovers. 'When Stow returns I shall ask him to shave you, but for now all I can do is to wash your face. Tomorrow, I hope to have a book to read to you. Lord Byron. *The Bride of Abydos*. Do you know it? I believe it is very popular, although I did not come across it until I came to Town this year. I have asked my aunt to send it to me, since I have not had chance to open it. I thought we might read it together—how will that be?'

She chattered on, eliciting no response from Garrick. She expected none, but more than one doctor had told her that patients often reported they had heard what was being said around them when they were unconscious. In Walter's case, sadly, she would never know, but Prudence would not give up hope.

# Chapter Twenty-Four

'Stow!' Prudence looked up in surprise when the bedroom door opened. 'Surely it is not yet time for you to relieve me?'

'No, ma'am, but Lady Borcaster and Mrs Clifford have come to see you. I have put them in the drawing room and asked for refreshments to be sent up.' He coughed. 'I thought you might like to go down immediately, ma'am.'

Pru nodded. She was not surprised to hear they had called, and could imagine their anxiety. She quickly made her way downstairs to the drawing room, pausing to take a deep breath before she opened the door.

She had barely uttered a greeting before Aunt Minerva fell upon her neck.

'Oh, my dear girl, we have been so worried about you!'

'I am very sorry, Aunt, but I thought it better to wait and write this morning, to tell you I was safe. The garbled words that were flowing from my pen in the early hours made no sense at all and would only have added to your fears.'

'But what happened?' demanded Lady Borcaster. 'And why are you now here, in the Duke of Hartland's residence?'

'Will you not sit down?' said Pru, conscious of her duty. 'Perhaps you would like to take a glass of wine?'

'I will do neither,' said Aunt Minerva, wiping her eyes.

'Nor I,' declared Lady Borcaster.

'I see,' said Pru. 'Have you brought the things I asked for in my letter, Aunt?'

'No, my love,' Mrs Clifford replied. 'We have come to take you back to Brook Street.'

'Ah.' Pru tried a smile. 'I'm afraid I cannot come back quite yet.'

Finding two pairs of eyes fixed on her with a mixture of horror and disbelief, she again suggested they should sit down.

'It will take some time to tell you everything,' she added.

Pru described all the events of the previous day, explaining that Sir Joseph and Lady Conyers's actions were the result of an ancient grievance. What that grievance might be she did not say and was grateful that the ladies were too stunned by her tale to enquire deeply.

'Well, well, it is all very shocking,' remarked Mrs Clifford, when Pru had finished. 'But now that His

Grace is back in his own house, my love, there can be no need for you to stay.'

'But there is, Aunt. The duke needs me to nurse him.'

'Nonsense!' declared Lady Borcaster. 'Hartland will have the finest doctors at his disposal. It is quite unnecessary for you to stay. And highly improper, too. Bad enough that you have been here since the early hours, but if you come back with us now, we can—'

Pru interrupted her. 'I beg your pardon, ma'am, but I will not leave the duke. He is unconscious, and I must look after him until I am sure he is recovered. Or...' Her clasped hands tightened until the knuckles glowed white. 'Or not.'

Her Ladyship looked outraged, but Mrs Clifford understood and said, by way of explanation, 'You know, Jane, that Pru's brother, Walter, died after falling from his horse. Pru tended him for several weeks. Until the end.'

'But that was her brother,' snapped my lady. 'Quite understandable that Prudence should nurse *him*. This however...' She began to fan herself vigorously. 'Why, every feeling is offended.'

'I will not leave him,' Pru repeated, stubbornly.

'I understand your concern, my dear,' said Aunt Minerva gently. 'But you must think of your reputation. Hartland has any number of scandals attached to him, to say nothing of this latest charge.'

'But that is now proved to be false, Aunt. The duke is no spy, as everyone will learn very soon.'

'Is that so? Well, well, I am relieved, but that is not all,' replied Mrs Clifford. 'It is common knowledge that he kept poor Miss Speke dangling for ten years and then abandoned her. And now someone has unearthed the rumour that he fought a duel with the husband of his mistress, and then ran off to France leaving his opponent for dead! What will people say when they know you are staying here in his house, unchaperoned?'

Pru shook her head. 'What they say of me is irrelevant. I have more knowledge of head wounds than anyone else in this house. I would never forgive myself if I did not do everything I can to aid the duke's recovery.'

Lady Borcaster gave an impatient huff. 'If you care nothing for your own reputation then pray consider your aunt! Do you not see how she too will be tarnished by this? She will be the object of ridicule and speculation. The best that people will say is she threw you at the duke's head. As for the worst...'

She broke off, spreading her hands in a gesture of despair. Mrs Clifford patted her friend's arm and turned again to Prudence.

'My dear, what do you expect to be the outcome of all this, if the duke recovers? Is there some understanding between you?'

'No, Aunt.'

'Perhaps you think he will offer for you out of gratitude?'

'I hope he will not,' replied Pru. 'I should never allow him to do that.'

'Then come away now, my dear, while it is possible for us to protect your good name.'

'I cannot.' Her fingers writhed together and she struggled to explain herself. 'I am not at liberty to explain everything to you, but the duke does not deserve his reputation. Any of it. The women he has known in his life have all betrayed or abandoned him when he needed them most. I cannot, will not do that. He is lying unconscious now because he was trying to help me and I will stay with him as long as I can be of some use.'

Lady Borcaster shook her head. 'Poor, deluded girl. You would be well served if your aunt disowned you.'

Pru ignored this and fixed her eyes on Mrs Clifford.

'I am aware I am flouting convention and I shall take the consequences. That is my choice, my decision and no blame should fall upon you, Aunt. We are only related by marriage, after all. If you feel you cannot support me in this, then I quite understand.'

'I will not abandon my late husband's niece, how can you think it, Prudence?' Mrs Clifford gave a long sigh. 'Very well, stay here, my love. If Jane will have me, I will remain at Brook Street, but I shall quite understand if that is not possible. I shall find myself a hotel where I may stay until I can carry you away

from town. I very much fear that you will not be able
to take up your life with me in Bath again, but the least
I can do is to see you safely restored to your parents.'

Lady Borcaster had listened closely to this interchange and now she surprised the others by declaring,
'Well, if you are going to show such Christian charity,
Minerva, then it behoves me to show some compas-
sion, too. There is no question but that you will remain
as my guest. We may yet be able to hush up all this.
We will put it about that Miss Clifford has been called
away. That man Stow appeared to be a very sensible
sort and assured us that the duke's household will not
gossip. I believe my own servants can be trusted to
stay silent on the matter, too.'

'Thank you, Lady Borcaster. And thank *you*, best
of my aunts.'

She kissed her aunt's cheek and the two ladies went
away, leaving Pru to consider all that had been said.
Despite the brave words at the end, both her aunt and
Lady Borcaster were convinced that by remaining in
Dover Street to nurse Garrick, her reputation would
be ruined. Sadly, she had to agree.

Prudence went up to her bedchamber. She needed
to rest if she was to nurse Garrick again in the evening and she tried to put the ladies' visit firmly to the
back of her mind. However, despite her exhaustion,
when she lay down on her bed sleep would not come.

She knew that her actions would reflect badly upon

both her aunt and Lady Borcaster if they stood by her, which made her doubly grateful for their support. Yet with that came guilt. It was one thing to risk her own reputation, but should she also risk theirs? But how could she not? Garrick's life was at stake. Yet the doubts persisted.

*You were not able to save your brother...what makes you think you can save the duke?*

Tears welled up and Pru forced them back. She could not be sure what she was doing would be successful, but she knew she must try. Her love for Garrick was so strong now she would do anything she could to help him.

Fatigue finally overcame Pru. She fell into a deep sleep, only waking when Betty came in to rouse her, late in the afternoon. Her trunk had arrived from Brook Street while she was sleeping and she was able to put on a fresh gown before making her way back to Garrick's room at the appointed hour. Stow greeted her with relief.

'His Grace is growing restless, Miss Clifford. I have not seen him like this before.'

'Let us hope it is a good sign.' She laid a hand on the duke's brow. 'He has a slight fever. I will try the lavender water again.'

'Aye, ma'am. If it's all the same to you I won't leave yet,' said Stow. 'He is very strong and you might need me to help you, if he grows too fidgety.'

Pru sat down at the bedside, the bowl of water infused with lavender oil at her elbow. At first she feared Garrick would not respond. He moved his head from side to side as if trying to avoid the damp cloth, but gradually he grew calmer. She thought he had sunk back into unconsciousness when he suddenly reached up and caught her wrist.

'Prudence.'

Her heart leapt, but she replied as calmly as she could, 'I am here, Your Grace.'

She thought her words woefully inadequate but they seemed to calm him. He released her and his hand fell back to his side.

'Well,' breathed Stow, standing beside her. 'That surely indicates an improvement, doesn't it, ma'am?'

'I hope so, Mr Stow.' Trying not to tremble, she wrung out the cloth again and applied it gently to Garrick's brow. 'I hope so.'

The remainder of Pru's vigil was uneventful but Garrick's speaking her name was heartening. When Stow returned at midnight she did not want to leave. She wanted to stay with Garrick, to be at his side if he should wake again, but she knew that was foolish. Stow was perfectly capable of keeping watch and she needed to be fresh and alert to relieve him again in the morning.

When Pru returned to the sickroom soon after dawn, Stow informed her that Garrick had shown no signs of waking again during the night. She was disappointed, but summoned a smile and agreed that the duke looked better now he had been shaved and dressed in a clean nightshirt. Stow went off to seek his bed and Pru settled down to while away the morning with her embroidery.

By ten o'clock her spirits had not improved. Garrick remained unresponsive to her occasional remarks, although she had managed to coax a few drops of lemonade between his lips. Sighing, she picked up the book she had brought in with her.

'I have the Byron to read to you, if you wish.'

No answer, but what had she expected? She opened the book at the title page.

'"*The Bride of Abydos. A Turkish Tale.*"' Her eyes moved down to four lines of a poem. 'It begins with a quote from Robert Burns... "*Had we never loved so kindly, Had we never loved so blindly, Never met or never parted, We had ne'er been broken-hearted.*"'

Her voice cracked on the final line and she put the book aside. It summed up how she felt today. Broken-hearted. Pru gave a sob and put her hands over her face.

'Oh, Garrick, please don't die,' she whispered. 'Please don't leave me in this world without you.'

Hot, silent tears ran through her fingers and she dashed them away, appalled at her own weakness. She quickly searched for her handkerchief to dry her cheeks.

'I beg your pardon,' she said to the motionless figure in the bed. 'I must be very tired. I am not normally
such a watering pot.'

Calming herself with a deep breath, she picked
up the book again and turned the pages until she arrived at the first canto. Then she cleared her throat
and began to read.

Pru was halfway through the second canto when
she heard the door open. Thinking it was Stow, she
carried on to the end of the stanza before looking up.

'Oh!' She almost dropped the book when she saw
the lady in the doorway. A tall, upright figure dressed
in black. She addressed Prudence in arctic tones.

'What in heaven's name are you doing with my son?'

Garrick's mother! Pru rose and curtsied.

'I am reading to him, Your Grace.'

She watched the duchess move closer to the bed.
Pru thought she must have been handsome once, but
her face was now pale and drawn, and the dark hair
beneath the black lace cap heavily streaked with grey.

'But he is unconscious. What good will that do?'

Pru tried not to feel angry at the duchess's cold tone.
She had not seen her son for ten years. Perhaps she
was shocked by his appearance now.

'One never knows if someone in this state can hear
anything, Your Grace,' she said calmly. 'But surely it
is better to try than not.'

The duchess turned and Pru found herself staring

into a pair of green eyes, so like Garrick's that she felt the breath catch in her throat.

'And what right have you to nurse him?'

Pru's chin went up. 'I have some experience of caring for persons with head injuries. My name is Prudence Clifford—'

'I know who you are.' The duchess cut her off. 'Stow has told me how you come to be here.'

'Nothing that has happened reflects badly upon the duke.' Pru was quick to assure her. 'Quite the opposite, in fact. He was being...recklessly brave.'

'I have never doubted his courage. Only his wisdom.'

The duchess stared down at Garrick, her countenance impassive.

Pru said quietly, 'Mr Stow and I share the task of keeping vigil at his bedside. He might wake at any time.'

'And he might not,' retorted the duchess. 'Stow told me the doctor was not encouraging.'

'He was afraid of raising false hopes.'

'And how long do you intend to carry on this vigil?'

'I shall stay as long as it is necessary, Your Grace.'

'What of your family? Do they support you in this?'

Pru hesitated. 'They do not, ma'am. However, I am of age and they cannot compel me to leave here.'

*But you could, Your Grace.*

She waited, wondering if the duchess would order

her to leave. After a long, nerve-racking silence, the older woman nodded. She looked around the room.

'Is that for my son?' she asked, indicating the tray bearing an empty cup and a plate of bread and butter.

'No, Your Grace. It was brought up for me to break my fast.'

'You did not want it?'

'I drank the coffee.'

Pru noted the duchess's frown and added quickly, 'Cook sends up nourishing broth for the duke. Stow tells me His Grace managed to swallow a little, to-night. We also keep lemonade and barley water for him, over there, on the side table. Stow and I administer a little every hour or so.' She added simply, 'It gives us hope.'

'Hope!'

The duchess looked unconvinced. She came back towards the bed and stared down at her son. It was impossible to read her countenance, but Pru did not think her uncaring. She suspected Garrick's mother did not like to display her emotions before a stranger. Finally, after another long silence, the duchess went out. With a sigh Pru sank down onto the chair and closed her eyes.

At noon, Stow came in to relieve her.

'Have you seen the duchess?' Pru asked him. 'Has she spoken to you about me?'

'Yes, ma'am, she has.'

'And...does she want me to leave?'

'Why no. Her Grace has requested your company at dinner.'

'Oh. I had not expected that! I would rather not...'

Stow coughed. 'If you will forgive my saying so, ma'am, I do not think it would be wise to refuse.'

'But I have to come back here at six o'clock this evening.' Pru was flustered. 'You cannot be expected to do it.'

'We can easily rearrange things, ma'am. Mrs Almond has said she will sit with His Grace while you are engaged this evening. She can summon me if needs be.'

'Very well.' There really was no choice. Pru realised the request from the duchess was in fact a summons. 'Perhaps you would help me turn the pillows before I go? I think it will make him more comfortable.'

The task was soon accomplished, but still she lingered, reluctant to leave.

'You should rest, ma'am.' Stow prompted her gently. 'You will need all your wits about you to dine with the duchess.'

'Yes. Yes of course.'

## Chapter Twenty-Five

At the appointed time, Prudence was shown into the dining room, where she found the duchess already at the table.

'Forgive me if we do not observe the niceties of gathering in the drawing room beforehand,' she remarked as Prudence sat down to face her at the only other place laid at the table. 'I realise your free time is limited. I understand you mean to return to the sickroom after dinner.'

Prudence inclined her head, relaxing slightly. It appeared the duchess had accepted her presence in the house.

'That is my intention, Your Grace.'

'Very well. However, I insist upon you dining with me each evening.'

'Oh, but I cannot—'

She was interrupted.

'Stow tells me you only pick at the food sent up to you. You cannot nurse my son properly if you do not eat.'

Pru felt a smile tugging at the corners of her mouth and accepted defeat.

'You are quite right, ma'am.'

The meal proceeded. Prudence was subjected to what amounted to an interrogation by her hostess. She answered questions about her family, her friends and her visit to London patiently and truthfully, but she found it most dispiriting. Almost every sentence she uttered emphasised the difference between her own world and that of the Duke of Hartland.

Not that it mattered, she told herself as the covers were finally removed and dishes of sweetmeats placed on the table between them. Her only purpose was to convince the duchess that she was a fit and proper person to nurse Garrick back to health.

She braced herself for more questions as the duchess dismissed the servants.

'Stow tells me this is not the first time you have come to my son's aid.'

'No, ma'am.'

'Since the duke is clearly not able to tell me what is going on, I should be obliged if you would do so.'

Pru countered with a question of her own.

'May I ask first, why Your Grace is in town?'

In the brief pause their eyes met across the table. Pru had the distinct feeling she was being judged. She kept her gaze steady and at last the duchess nodded, apparently satisfied.

'I heard that my son is accused of treason. You look surprised, Miss Clifford. I may live retired in Devon, but I have friends here who keep me apprised of current gossip.'

'You may also know, then, of the other accusations that are levelled at the duke.'

'That he rejected the lady who has waited faithfully for him for the past ten years? That does not surprise me. His profligate ways have long been a source of dismay to me.'

'I do not believe he *is* profligate,' replied Prudence, surprised at her own daring.

'You presume to know him better than his own mother?'

'I know him to be a kind, brave and honourable man.'

'Do you indeed? Then you interest me, Miss Clifford. Pray explain yourself.'

'He has told me something of his earlier life.' How much should she say? 'His unfortunate *affaire* with a married lady—'

'Helene Conyers. Yes, I know of that!' The duchess interrupted her. 'If we are to discuss these matters then we should speak plainly, so there can be no misunderstanding.'

'Very well, ma'am. Lady Conyers seduced your son, as she had done with several young men before and still does. Her husband then gave Garrick the choice of paying a substantial sum to keep the affair from his family or facing him in a duel.'

'My son confided all that to you?'

The duchess looked shocked, but she had asked for plain speaking and Pru was not going to avoid it.

'Yes, although he was rather drunk at the time. I believed him then, and having since met Sir Joseph and his wife, I see no reason to doubt it is the truth.' She looked across the table at the duchess. 'Your son chose honour over extortion.'

'And was obliged to fly the country!'

'He told me he did not expect to hit his man. He believed *he* would be the one to perish.'

'Do you think his death would have been more acceptable to me?' exclaimed the duchess, high spots of colour appearing on her wan cheeks.

Prudence said gently, 'No, ma'am, but can you deny that he was reared to think the honour of the family of more importance than his life?'

She wondered if she had gone too far. The duchess reached towards the dish of sugared almonds then thought better of it and picked up her wine instead.

'You are quite right,' she said at last. 'Garrick has as much of the Chauntry Pride as any of his forebears. I can quite believe he risked his life to uphold the family honour. He broke his father's heart. And now he is going to break mine.'

Her voice shook. She dabbed at her mouth with her

napkin and Pru felt a rush of sympathy for the old woman.

'He is not going to die, Your Grace, I will not let him.' Pru pushed back her chair. 'Now if you will excuse me, I had best return to my patient.'

Silence had fallen over the house. Pru heard the hall clock chiming the hours as she sat beside Garrick's bed. She had tried reading to him, but her mind was too distracted by her conversation with the duchess.

She had said she would not let him die and at that moment she had meant it, but now, sitting in the lofty, silent room, her conviction wavered. She could not see into the future. She did not know what state of mind Garrick would be in when he recovered. She could not even be sure that he *would* recover. But she must not think of that.

The eminent physician Sir Henry Halford arrived the following morning, summoned by the duchess, but his assessment was little different to that of Garrick's own doctor. There was nothing more to be done at present, and he could not fault the care the duke was receiving.

The days took on a familiar pattern. Stow and Prudence continued their vigil, both determined that one or the other of them would be on hand, should Garrick regain consciousness. Other members of his household were brought in when he needed to be moved while his bedding and nightshirt were replaced. Stow shaved his master at regular intervals, maintaining that the duke would not wish for anyone to see him looking less than his best.

'Especially now he is receiving visitors,' he added with a twinkle.

The only visitor was in fact Lord John, who called each day and stayed an hour talking with Garrick.

The duchess did not appear in the sickroom again, which saddened Pru until it occurred to her that the older lady might not be able to endure the sight of her only son lying still and unresponsive. Heaven knew it was hard enough for Pru! When they met at dinner each evening, she made sure she reported the duke's progress, or lack of it. Society manners prevailed in the dining room and, although their conversation was stilted at first, it gradually became easier. Pru grew more accustomed to her hostess's abrupt manner and was not afraid to disagree when she thought it necessary.

The duchess might not be pleased with her candid replies, but Pru saw no reason to dissemble. She was not trying to impress the older woman and there was no doubt it enlivened their discussions. Afterwards she would retire to her room, exhausted but well-fed, and sleep until she was roused in the early hours to sit with Garrick.

With a good meal each evening, Pru's energy and her spirits improved, although she still found the night-time vigil the most difficult. She stretched out on the daybed beneath the window, resting but alert for the slightest sound from Garrick. During the day she read to him, fed him with broth and teased drops of lemonade or barley water between his lips. She took courage from the fact that each day the bruises on his face were fading. He was looking better, but still he did not wake.

It was six o'clock on Monday morning and the household was already stirring when Prudence left the sickroom and returned to her bedchamber. In her pocket was the letter that had arrived late the night before and she had scanned it briefly, while sitting with Garrick.

Its contents had distressed her, but she had quickly hidden her anguish while she had tended Garrick. Now, however, in the privacy of her own room, she knew she must read it again.

It was from her Aunt Minerva, and after a brief hope that the duke was recovering she launched into the real reason for writing. The scandal had broken.

Heaven knows Lady B and I have not mentioned the matter to a soul, merely saying you were away on family business, but somehow word has got out that you are installed in Dover Street! It was the only subject on everyone's lips after morning service today, although no one was bold enough to quiz me directly about it.

*The stories are wild and varied. Everything from the duke abducting you to be his mistress, to your being his nurse after he was fatally wounded in a duel and not expected to live.*

*My dear Prudence, I fear it is too late now to save your good name. All I can do is beg you to let me know as soon as you mean to quit Dover Street and I shall call for you. If I do not hear from you then I shall remain in London until the end of August, as planned.*

*Lady B is very good and insists I continue to live here as her guest. She still goes out into society, but I have quite given it up. Dear Jane is, of course, a diplomat's widow. She is accustomed to saying nothing and depressing pretension with a stare, but I cannot bear the sly looks and innuendo, for which I have no reply!*

If you are still needed in Dover Street when I leave London, then you must come to me at Bath as soon as you can. Even if everyone there knows the scandal, I shall not desert you. From there we can write to your parents and arrange for you to go back to Melksham until this sorry business is forgotten…

There was more of the same. When she had first read it, Pru had shed tears for the hurt and disgrace she had brought upon her family. Word of the scandal could not yet have reached Dover Street, because the duchess had not mentioned it at dinner, and Pru was convinced she would not keep her thoughts on the subject a secret.

Pru was determined nothing should hinder a reconciliation between Garrick and his mother, but that could not happen until he regained consciousness. She could only pray she would be allowed to stay and nurse him until then.

Sleep was impossible, knowing that at any moment she might be summoned by an outraged duchess and thrown onto the street, and Pru merely dozed away the morning. However, by noon no such catastrophe had occurred and she took her place at Garrick's bedside. Stow went off after reporting that the duke had passed a peaceful night, which meant he had not stirred, there had been no sign of waking. And yet he breathed. She clung onto that one, fragile thread of hope.

Prudence sat down beside the bed. Her eyes were gritty from lack of sleep. She felt too tired to read and decided she would just sit there and keep watch. She reached out and took Garrick's hand—it was warm but unresponsive. Through the open window she could hear the traffic, the sounds of carriages rattling by, hawkers crying their wares, but in the room itself there was silence. Pru leaned forward and rested her cheek against Garrick's hand and closed her eyes.

'Pru.'

She heard him calling to her, very softly, and raised her head. He smiled, his green eyes warm with love.

'Come and lie with me.'

She walked around to the empty side of the bed and climbed in, measuring her length against him, sighing at the comfort it gave her just to be close to him.

'Darling Pru.'

He turned, folding her in his arms, kissing away all the pain and unhappiness. Desire stirred and her body came alive as his hands roamed over her breasts. They were both naked now, their skin touching, legs tangling. She moaned softly, her body aching with longing for him to hold her closer and feed the desire rippling through her.

A sudden crash and raised voices from the street jerked Pru to consciousness and her eyes flew open. She was still sitting beside Garrick's bed, still holding his hand and he was lying perfectly still, eyes closed. Dear heaven, it had all been a dream!

Yet her body was on fire for him. One night. One night she had spent in his bed and the memory was so strong it had infused her very bones! Tears of anguish and frustration welled up and Pru was obliged to blink them away. She went over to the wash stand and bathed her face. Was this what it would be like once she had left Dover Street? Would Garrick haunt her dreams as well as her waking hours?

*I shall manage. I can live without him. Only please, please, let him recover!*

She turned quickly as the bedroom door opened and the housekeeper bustled in.

'Well, ma'am, I beg your pardon for being so late with your refreshments today. The brewer's dray collided with a milk cart directly outside the door and the kitchen maid was too busy a-gawping at the mess to notice that the kettle had boiled dry. What a to-do! I hope the noise didn't disturb you or the master?'

'No.'

That must have been the crash that woke her. Pru looked at the motionless figure in the bed and her throat constricted.

'No,' she repeated. 'It did not disturb His Grace.'

## Chapter Twenty-Six

By the time she had drunk a cup of tea and fed Garrick a few spoonsful of broth Prudence was once more in command of herself. Whatever the future held for her she would face it. If she could not return to Bath to live with Aunt Minerva then she would go back to Melksham and make a life for herself there with her parents. But for now, she must work at making Garrick well. She would read to him.

She had finished almost all of the books Lord John had procured for her. Having read several of Lord Byron's works and a rather improving tale by Maria Edgeworth she decided upon a three-volume novel handsomely bound in red leather.

'It is called *Pride and Prejudice*,' she told Garrick, keeping her tone cheerful. 'I think you were looking at it in Hatchards when I met you there with Lord John. Do you remember?'

She recalled that day only too well. How angry he had been with her and Jack for interfering. How she had found him later, beaten and bloodied. Pru quickly shook off that memory. She would not give in to any more melancholy thoughts today.

'I have heard good reports about this,' she went on. 'I hope we will enjoy it, Your Grace.'

It proved a good choice. The lively style and engaging character gripped Pru from the start. An hour flew by before she stopped and begged his pardon.

'My throat is too parched to carry on,' she told him, getting up and going across to the side table. 'The teapot is cold now...do you mind if I pour myself a glass of the barley water Mrs Almond brought up for you?' It had become second nature to carry on a one-sided conversation and she continued once she had filled a glass and taken a sip.

'Mmm,' she said, turning back. 'It is very good. I must ask her for the...'

The words died on her lips. Garrick's eyes were open and fixed upon her.

'Good day, Your Grace.'

Pru's cautious greeting was very much at odds with the ferocious pounding of her heart. She had longed for this moment, prayed for it, but now she did not know quite what to do. Garrick's eyes followed her as she started back across the room towards him.

'Pru.'

Her name. He murmured just the one word but it was her name! Relief and happiness flooded through

her. It was a good start, but she must not be too com-
placent. She hurried over and took his hand.

'Yes, I am here.' His eyelids drooped and she felt
a moment's panic. 'No, no, do not go back to sleep!'

She saw him frown a little, and although he did
not open his eyes again, she felt the pressure as he
squeezed her hand.

Over the next few days Garrick showed more signs
of recovery. He was awake for longer periods and even
managed to eat some of the succulent delicacies con-
cocted by his chef to tempt his appetite. Between them,
Stow and Pru watched him constantly, heartened by
Sir Henry Halford's assurances that the patient was on
the mend, even though he was dazed and confused,
and only spoke the odd word.

Pru continued to read to him. The lively tale was
so engrossing that at times she was even able to forget
the weight of anxiety pressing down upon her spirits.
She was halfway through the third volume, a few days
after that first waking, when she looked up to find
Garrick watching her.

Her heart leapt. Surely his eyes looked more alert
this time.

She smiled. 'Are you thirsty?'

A slight nod. She picked up the glass of lemonade
at the bedside and held it to his lips.

'Thank you.'

His voice was stronger, she thought, although as she

turned away to put down the glass, she cautioned herself not to be too hopeful. Experience had taught her that indulging in fanciful imaginings only led to more pain. However, when she turned back, Garrick was holding out his hand and a surge of emotion rocked her. She could no longer deny the overwhelming love she felt for this man, nor the relief that he was awake and recovering.

She took his hand, saying as calmly as she could, 'What is it, Garrick, what can I do for you?'

His eyes closed and all her fears came rushing back. She watched anxiously, desperate to stop him slipping away again.

'Would you like to talk, Your Grace?'

'No,' he murmured. 'Read to me. I am enjoying it.'

'There.' Prudence closed the book. 'That is enough for today. We have only a few chapters left and we shall keep them for tomorrow.'

He had not opened his eyes since she had started reading and she thought he was sleeping. It was something of a shock when he spoke to her.

'What happened to me? How did I get here?'

'You passed out in Lady Conyers's carriage.' She wanted to touch him, to pick up his hand and press her lips against it, or to gently caress his cheek, but it would not do. She was his nurse, not his lover. Instead, she straightened the sheet covering his chest. 'Do you not remember?'

'No.'

'No matter. That is often the case, I believe.' She studied his dear face, noting the faint crease in his brow. 'Shall I fetch Stow? He will be delighted to know you are awake—'

'No.' He reached out and caught her fingers. 'Not yet. What day is it?'

'Thursday, your Grace. You have been here for ten days.'

'And you were here all that time. Nursing me.'

'Yes.'

*Nursing you, loving you, knowing our worlds are so far apart that this is all the time we can ever have together.*

He was silent, but she thought he looked content and she was happy to sit down again, her hand snugly in his, storing up the memory for the dark, lonely days that stretched ahead of her.

The arrival of the duchess with her entourage had brought home to Pru the hopelessness of her situation. Garrick was a duke. His mother wanted a reconciliation and she would expect him to marry a lady of equal status, not an inconsequential spinster from Bath. Pru had no grand relations and no vast fortune to enhance the ducal coffers. If he had loved her, perhaps these things might not have mattered, but he did not. He liked her and he had taken her to his bed. He had even proposed to her, but that had been out of a sense of duty.

She hoped he was no longer in love with Helene Conyers, but there were other beautiful women in his world, women far more suitable to be his duchess than dull, plain Prudence Clifford.

The duke continued to be wakeful for the rest of the day and the following morning he insisted Stow should help him into a chair. He felt as weak as a cat and his mind was still fogged, but memories were returning. Stow fussed about him like a mother hen, banning all visitors except the duchess until Sir Henry had examined his patient and given his approval.

Garrick submitted meekly to everything, including the visit from his mother, who insisted on coming to see him shortly before the dinner hour. The meeting lasted only a few minutes, but it exhausted him. Not that they spoke much, mere platitudes, but there was true warmth in her eyes and she gripped his shoulder before leaving him and her touch conveyed a great deal. They both knew there was much to be discussed, but that could wait until he was stronger.

He felt too weak to argue with his man, except on one point. When Stow suggested that Miss Clifford should return to Brook Street he refused to allow it. He persuaded Sir Henry to support him, when the physician called to see him later the same day, and that brought an indignant Pru into his room within minutes of Sir Henry's departure.

He was at least sitting upright in a chair, but his

weakness frustrated Garrick. He managed a smile and waved a hand towards the garish banyan he was wearing.

'Forgive my informal dress, ma'am, and the fact that I am unable to rise to greet you.'

'It is time I went back to my aunt,' she said, ignoring his attempts at gallantry. 'I am no longer needed here.'

'You are wrong. *I* need you.' He smiled. 'Sir Henry agrees with me.'

'He does not. I asked Stow to tell me *exactly* what was said,' she retorted. 'Sir Henry advised that you were not to be upset.'

'Yes. It will upset me if you go now.'

'Nonsense. You have plenty of people to wait upon you.'

'But you have proved yourself a fine nurse.'

A becoming flush mantled her cheeks, but she shook her head.

'It is no longer necessary for you to have someone with you at all times. Mr Stow is quite capable of looking after you now. He is going to sleep in your dressing room, in case you wake during the night.'

His eyes searched her face. He said bluntly, 'Has my mother suggested you leave?'

'No. The duchess has been…most gracious to me.'

'I am glad of it. She can be rather outspoken.'

'I know it. I am only surprised she—' Pru stopped, giving her head a little shake before returning to her reason for being there. 'Sir Henry says you are recovering well. You no longer need me to nurse you, Your Grace. My work in the sickroom is done.'

He frowned. 'Is that all I ever was to you, a patient, someone to be nursed back to health?'

'Why, of course,' she said brightly. Too brightly in Garrick's opinion. 'Now I can go back to my life's work of helping the poor.'

She met his eyes; her gaze was steady, determined. Something was not right, although Garrick could not work out what it was. He must keep her at Dover Street a little longer. Until his faculties had recovered sufficiently for him to break through the barrier she had erected around herself.

'Give me your word you will not leave without telling me.'

'I must go today.'

'No! Damnation, you cannot go before I am on my feet again!'

Pru's heart ached for him. He looked so vulnerable, the black hair falling over his brow, his face still showing grey traces of the fading bruises. She wanted to stay with him. Not just until he was on his feet again but for ever. But it was impossible. Her reputation was already tarnished, it would be ruined completely if she remained in Dover Street. Garrick was still weak, but once he was stronger, he might want her for his mistress and she did not trust herself not to fall into his arms. To give herself up to the passions that she knew would be far stronger than her resolve.

The duchess never mentioned it, but she must know how Pru felt. Only last night Her Grace had talked about Hartland, which she had now vacated, having moved to the nearby Dower House. It was clear she expected the duke to marry soon and live at Hartland with his bride.

Pru guessed it was the duchess's way of warning her off. Quite rightly. Much better that she left him now.

'Excuse me,' she said at last, knowing she would not hold out if he continued to question her. 'I have arrangements to make. My aunt is anxious to return to Bath and I have to admit, I am, too. I miss my friends, and especially my work at the infirmary!'

It was not quite a lie. It might not be possible for her to remain in Bath but she could carry on her charity work in Melksham. The poor would always need her.

'No, stay.' Garrick's hands were gripping the arms of the chair. 'Stay and marry me.'

# Chapter Twenty-Seven

Garrick held his breath. He had not wanted to utter those words until he was well again. Until his mind was sharp enough to refute any arguments she might come up with and he was physically strong enough to protect her from the world.

Pru was staring at him, horrified.

'I beg your pardon,' he said now. 'That was not right. What I mean is—' he put up a hand, raking back his hair. 'Pru—'

'I know exactly what you mean, Your Grace.' She was very pale, but she was calm enough, and at least she was smiling at him. 'This is not the time to discuss such matters. You need to rest.'

His mouth twisted. 'I have been *resting* for the past ten days!'

'Sir Henry said you must not overtire yourself.'

'I know, but.' He reached out to her. 'Pru, at least consider my offer.'

She came over and took his hand. 'I promise you I shall.'

She bent and placed a gentle kiss on his brow before turning and walking away.

It took an enormous effort but Pru managed to keep up the pretence until she had closed the door behind her. Then her smile disappeared. She felt quite sick. Jack Callater was coming up the stairs and she greeted him with relief.

'Lord John, the very person.'

'Good day to you, Miss Clifford. Stow had told me I may see the duke today.' He grinned at her. 'Veritable guard dog, ain't he? But what's this?' He looked at her more closely. 'Something has upset you. Has Garr taken a turn for the worse?'

'No, no, nothing like that. He goes on very well, but I would like a word with you, if you could spare me five minutes?'

'Yes, yes of course, ma'am.'

He followed her into the morning room and she invited him to sit down.

'I will, of course, but not if you are going to pace the floor,' he retorted. He took her hands and drew her down onto a sofa. 'We are good friends now, Pru, are we not? Tell me what is troubling you.'

'I...' Another steadying breath was required. 'I understand from my aunt that everyone knows I am living here.'

'Ah.'

Her throat felt constricted and she swallowed painfully. 'It is true, then. I am ruined.'

'No such thing,' he said stoutly. 'There has been the odd comment, but the official story is still that you have gone out of town. No one of any consequence has admitted to anything different.'

'I have not left the house since I arrived here with the duke,' she said, slowly. 'But surely, if there is gossip, everyone in the household must *know*?'

'One would have thought so, yes. Except Garrick, of course.'

'I agree. Stow would not have mentioned it to him. But would the duchess be aware of it?'

He frowned. 'I cannot believe she does not.'

'Then why has she not said anything? Why has she not ejected me?'

'Possibly because she will do nothing to jeopardise Garr's recovery. The duchess loves him dearly, you know, although she would never say so. I think she now regrets keeping him away for all those years.'

'I am glad they have found each other again. I would not for the world have anything come between them.' Pru was silent for a while, then she smiled. 'Thank you, Lord John.'

'For what? I have done nothing.'

She fluttered one hand and shook her head, as if it was no matter. 'You should go to the duke now. No doubt you have news for him, about the Conyerses?'

'Aye. The home secretary now has them both

clapped up. As if perverting justice was not enough, Stow and I also made sure they were accused of your abduction. I have taken the liberty of engaging a lawyer for you. He will need to speak with you soon.'

'Thank you.' Pru nodded, but did not linger on the subject. She would deal with that matter at a later date. 'Go and talk with the duke, my lord. You will see for yourself that he is very much recovered. He no longer needs constant nursing, whatever Sir Henry Halford might say. Perhaps you would be good enough to persuade him of that.'

'I shall do nothing of the sort. I certainly cannot go against his physician.' Jack rose and stood, feeding the brim of his hat between his fingers. 'Garrick owes you a great deal, Pru. We both do, and—'

'Then you will repay me by saying nothing of this conversation to the duke.' She crossed to the door with him. 'Look after Garrick, Lord John.'

With that she slipped away to her room.

Garrick did not return to his bed until it was dark, when he fell into a deep sleep from which he did not wake until sunlight was filling the room the next morning. Who would have thought sitting in a chair could be so exhausting? However, for the first time since he had collapsed he felt hungry and was glad when Stow came in with his breakfast.

After that he submitted to being shaved and only

when Stow had finished did he ask the question that had been on his mind all morning.

'Where is Miss Clifford?'

'I have not seen the young lady, Your Grace. If you remember, we decided last night that it was not necessary for anyone to sit with you during the night hours, now I am sleeping in your dressing room.'

'*You* decided that! But—' A knock at the door made him sit up eagerly. It was only a servant, announcing that Sir Henry Halford had arrived. 'Show him up.'

Garrick eased himself back in his chair. There was no time now to talk to Pru before he had seen the physician.

'Garr? Can I come in? I met Halford on the stairs and he said you were well enough to see me.'

Garrick opened his eyes. Jack Callater stood in the doorway, looking uncertainly across the room at him.

'Aye, Jack come in. I am feeling much better today and Sir Henry says I should begin taking a little exercise.'

Perhaps he would ask Pru to come for a drive with him in the park. The fresh air would do them both good.

'Excellent,' said Jack. 'We will soon have you back on your feet. And you will want to know what is happening with Conyers…'

Garrick listened, but he took little interest now he knew that Sir Joseph and Helene were no longer a threat. He had not seen Prudence this morning and his head was full of her. She thought she could fool him with her talk of charitable deeds, but he knew she cared for him, far more than she was admitting. He remembered her voice, when she had been sitting at his bedside. Not just reading to him. He had heard her weeping, begging him not to leave her. She had held his hand, too. Pressed her soft cheek against it...

He shifted restlessly in his chair.

'I am sorry to cut you off, Jack, but I need to see Pru. Now. Would you send for her?'

'Why of course, I'll go and find her.' He lounged out and Garrick waited impatiently. Something was nagging at his mind and he knew he would not be content until he had spoken her.

At last Jack returned, but one look at his face told Garrick something was wrong.

'She is gone.' Jack closed the door carefully behind him. 'She left while Sir Henry was here. Said she did not want you to be disturbed.'

'The devil!' Garrick pushed himself to his feet, swaying unsteadily and Jack quickly took his arm.

'Sit down, you fool, you are in no state to go after her.'

'But I must. I have to tell her.' He rubbed his temples. 'I made a mull of it, Jack. Yesterday. I asked her to marry me.'

'The devil you did.' Jack looked closely at him. 'Was that before my visit?'

'Aye. She was talking of leaving and I... Hell and confound it!' He looked up. 'Did you see her, Jack, did she say anything to you?' He frowned when he saw the consternation in his friend's face. 'Out with it, man!'

'She asked me about the rumours.'

'Rumours?

'Damn it all, Garr. She has been here all this time, nursing you. Tongues were bound to wag.'

'But that won't matter once it is known we are to be married.'

'I think it matters to Pru.'

'What do you mean?

Jack paused. Garrick could see he was choosing his words carefully. At last he said, 'I think Pru believes she is not worthy of you.'

'Nonsense!'

'Perhaps she thinks your mother would object to the union.'

Garrick waved a dismissive hand. 'And what if she does?'

'Something Pru said to me yesterday. About not allowing anything to come between you and the duchess.'

'Did I hear my name?

Both men looked up.

'Mama! Pru has gone,' Garrick barked out the words, trying to stay calm. 'Did you know of this?

'No, but it does not surprise me.' She held out a

letter. 'Mrs Almond found this in her room. It is addressed to you.'

Garrick snatched the paper and unfolded it, frowning over the script.

'She says she is gone back to Bath today, with her aunt. I am not to worry about her.' Muttering, he threw down the paper. 'How can I not worry? I must go after her!'

'Do not be so foolish, my son.'

'Is it true, then?' He glared at the duchess. 'You knew of the rumours about Prudence?'

'I had heard them, yes.'

'Of course.' He slumped back in his chair. 'She was already here when you arrived, was she not? She saved my life, but you have decided she is not the wife for me.'

'On the contrary,' retorted Her Grace. 'I think she is the *only* wife for you!'

# Chapter Twenty-Eight

September had started with rain and it threatened to continue. Pru gazed out of the window and thought there was no place as depressing as Bath in wet weather.

She had been in Kilve Street for almost two weeks and would be here for some time yet. Her youngest sister, Jemima, was to be married at the end of the month and Pru had decided to postpone her return to Melksham. The presence of a prodigal daughter would cast a shadow over the nuptials and she had already caused enough upset to her family.

With a sigh she turned away from the window and went back to the little writing desk, where she was trying to compose a letter for Mama. She had been putting it off, but she needed to write now, as a matter of urgency, to explain why she would not be attending Jemima's wedding. Aunt Minerva was sure the gossip would not penetrate deepest Wiltshire, but Pru could not be so sanguine.

There was already speculation in Bath as to why

Mrs Clifford and her niece had returned from London
two weeks early. Soon other residents would be returning to Bath for the winter and some of them were
bound to know the scandal surrounding Miss Prudence Clifford. Then there were the wedding guests.
At least some of them would be from London. It could
only be a matter of time before the rumours reached
Melksham. Pru had made up her mind to write and
tell her parents everything. They deserved to know
the truth, however painful.

Her dismal thoughts were interrupted by the thud
of the street door, then voices in the hall and a light
step on the stairs. Moments later Aunt Minerva came
into the room.

'My dear, how wise you were not to come to Milsom Street with me this morning. The rain was tor-
rential and my dress is quite *sodden*! I am going up
and change immediately, but a runner arrived with a
note, just as I was giving my hat and pelisse to Norris,
and I thought I would bring it up to you on my way.'

Pru took the sealed letter and stared at the unfamiliar handwriting.

'Who is it from, dear?' asked Minerva, pulling the
muddy hem of her skirts away from her ankles.

'I do not know…oh!' Pru put a hand up to her cheek.
'It is f-from the Duchess of Hartland.'

Minerva gave a little shriek and ran over, her wet
clothes forgotten. 'Let me see!'

'She is in Bath,' said Pru, handing her the letter.

'At York House.' Minerva nodded. 'And she has invited you to call. Today.'

'I cannot go!'

'You must,' replied her aunt. 'She is sending her carriage for you at four o'clock. Goodness me, that is only an hour!'

'Oh, heavens!' Pru jumped up and began to pace back and forth across the carpet. 'What can she want with me? Why will she not leave me in peace! I am sure I did not come away with anything inadvertently packed in my bags. I distinctly remember giving back the shift I borrowed from Mrs Almond!'

'My dear, I really do not think the duchess would be interested in that,' replied Mrs Clifford, regarding her with fond amusement. 'If she suspected you of stealing I am sure she would have engaged the runners to come after you.'

'Then what can it be?' Pru put both hands to her cheeks. 'Unless the duke has taken a turn for the worse.'

'Now stop that. You are working yourself up quite unnecessarily. You will only find out what Her Grace wants by going to York House, so you had best get ready.' She shepherded Pru out of the room, saying, 'What a pity you did not engage Meg as your dresser after all.'

'How could I, when I was leaving town in disgrace? It would hardly help the poor girl's prospects.'

'Well, no matter. Norris will have to look after you and I shall make do with the housemaid's services. I suggest you wear the new pelisse you bought from Mrs Bell. You wore it but once in London, the weather being so warm, but it makes you look quite dashing.'

'I do not want to look dashing.'

'Nonsense! If you are visiting a duchess, you want to look your best. And do not look so frightened, she cannot eat you. Now come along and get changed.'

When the duchess's carriage arrived in Kilve Street, Pru was ready in her new and fashionable Pomona green pelisse with the matching bonnet. The journey to York House was not long enough to calm her nerves and her knees felt dangerously weak as she followed a liveried servant up the stairs.

She was shown into an elegant sitting room where a small fire burned in the hearth. Not that the heat was needed, but it did add some cheer to the dismally wet day. The duchess, however, looked as cold and stern as ever.

'Thank you for coming, Miss Clifford. Please sit down.'

Pru obeyed, resisting the urge to perch on the edge of the chair, but she sat up very straight as she faced her hostess.

'You left London before we had an opportunity to talk,' remarked the duchess. 'Why was that? And pray do not give me any of the nonsense you gave my son about wishing to return to your charity work in Bath.'

'I was no longer of use in the sickroom. I thought it

best to leave before—' she drew in a breath '—before I was asked to do so.'

'You thought that a possibility?'

'Yes.' Pru looked down and smoothed a crease from her skirts. 'Perhaps Your Grace is not aware of the gossip.'

'Of course I am aware of it,' snapped the duchess. 'Good heavens, girl, I am not in my dotage yet! I believe Garrick offered to give you the protection of his name.'

'He did, and I was very grateful for the offer, but—'

'But you could not bring yourself to accept a man with such a tarnished reputation, even to save your own.'

'No!' Pru looked up, shocked. 'That is not it at all.'

'Then tell me, truthfully, why you ran away, when you are clearly in love with him?'

Pru blushed. Was it so very obvious? She bit her lip. 'I am not of his world.'

'And yet you do love him.'

'Yes.' Pru did not hesitate.

'But not enough to fight for him.'

'I did not want to cause another rift between you.'

'Hmmph.' The duchess cast her eyes to the ceiling. 'I have no patience with you young people! In my day a duke would have carried you off and married you out of hand, none of this shilly-shallying. However, Garrick insisted I should come and speak with you first, to assure you I have no objection to the match.

Of course, if you would rather not marry him, then I shall ensure no blame will be attached to you—you have my word on that. Now, I have said enough.'

She picked up a small hand bell resting on the table and shook it. Barely had the chimes died when a door behind her opened and the duke walked in.

Pru jumped to her feet and the duchess said, testily, 'Now pray do not run away again until you have spoken to my son. You owe him that, at least!'

Pru was rooted to the spot. She watched as Garrick held the door for his mother to withdraw, then he closed it gently and stood, looking across at her.

'Well,' he said at last. '*Will* you talk to me?'

She cleared her throat. 'Th-there is nothing to say.'

'When I saw you last, I asked you to consider my proposal of marriage.'

'I did consider it.' With an effort she turned away from his searching gaze and walked to the window.

'But you never gave me your answer.'

A hand fluttered. She said sadly, 'My leaving should have told you everything.'

'No. It raised a great many questions.'

She heard his soft tread coming closer and felt panic rising. What would she do if he pulled her into his arms? The small part of her brain that was still working said she must resist, but oh, how she wanted to give in! How she wanted to stop fighting and take the comfort she knew she would find there. Pru braced herself to be strong.

He did not touch her.

'Will you not sit down and take a glass of wine with me?' he said, politely. 'There is a rather fine claret on the tray that I would like you to try.'

'I know nothing about wine.'

'But you drink it, and I want to know your opinion before I stock our cellars.'

'I think it is your mother's opinion you need.'

'No, it is yours. I want to have the wine sent to Hartland before I take you there. As my duchess.'

'Pray do not tease me, Garrick!' She swung around to face him. 'You know I cannot marry you.'

'I know nothing of the sort,' he said smiling at her so fondly that she wanted to weep. 'Tell me why. Is it my reputation?'

'No, *mine*!' she hunted for her handkerchief and buried her face in it.

'Oh, my darling girl.'

Garrick's gentle endearment made the tears come even faster. He guided Pru to a sofa and he sat down with her, one arm about her shoulders.

'Here,' he said, handing her his handkerchief. 'That silly scrap of lace is soaked through.'

'Th-thank you.' She took the linen square he pressed into her hand and dried her cheeks. 'It is no good, Garrick. I have made up my mind not to marry you.'

'Even if I don't care a jot for your reputation? Why should I, when mine has never concerned *you*?'

'But it will concern our families,' she said, trying

to make him understand. 'P-people will say I tricked you into offering for me, or that you were so grateful for my nursing that you felt you had no choice.'

'Does it matter what others think?' he asked as she gave her eyes a final wipe.

'Not in general, perhaps, but...' She was about to return his handkerchief, then thought better of it.

'But what?' he prompted.

Pru took a long breath.

'I am not the wife for a *duke*,' she said in a rush. 'Despite everything the duchess said, I cannot be the bride she had in mind for you! I w-would not have you fall out with her again when you have only just been reunited.'

Garrick was silent and Pru stared down miserably at the handkerchief clasped between her fingers, smoothing her thumb over the elegantly embroidered monogram. Could she keep it? A small, precious reminder of what might have been.

'So,' he said at last. 'You would have me marry a bride of my mother's choosing?'

'Yes!'

'Then let me tell you, my beautiful idiot, that is *exactly* what I am going to do.' His arm tightened around her shoulders. 'Why do you think she agreed to come to Bath with me? She is giving our marriage her blessing.'

'But, but she can't! I mean, everyone knows I was in your house alone with you...'

'As my nurse.'

'Many say I was there as your mistress,' she muttered, hanging her head.

This did not appear to shock Garrick at all, but neither did it appear to anger him, which it surely would, if he truly cared for her? She tried to shrug off his arm, but he tightened his hold.

He said, 'After you left town so precipitately, my mother went to see Lady Borcaster. They are both formidable women who know a thing or two about society. They have arranged everything between them.

'It is now common knowledge in town that you and I have been secretly engaged for some time, and that my mother was already in Dover Street the night you rescued me and brought me back there.'

'But—' She looked up and he laid a finger across her lips.

'It was the duchess who insisted that you stay to look after me,' he went on. 'Your aunt and Lady Borcaster were sworn to secrecy about the engagement, which led to a little embarrassment for them when the rumours began to circulate.'

His finger was tracing her lip and Pru felt a strong desire to kiss it. Instead she reached up and pulled his hand away. She needed to concentrate.

She said, 'But why should the duchess do this for *me*?'

'Because she wants you to marry me.'

That could not be right. And yet he looked and sounded perfectly serious.

'Mama told me herself she considers you the only suitable wife for me.' He paused. 'Of course, I realise that we have to consider your family, as well, which is why I stopped at Melksham on my way here.'

'M-Melksham?'

'Why, yes. I called on your parents and explained everything to them. They are up to their eyes in wedding preparations for your sister at present, but your father was good enough to listen to my proposal and give me permission to pay my addresses to you. He did suggest we should announce the engagement at your sister's wedding, but I thought that might overshadow her nuptials somewhat. I thought a special licence might be better. The ceremony to take place in Bath, as soon as possible.'

'Because you are ashamed of me?' she murmured.

'No! Damnation, Pru, because I cannot bear to live without you a moment longer.'

His hand twisted beneath hers and he gripped her fingers.

'If you want all the pomp and grandeur of a London wedding next year then it shall be arranged,' he told her, his voice ragged with emotion. 'The ceremony can take place whenever and however you wish it, my darling Prudence, only please say you will marry me!'

'For your mother's sake?'

'Because you love me.'

'I do, Garrick.' Hot tears threatened again. 'But do you love *me*?'

'Oh, my nonsensical darling, I love you more than life itself.' He pulled her onto his lap and kissed her, so deep and fierce that she was left breathless and dizzy.

'In fact,' he murmured as his lips dropped butter-fly kisses over her cheeks, 'I do not think I can live without you.'

'Oh, Garrick!'

She caught his dear face between her hands and captured his mouth with her own, giving herself up to the pleasure of being in his arms, their tongues dancing together. She was filled with sensations new to her, but as old as time. He unbuttoned her pelisse, his mouth seeking out the bare skin of her neck as he pushed the cloth from her shoulders. Pru scrabbled with the buttons of his own blue coat and it quickly followed the pelisse to the floor.

Garrick was easing her down onto the sofa when she recovered her senses sufficiently to protest.

'Wait, wait! What if the duchess should return and find us like this?'

'My mother has gone to Kilve Street, to explain everything to your aunt. She has also given instructions that *upon no account* are we to be disturbed.' His eyes glinted. 'She would tell you herself that in *her* day, lovers did not have such namby-pamby notions of propriety.'

His face was so close, his forest-green eyes so dark

that her insides were melting under their gaze. She tried to fight the rapid beating of her heart.

'I suppose these things are quite normal in ducal households,' she murmured.

'They will be in ours.'

The wicked smile that accompanied his words were Pru's undoing. The last shreds of resistance fell away. She pulled him down to her, closing her eyes as he lowered his head and trailed kisses over the column of her throat while his hands expertly freed her breasts from the muslin bodice, ready for his lips to continue their relentless onslaught. All the longing and desire that had been pent up since her one night in his bed exploded and Pru gave herself up to it. They discarded clothes as necessary to allow them to touch and caress each other.

Garrick had never known anything like it. Pru abandoned was a delight, swift to learn and eager to please. She was excited, wondering. Her soft fingers explored his body, repeating the lessons she had learned in his bed and rousing him to the very edge of ecstasy.

The sofa was too restricting and he eased her down onto the floor before running his mouth across the soft skin of her thigh, just above the garter. She moaned softly and he continued to kiss and stroke the soft skin with his tongue, gradually moving upwards to the warm hinge of her thighs. She was opening to him like a flower, offering herself to his touch. Garrick ignored the demands of his own body until she

was almost thrashing beneath him, her fingers claw-
ing at his shoulders. She began to buck wildly, sending the blood pumping through him, hot and urgent.
He covered her, thrusting hard and fast until they both
juddered with the final ecstatic release and clung together, bodies locked, gasping for breath.

Later, much later, they were sitting together on the
sofa, Pru wrapped safely in Garrick's arms and with
her head resting on his shoulder. He dropped a kiss
onto her hair.

'You still have not given me your answer. Will you
marry me, my darling Prudence?'

She chuckled, the soft, melodious sound filling him
with hope.

'I believe I shall have to do so, or people will say I
ran away from you, like poor Miss Speke.'

'Ah.' He settled her more comfortably against his
shoulder. 'There has been an interesting development
with the lady. It seems it was not just me that Annabelle was rejecting. She has renounced all men.'

'What? I do not understand.'

'Annabelle and her friend Miss Emily Undershaw
have set up a permanent home together. They have
both declared they have no intention of ever marrying.
Upon learning of it, the Tirrills recently travelled into
Wales to bring their daughter home, but she refused
to leave.' He grinned. 'The best part, my darling, is
that Annabelle admitted to her parents that she only

remained faithful to me for all those years in order to avoid them making any other marriage plans for her.'

'But how can you know all that?'

'Lady Tirrill was angry and foolish enough to take her close friends into her confidence. Those same friends who spread the original rumours about me. Word has gone around London like wildfire, and society now believes that rather than being a jilt, I am well out of a bad bargain.'

Pru sat up and looked at him, her eyes searching his face. 'And you do not mind that?'

'Why should I? The match was suggested by our parents when we were children. We were friends, but I do not think we ever really loved one another.'

'And... Helene Conyers.' Her gaze shifted to somewhere below his chin and she began to fasten the buttons of his shirt.

'Ah, *la belle* Helene. She was my first real passion.' He brushed her hand away and drew her back into his arms. 'But that was mere boyish lust, not the enduring love I have found with you.' He kissed her. 'I do love you, you know. Beyond life itself.'

'Truly?' she asked, smiling up at him mistily.

'Truly. I want you here with me for ever. Dearest, loveliest Pru.'

'Oh,' she buried her face in his shoulder. 'That is so beautiful. Like something from a book.'

'It is. The one you never finished reading to me. I read it last night, when I could not sleep for fear you might reject me.' He added, 'You might still, since you have yet to give me your answer.'

'Do you doubt what it will be?'

'You are an independent and high-minded woman. I have no idea what you will do.' He paused. 'And I am still not strong enough to prevent you walking out on me.'

'Oh, I had quite forgotten your poor ribs!'

She tried to move away and his arms tightened. 'My poor ribs are doing very well, thank you. Although I am shocked that you should have forgotten so quickly.'

'You distracted me!'

'Did I?'

'You know you did,' she replied, blushing hotly. 'How can I think of anything else, when you are doing *such* things to me?'

'Think about it now,' he commanded. 'I must have an answer, madam.'

'Very well, then.' She lowered her eyes. 'If you are sure you want me for your duchess.'

'For my duchess, my wife, my lover and my friend,' he said, marking each word with a kiss. 'Now say it and put me out of my misery. Will you marry me?'

And Prudence, abandoning all reason, listened to her heart and gave him his answer.

'I will, Garrick. Yes, please.'

\* \* \* \* \*

# COMING SOON!

We really hope you enjoyed reading this book. If you're looking for more romance be sure to head to the shops when new books are available on

# Thursday 25<sup>th</sup> May

MILLS & BOON

# MILLS & BOON®

## Coming next month

### LADY AMELIA'S SCANDALOUS SECRET
### Eva Shepherd

Be brave, Amelia, be brave. You're a fearless journalist, remember? The owner of a soon-to-be successful publication. You will not be intimidated by anyone, even a man like Mr Devenish.

Her smile became strained as she desperately tried to think of something to say that would cause him to share some titbits of gossip which would entertain her readers.

But her mind remained a blank.

'I have not seen your father tonight,' he said as she fought to get her mind to actually start working. 'I was hoping to talk with him,' he added.

Amelia's stomach clenched tighter. It was not her that Mr Devenish wished to talk to but her father. Of course. Men like him did not speak to young women like her. They went in pursuit of women like Lady Madeline.

'He is here, but I'm afraid he seems to have disappeared. It looks like you're stuck with me.' She gave a little laugh, but he neither smiled nor laughed in response.

'That will be no hardship.' His dark eyes swept quickly over her and Amelia swallowed a gasp as heat rushed to her cheeks and radiated throughout her body. Never before had she been more conscious of her appearance, more aware of her feminine shape, and more in need of a man's approval.

She blinked to brush away such silliness. She needed no man's approval, and Mr Devenish's less than most.

'You are looking particularly lovely this evening, Lady Amelia,' he said.

She gave a forced smile, as if it were merely a compliment made out of politeness that meant nothing, which it surely was.

He did not smile back. Did this man ever smile?

'Thank you.' She bit her lip, racking her brain for some meaningless conversation that would give her time to regain her composure. 'And you're looking...I mean, the ballroom is also looking particularly elegant this evening.' She gazed around the room, smiling inanely, then back at Mr Devenish.

He raised his eyebrows and Amelia blushed brighter. She really was burbling. And she had never seen this ballroom before so didn't know whether it was looking particularly elegant or not. For all she knew, the large central chandelier with its myriad candles always sent light sparkling around the room, the parquet floor always shone to perfection, and the enormous bouquets of scented lilies, lavender and gardenia were a regular feature.

'Perhaps you'd do me the honour of the next dance. Then you can familiarise yourself with the room,' he said, offering her his arm. He was making fun of her, but as she could think of no witty comeback, she mutely placed her hand on his and let him lead her out to the centre of the dance floor.

*Continue reading*
LADY AMELIA'S SCANDALOUS SECRET
Eva Shepherd

*Available next month*
www.millsandboon.co.uk

# LET'S TALK

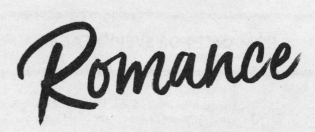

For exclusive extracts, competitions
and special offers, find us online:

 facebook.com/millsandboon

 @MillsandBoon

 @MillsandBoonUK

@MillsandBoonUK

Get in touch on 01413 063 232

For all the latest titles coming soon, visit
**millsandboon.co.uk/nextmonth**

# MILLS & BOON

## THE HEART OF ROMANCE

---

### A ROMANCE FOR EVERY READER

---

**MODERN** — Prepare to be swept off your feet by sophisticated, sexy and seductive heroes, in some of the world's most glamourous and romantic locations, where power and passion collide.

**HISTORICAL** — Escape with historical heroes from time gone by. Whether your passion is for wicked Regency Rakes, muscled Vikings or rugged Highlanders, awaken the romance of the past.

**MEDICAL** — Set your pulse racing with dedicated, delectable doctors in the high-pressure world of medicine, where emotions run high and passion, comfort and love are the best medicine.

**True Love** — Celebrate true love with tender stories of heartfelt romance, from the rush of falling in love to the joy a new baby can bring, and a focus on the emotional heart of a relationship.

**Desire** — Indulge in secrets and scandal, intense drama and sizzling hot action with heroes who have it all: wealth, status, good looks…everything but the right woman.

**HEROES** — The excitement of a gripping thriller, with intense romance at its heart. Resourceful, true-to-life women and strong, fearless men face danger and desire - a killer combination!

---

To see which titles are coming soon, please visit

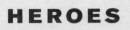

**millsandboon.co.uk/nextmonth**